Download the Gunner Goggles App Now!

Go to the App Store from your iPhone or iPad and search for **Gunner Goggles**

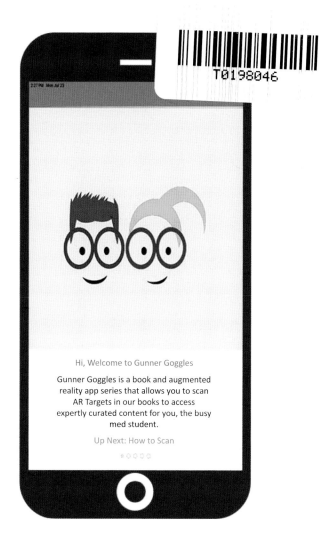

Each Gunner Goggles specialty has its own app; you can purchase other titles at:
ElsevierHealth.com/GunnerGoggles

GUNNER GOGGLES

Pediatrics

HONORS SHELF REVIEW

EDITORS:

Hao-Hua Wu, MD
Resident, Department of Orthopaedic Surgery
University of California–San Francisco
San Francisco, California

Leo Wang, MS, PhD
Perelman School of Medicine
University of Pennsylvania
Philadelphia, Pennsylvania

FACULTY EDITOR:

Rebecca Tenney-Soeiro, MD, MSEd
Associate Professor of Clinical Pediatrics
Children's Hospital of Philadelphia
Perelman School of Medicine
Philadelphia, Pennsylvania

ELSEVIER

ELSEVIER

1600 John F. Kennedy Blvd.
Ste 1800
Philadelphia, PA 19103-2899

GUNNER GOGGLES PEDIATRICS, HONORS SHELF REVIEW ISBN: 978-0-323-51038-7

Library of Congress Cataloging-in-Publication Data
Names: Wu, Hao-Hua, editor. | Wang, Leo, editor. | Tenney-Soeiro, Rebecca, editor.
Title: Gunner goggles pediatrics : honors shelf review / editors, Hao-Hua Wu, Leo Wang ; faculty editor, Rebecca Tenney-Soeiro.
Description: Philadelphia, PA : Elsevier, [2019] | Includes bibliographical references.
Identifiers: LCCN 2017051681 | ISBN 9780323510387 (pbk. : alk. paper)
Subjects: | MESH: Pediatrics | Test Taking Skills | Study Guide
Classification: LCC RJ61 | NLM WS 18.2 | DDC 618.92--dc23 LC record available at https://lccn.loc.gov/2017051681

Executive Content Strategist: Jim Merritt
Senior Content Development Specialist: Dee Simpson
Publishing Services Manager: Patricia Tannian
Senior Project Manager: Cindy Thoms
Senior Book Designer: Maggie Reid

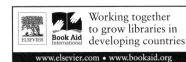

Printed in China

Last digit is the print number: 9 8 7 6 5 4 3 2 1

Gunner Goggles Honors Shelf Review Series

Gunner Goggles Family Medicine   978-0-323-51034-9

Gunner Goggles Medicine   978-0-323-51035-6

Gunner Goggles Neurology   978-0-323-51036-3

Gunner Goggles Obstetrics and Gynecology   978-0-323-51037-0

Gunner Goggles Pediatrics   978-0-323-51038-7

Gunner Goggles Psychiatry   978-0-323-51039-4

Gunner Goggles Surgery   978-0-323-51040-0

Contributors

SECTION EDITOR

Sila Bal, MD, MPH
Resident Physician
Massachusetts Eye and Ear
Boston, Massachusetts
Immunologic Disorders
Diseases of the Blood and Blood-Forming Organs
Cardiovascular Disorders

QUESTIONS EDITOR

Daniel Gromer, MD
Resident Physician
Internal Medicine
Massachusetts General Hospital
Boston, Massachusetts

CONTRIBUTING AUTHORS

Atu Agawu, MD, MPH
Resident Physician
Children's Hospital of Philadelphia
Philadelphia, Pennsylvania
Diseases of the Musculoskeletal System and Connective Tissue

Anup Bhattacharya, MD
Resident Physician
Mallinckrodt Institute of Radiology
Washington University School of Medicine in St. Louis
St. Louis, Missouri
Cardiovascular Disorders

Lauren Briskie, MD
Resident Physician
Emergency Medicine
Christiana Care Health System
Newark, Delaware
Diseases of the Respiratory System

Morgan Brown, MD
Resident Physician
Children's Hospital of Philadelphia
Philadelphia, Pennsylvania
Disorders of Pregnancy, Childbirth, and Puerperium

Peter Capucilli, MD
Resident Physician
Children's Hospital of Philadelphia
Philadelphia, Pennsylvania
Immunologic Disorders

Sierra Centkowski, MD
Resident Physician
Department of Dermatology
Stanford University School of Medicine
Palo Alto, California
Endocrine and Metabolic Disorders

Jacob Cox, MD
Resident Physician
Department of Ophthalmology
Harvard Medical School
Boston, Massachusetts
Diseases of the Nervous System and Special Senses

Joanne M. Cyganowski, MD
Resident Physician
Children's Hospital of Philadelphia
Philadelphia, Pennsylvania
Gynecologic Disorders

George Dalembert, MD
Resident Physician
Children's Hospital of Philadelphia
Philadelphia, Pennsylvania
Mental Disorders

Nina Fainberg, MD
Resident Physician
Children's Hospital of Philadelphia
Philadelphia, Pennsylvania
Disorders of the Skin and Subcutaneous Tissues

Anne Fallon, MD
Resident Physician
Children's Hospital of Philadelphia
Philadelphia, Pennsylvania
Diseases of the Nervous System and Special Senses

Jacques Greenberg, MD
Resident Physician
Department of Surgery
Cornell University
New York, New York
Renal, Urinary, and Male Reproductive System

Kishore Jayakumar, MD, MBA
Resident Physician
Department of Dermatology
Hofstra Northwell School of Medicine
Hempstead, New York
Disorders of the Skin and Subcutaneous Tissues

Garrett P. Keim, MD
Resident Physician
Children's Hospital of Philadelphia
Philadelphia, Pennsylvania
Diseases of the Respiratory System

Omar Khan, PhD
Perelman School of Medicine
University of Pennsylvania
Philadelphia, Pennsylvania
Immunologic Disorders

Marissa J. Kilberg, MD
Resident Physician
Children's Hospital of Philadelphia
Philadelphia, Pennsylvania
Endocrine and Metabolic Disorders

Diana Kim, MD
Resident Physician
Department of Ophthalmology
University of Pennsylvania
Philadelphia, Pennsylvania
Nutrition and Digestive Disorders
Renal, Urinary, and Male Reproductive System

Rafael Madero-Marroquin, MD
Johns Hopkins School of Medicine
Baltimore, Maryland
Diseases of the Musculoskeletal System and Connective Tissue

Susan McClory, MD
Resident Physician
Children's Hospital of Philadelphia
Philadelphia, Pennsylvania
Diseases of the Blood and Blood-Forming Organs

Erika Mejia, MD
Resident Physician
Children's Hospital of Philadelphia
Philadelphia, Pennsylvania
Cardiovascular Disorders

Elana B. Mitchell, MD
Resident Physician
Children's Hospital of Philadelphia
Philadelphia, Pennsylvania
Nutrition and Digestive Disorders

Alejandro Suarez Pierre, MD
Johns Hopkins School of Medicine
Baltimore, Maryland
Nutrition and Digestive Disorders

Eloise Salmon, MD
Pediatric Nephrology Fellow
Children's Hospital of Philadelphia
Philadelphia, Pennsylvania
Renal, Urinary, and Male Reproductive System

Acknowledgments

"If I have seen further than others, it is by standing upon the shoulders of giants."

– Isaac Newton

We would like to thank the many exceptional innovators who helped transform our vision of *Gunner Goggles Pediatrics* into reality.

To our editorial team at Elsevier, thank you for your unrelenting support throughout the publication process. Jim Merritt believed in *Gunner Goggles* from day one and used his experience as an executive content strategist to point us in the right direction with respect to book proposal, product pitch and manuscript development. Dee Simpson and Lucia Gunzel expertly guided us through manuscript submission and revision, no easy feat with two first-time authors. Maggie Reid collaborated with us closely to create the layout design and color schemes. Cindy Thoms and the copy editing team made sure our written content adhered to a high professional standard.

To the editors, authors, and student reviewers of *Gunner Goggles Pediatrics*, thank you for your scholarship and unwavering enthusiasm. Dr. Rebecca Tenney-Soeiro took time out of her busy academic schedule to meticulously edit each chapter, and she provided numerous invaluable insights on how we could improve quality and accuracy. A number of outstanding residents and medical students contributed to the content of this textbook and provided us feedback on high-yield topics for the NBME Pediatrics Subject Exam, notably Dr. Sila Bal, Dr. Anup Bhattacharya, Dr. Jacob Cox, Dr. Jacques Greenberg, Dr. Daniel Gromer, Dr. Kishore Jayakumar, Dr. Omar Khan, Dr. Diana Kim, Dr. Rafael Madaro-Marroquin, and Dr. Alejandro Suarez-Pierre. We would also like to thank the Chief Residents and Fellows from the Children's Hospital of Philadelphia for lending their expertise to these chapters, including Dr. Atu Agawu, Dr. Morgan Brown, Dr. Peter Capucilli, Dr. Joanne Cyganowski, Dr. George Dalembert, Dr. Nina Fainberg, Dr. Anne Fallon, Dr. Garrett Keim, Dr. Marissa Kilberg, Dr. Susan McClory, Dr. Erika Mejia, Dr. Elana Mitchell, and Dr. Eloise Salmon.

To our augmented reality (AR) team, thank you for your creativity and dedication during the development of the *Gunner Goggles* AR application. Nadir Bilici, Brian Mayo, Vlad Obsekov, Clare Teng, and Yinka Orafidiya helped us develop and test the initial *Gunner Goggles* AR prototype. Tammy Bui designed the *Gunner Goggles* logo and AR app icon.

We would also like to thank the Wharton Innovation Fund for awarding us seed money to help pursue development of *Gunner Goggles* AR.

You all continue to inspire us, and we are incredibly grateful and deeply appreciative for your support.

– Hao-Hua and Leo

Contents

Introduction

Hao-Hua Wu, Leo Wang, and Rebecca Tenney-Soeiro

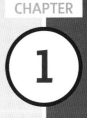

I. Gunner's Guide to a Better Test Score

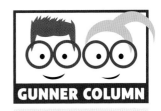

GUNNER COLUMN

Curious why certain classmates perform well on every exam? Frustrated by how few of these "Gunner" peers share study secrets?

At *Gunner Goggles*, our goal is to reveal and demystify. By integrating *augmented reality* (AR) into this review book, we **reveal** how the best students approach topics, conceptualize complex disease, and allocate study time efficiently. By organizing each topic according to the National Board of Medical Examiners (NBME) format, we **demystify** exam content and the types of questions one can expect on test day.

Of all the tests medical students strive to conquer, shelf exams boast the highest ratio of importance to the quality of study resources. For instance, performance on shelf exams typically informs final clerkship grades, which are the most important criteria on the medical school transcript for residency application. Yet there is no single authoritative study resource for the shelf across all disciplines. Most importantly, no current book specifically targets shelf exam prep, so that students must rely on miscellaneous resources and anecdotal advice to get the job done.

In light of this void in authoritative test prep, we have created the *Gunner Goggles* series to provide you with the most effective shelf exam testing resource. *GG* stands out for three important reasons:

First, readers have the opportunity to enhance their understanding of important shelf topics by utilizing the **AR** features on each page. With an iPhone or iPad, users can download the *Gunner Goggles* AR iOS app and use it to turn book figures into three-dimensional (3D) images, access high-yield videos and view pertinent digital media. More on how AR technology works can be found on page 2.

Second, *Gunner Goggles* provides a plethora of tips on how to manage time efficiently when studying for the shelf. Mnemonics and strategies for how to approach difficult concepts can be found in the blue "Gunner Column" at the right of each page. We also tell you how to *think* about these concepts, so that Pediatrics never feels like a laundry list of items you simply have to memorize.

Third, this review book is written and organized optimally for shelf exam test prep. Each chapter is organized according to the NBME Clinical Science Subject Examination and USMLE course content outlines. In addition, a concise summary of how topics are tested prefaces each chapter.

As experts on the shelf exam, we understand how difficult it is to carve out time to study while juggling clinical responsibilities during your clerkship rotation. We also know that each student's learning curve is different based on timing of the rotation (first block vs. last block), year in medical school (MS3 vs. MD/PhD returning after graduate school), and future career interests (e.g., an aspiring orthopedic surgeon learning about obstetrics and gynecology). However, we believe that any student can perform well on the shelf with the right strategy and study resources.

We created this book anticipating the needs of all types of students, and we hope that *Gunner Goggles* will be the most comprehensive, authoritative shelf exam review book that you will ever use. We are confident that *Gunner Goggles* will enable you to achieve your test performance goals and stick it to your "Gunner" classmates, whose advice, or lack thereof, you won't be needing after all.

II. Augmented Reality: A New Paradigm for Shelf Exam Test Prep

Think of AR as your best friend.

To use it, download the free *Gunner Goggles Pediatrics* application on your iPad or iPhone and create your own optional profile. Now, with the application open, point your smart mobile camera at this page.

Notice how there are now links on your camera on which you can click, 3D figures you can rotate, and a video you can watch. You have just unlocked the AR features for this page!

Take a moment to play around with these AR features on your smart mobile device. The way this works is that anytime you see the *Gunner Goggles* icon 𝐠𝐠 in the blue Gunner Column at the left or right of each page, there is an AR feature accompanying the text with which you can interact.

Still not convinced? Here are three reasons why AR is your ideal study companion:

Presentation

AR breaks the boundaries of how information can be presented in this textbook.

𝐠𝐠 AR
Gunner Goggles Introduction Video

𝐠𝐠 AR
Gunner Goggles Contact

Traditionally, if you wanted to learn about a disease in a review book, you would be expected to read and memorize a block of text similar to the following:

"Huntington's disease (HD) is a GABAergic neurodegenerative disorder that is caused by an autosomal dominant mutation leading to CAG repeats on chromosome 4. Patients typically present in the fourth and fifth decade of life with chorea, memory loss, caudate atrophy on neuroimaging and motor impairment, depending on the variant. Although there is no cure for Huntington's, the movement disorders associated with the disease, such as chorea, can be treated with drugs like tetrabenazine and reserpine to decrease dopamine release."

Having read (or most likely glazed) through that paragraph, do you feel comfortable enough to answer questions about the genetics, presentation, and treatment of Huntington's right now? A week from now? Or 3 weeks from now when you have to take your shelf exam?

Here's where AR comes in. Use your *Gunner Goggles* app to check out how we're able to present Huntington's disease in different, memorable ways.

For visual learners, here's a video of an effective HD mnemonic→

AR

Huntington's Disease Mnemonic

If you are an audio learner, here's a link to key points about Huntington's for the shelf→

AR

Huntington's Podcast

Forgot your neuroanatomy? Here's where the caudate is →

AR

The caudate nucleus is part of the basal ganglia

What's the difference between chorea, athetosis, and ballismus again? Chorea looks like this →

AR

Chorea Patient Example

Now write a one-line description of Huntington's in your own words in the margins of this page for future reference. It's much easier with AR right? Like we said, it's your best friend.

Evaluation

The GG Pediatrics app has the potential to exponentially enhance how you can evaluate your own understanding of the material. Although not available with the first edition, we are in the process of developing a personalized question bank as well as a flashcards feature. Our vision is to allow you to scan a topic on the page for immediate access to relevant practice questions and flashcards. In future versions, you will also be able to create your own flashcard deck and track your mastery.

In addition the GG app can keep track of the AR Targets scanned and the Learning links viewed. These links are saved to a Link Library which you can view at any time. You

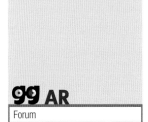

can also like or dislike a Learning Link with an opportunity to provide us feedback for better resources available.

As development of the GG Pediatrics app is an ongoing process, we encourage and welcome your feedback. If you like the idea of having a personalized question bank and flashcard feature or have an idea for how we can improve the GG app to better serve your studying needs, please provide us feedback through an in-app message. You can also email us at GunnerGoggles@gmail.com.

Community Engagement

Studying for the shelf can be isolating. Our vision is to develop a feature in the GG Pediatrics that would allow you to connect with chapter authors and fellow readers. We are in the process of developing a medium in which shelf-related inquiries can be discussed among authors and readers through an optional short message system (SMS) feature.

Given that the community engagement feature is in development and unavailable for the first edition, we welcome your input on how we can connect you with the people who will enable your test day success.

To provide feedback, please scan the page and vote. You can also email us GunnerGoggles@gmail.com for any comments or suggestions.

Augmented Reality Frequently Asked Questions

"Since augmented reality is integrated into *Gunner Goggle Pediatrics*, does this mean I have to pull out my iPad or iPhone for every page of the book?"

No, only if you need it. Some may use AR more than others, depending on background and level of comfort with Pediatrics. For instance, you may already have a solid understanding of Huntington's and only need to read the text as a refresher. On the other hand, if you are less comfortable with Huntington's, the AR features are there just in case.

"Can't I just look up everything I don't know on my own? Why do I have to use the *Gunner Goggles* app?"

You can absolutely look things up on your own. But that takes time. And sometimes you can't find the best reference or mnemonic. Our team of experts has already gone to the trouble of identifying potential sources of confusion and found the perfect resources. In the *Gunner Goggles* app, we have compiled the slickest and most concise resources you could use to better understand a topic. Videos, audio files, and images are first vetted by subject experts for accuracy of content. They are then evaluated by students like yourself for utility of content to enhance test performance. Only resources with the most Gunner votes are embedded into each page.

"What if a link doesn't work or I want something on the page to change?"

Please tell us! Another advantage of AR is that we can immediately receive and implement your feedback. Just use the *Gunner Goggles* app to text us your concerns and our tech support team will respond ASAP!

III. Study Smart: Mnemonics and Gunner Study Tips

Even with incredible AR features at your disposal, you won't be able to optimize exam performance unless you know how to study. Below are the four most important things one can do to study for the Pediatrics shelf under the time restraints imposed by clerkships.

Understand the Organizing Principle

The easiest way to save time and perform well on the shelf is to understand how a specific disease or concept fits into the big picture. For instance, knowing the Buzz Words for physiologic jaundice of the newborn will likely lead to only one correct answer on the test. However, understanding the spectrum of diseases that can cause jaundice as well as the associated workup can help you to identify any hepatobiliary complaint more easily.

Create Effective Mnemonics

If you have a photographic memory, skip this section. For the rest of us mere mortals, the list below outlines the organizing principles (OP) of what constitutes a Gunner mnemonic.

Mnemonics are important when:
1. You have to learn a lot of material.
2. You want to teach something to your colleagues during morning rounds. Attendings and residents are always impressed when they can learn something from a medical student.
3. You want to remember something 15 years from now when you are working the thirtieth hour of a busy call day.

OPs for mnemonics are as follows:

1. Use the spelling of a name to your benefit (**Spell**)
Examples:
   a. "8urk14tt's" lymphoma (Burkitt's lymphoma), lep"thin" (leptin), "supraoptiuretic" nuclei (supraoptic nuclei that produce antidiuretic hormone)
   b. Tenofovir is the only NRTI [nucleoside reverse transcriptase inhibitor] nucleoTide
   c. We "C"ener's granulomatosis (GPA) for C-ANCA and Cyclophosphamide tx
2. Create an acronym that contains distinguishing syllables or letters of names (**Distinguish**)
Example:
   a. Chronic Alcoholics Steal PhenPhen and Nevar Rifuse Grisee Carbs (Chronic alcohol abuse + St John's wort + phenytoin + phenobarb + nevaripine + rifampin + griseofulvin + carbamazepine)
      • reinforce mnemonic by spelling the name of an item to be memorized accordingly
      • For example, "Refus"ampin, "Never"apine, "Greasy"ofulvin, "Carb"amazepine, etc.
      • This ties mnemonic OP 1 with mnemonic OP 2
3. Drawings help (**Draw**)
Example: Trisomy 13 looks like polydactyly + cleft lip when the number 13 is rotated 90 degrees clockwise (the horizontal 1 is the extra digit, and the cleft of the horizontal 3 is the cleft lip)
4. Counting the letters of a word (**Count**)
Example: Patau syndrome = 13 letters = Trisomy 13
5. Arrange acronym in alphabetical order (**Arrange**)
Example: ABCDEF for diphtheria (ADP ribosylation, beta prophage, C Diphtheria, elongation factor 2)
Examples of instructors who practice this concept well are Dr. John Barone of Kaplan and Dr. Husain Sattar of Pathoma.
On the flip side, here are examples of poor mnemonics (although you may remember them now, given that they were highlighted in this text):
   a. Blind as a bat, mad as a hatter, red as a beet, hot as Hades, dry as a bone, the bowel and bladder lose their tone, and the heart runs alone = poor mnemonic for anticholinergic syndrome:
      • This mnemonic forces you to memorize extra and extraneous things (like bat, beet, Hades, and bone) that have nothing to do with anticholinergic syndrome.

b. WWHHHHIMP (withdrawal + wernicke + hypertensive crisis + hypoxia + hypoglycemia + hypoperfusion + intracranial bleed + meningitis/encephalopathy + poisoning) = poor mnemonic for causes of delirium:
- Wait—how many H's does this mnemonic have again?

A good rule of thumb: if you can still remember a mnemonic in a high-pressure situation (attending pimps you) or after a 7-day period, then you have a winner.

Ultimately, the best mnemonics are the ones you invent and apply repeatedly, so use these mnemonic principles to give yourself a solid head start.

Devise a Study Schedule and Stick to It

The third most important piece of advice for the shelf is to create a study schedule at the beginning of the rotation and follow it. Rotations such as Pediatrics are particularly draining. Often you may find yourself coming home after a 12-hour shift not wanting to study, especially when prerounds are the next day at 6 a.m. However, if you are mentally committed to following a schedule, you will find creative ways to get your studying done. For example, some students wake up an hour early to read before prerounds. Others fit study material into their white coats and read during downtime. Pediatrics is unique because you will likely spend significant time in an outpatient setting, meaning easier hours than in an inpatient rotation and more time for study.

Distinguish Rotation Knowledge From Shelf Knowledge

Most things you learn on rotation do not apply to the shelf exam, and vice versa. For example, you may be able to impress your Pediatrics attending by committing the components of the Apgar test to memory. However, with only 150 minutes to answer 100 lengthy questions on the shelf, details like that have no real utility.

Thus, learn to compartmentalize. Know exactly what is needed for your Pediatrics rotation and what is expected on the shelf to save yourself precious study time. If your Pediatrics clerkship allows you to do a subspecialty rotation, keep in mind what material you can learn from your attendings that would help you for the shelf (e.g., how to differentiate eating disorders on an Adolescent Medicine rotation).

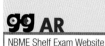

NBME Shelf Exam Website

IV. Intro to the National Board of Medical Examiners Clinical Science Pediatrics Subject Exam

The Clinical Science Pediatrics NBME Subject Exam is a 100-question computerized exam administered over a recommended course of 2 hours and 30 minutes, typically at the conclusion of the Pediatrics clerkship rotation. The test questions come from either retired Step 2 CK questions or are written by a committee of faculty across the country. Thus, it is important to master shelf exam–style questions to set yourself up nicely for Step 2 CK.

Unlike Step 1, shelf exam questions focus almost exclusively on disease processes rather than normal processes. That being said, the most high-yield principles to know for the Pediatrics shelf are normal lab values. Knowing what values to expect for the basic metabolic panel will help you quickly identify abnormal processes, such as hyper/hyponatremia, anion gap metabolic acidosis, or acute kidney injury.

According to the NBME, the exams are curved to a mean of 70 with a standard deviation of 8. The curve does not take into account timing of rotation. For instance, students who take the exam during their first clerkship block will be held to the same statistical standard as those who take the exam during their fourth block. However, the NBME does release "quarterly norm information" to medical schools in order to make clerkship directors aware of the relationship between exam score and rotation timing. Importantly, as of now, shelf exam scores are sent to the school directly; students cannot request their shelf exam score independent of their school.

Although different Pediatrics clerkships have different standards for determining grades, in general each program has its own internally generated shelf exam cutoff score that must be achieved in order to be eligible for the highest clerkship grade (e.g., Honors). If this is the case, confirm the cutoff score with your clerkship director so that you have a reasonable performance goal to shoot for.

Students are expected to master content organized within the following categories:

Pediatrics Outline

System

General Principles, Including Normal Age-Related Findings and Care of the Well Patient	3%–7%
Immune System	3%–7%

Blood and Lymphoreticular System	3%–7%
Behavioral Health	1%–5%
Nervous System and Special Senses	5%–10%
Skin and Subcutaneous Tissue	1%–5%
Musculoskeletal System	3%–7%
Cardiovascular System	5%–10%
Respiratory System	5%–10%
Gastrointestinal System	3%–7%
Renal and Urinary System	5%–10%
Disorders of the Newborn and Congenital Disorders	5%–10%
Female Reproductive System and Breast (Infectious, immunologic, and inflammatory disorders; Menstrual and endocrine disorders)	3%–7%
Male Reproductive System	1%–5%
Endocrine System	5%–10%
Multisystem Processes and Disorders	10%–15%
Social Sciences, Including Medical Ethics and Jurisprudence	1%–5%

Currently, the NBME Pediatrics Content Outline breaks down question types into three categories:
- Applying Foundational Science Concepts (13%–17%)
- Diagnosis: Knowledge Pertaining to History, Exam, Diagnostic Studies, and Patient Outcomes (55%–60%)
- Health Maintenance, Pharmacotherapy, Intervention, and Management (20%–25%)

However, devising a study plan from these three categories can be confusing. "Applying Foundational Science Concepts," for instance, is vague and difficult to prepare for. Instead, many students prefer to study according to Physician Tasks provided in older content outlines. Since every subject exam question asks about one of four things – 1) protocol for promoting health maintenance (Prophylaxis [**PPx**]), 2) the mechanism of disease (**MoD**), 3) steps to establishing a diagnosis (**Dx**), and 4) steps of disease management (**Tx/Mgmt**) – we recommend studying according to Physician Tasks from the 2016 Content Outline.

Physician Tasks (from 2016 Content Outline)

Promoting health and health maintenance	5%–10%
Understanding mechanisms of disease	25%–30%
Establishing a diagnosis	40%–45%
Applying principles of management	10%–15%

In addition, the NBME breaks down questions by Site of Care, including
- Ambulatory (65%–70%)
- Emergency Department (25%–25%)
- Inpatient (12%–16%)

Our recommendation is to not worry about site of care and focus on studying content related to Physician Tasks.

Gunner Goggles Pediatrics presents material to reflect how the NBME structures its subject exams. Each chapter covers at least one of the main testable categories above. For instance, topics pertaining to "Disorders of the Newborn and Congenital Disorders" is covered under Chapter 12. Topics from "Multisystem Processes and Disorders," such as Down syndrome and fragile X syndrome have been divided throughout the textbook based on the most likely presenting complaint Each disease is presented in a "PPx, MoD, Dx, and Tx/Mgmt" format, which represents the four physician tasks the NBME can test you on. Since establishing a diagnosis is weighted especially heavily (40%-45%), the "Buzz Words" category shows readers how to quickly identify the disease process from just a few key words. The "Clinical Presentation" section serves to more thoroughly describe the disease. However, it is important to note that Buzz Words are sufficient in correctly identifying the corresponding disease on the shelf. The detail provided in the Clinical Presentation section is only meant to augment your understanding, particularly if it is your first pass and you are unfamiliar with the material. However, by the end of studying, the focus should primarily be on Buzz Words.

Finally, here are four things to keep in mind while studying for the Pediatrics shelf:

1. If pressed for time, practice identifying disease processes only through Buzz Words. For instance, a patient with a strawberry tongue and a high fever lasting 5 or more days has Kawasaki's disease.

2. Don't get sick! Be vigilant about hand hygiene and avoid ingesting anything without having washed your hands first. You will likely treat many kids with contagious colds, and it behooves you to take the appropriate precautions so that you can stick to your study schedule.

3. Make sure to begin doing questions early (e.g., 10 questions a day starting from day 1). Ideally you should make a second pass of the most high-yield questions before test day.

4. For each question, write a one-line take-home point in an Excel spreadsheet. This makes for quick and easy review in the days leading up to the exam.

If any questions arise while you are studying, use the *Gunner Goggles* app to access the AR features embedded on each page.

Good luck and happy hunting!

—The *Gunner Goggles* Team

Normal Development

Hao-Hua Wu, Daniel Gromer, Leo Wang, and
Rebecca Tenney-Soeiro

Introduction

Five to ten questions on the Pediatrics shelf will be about normal development. This covers the normal neonate exam, developmental milestones, and normal puberty. The most high-yield concept for the Peds exam is knowing the developmental milestones. What to expect during puberty is also important to understand, as it may show up on your Ob/Gyn and Family Medicine exams as well. Of note, topics related to normal development—such as autism, attention deficit hyperactivity disorder (ADHD), developmental delay, and enuresis/encoperesis—are covered in Chapter 5.

This chapter is divided into (1) Normal Neonate Exam, (2) Normal Developmental Milestones, (3) Neonatal Skin Exam, (4) Puberty, and (5) Gunner Practice.

Normal Neonate Exam

Since the Pediatric shelf focuses on abnormal processes, it is unlikely that you will be tested directly on the normal neonate exam. Thus, if pressed for time, skip to developmental milestones. The most high-yield concept to learn in this subsection is the APGAR score (Table 2.1). The APGAR score is a tool used by health care professionals in evaluating a newborn at 1 and 5 minutes after delivery. The maximum score is 10, therefore 8 to 10 means healthy, whereas 7 or less means that there is cause for further workup. You do not need to know how to add up the APGAR score for the Pediatrics shelf; instead, like the Glasgow Coma Scale (GCS), just know generally what's healthy (e.g., everything that gives baby a score of 2) and what's bad (e.g., signs that lead to a score of 0). That gestalt (i.e., pink is good; blue is bad) will be enough to steer you in the right direction on test day.

Other key features of the normal neonate exam that you may be asked about on your clinical rotations include the following:

- General appearance and measurements/growth charts
- Head and neck (e.g., sutures, fontanelles, red reflex, corneal light reflex, palate)

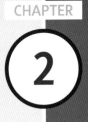

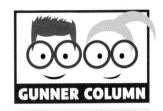

AR

Video about APGAR scoring

TABLE 2.1 APGAR Scoring System

Score	Appearance	Pulse	Grimace	Activity	Respiration
0	All blue	Absent	None	Limp	Absent
1	Blue extremities, pink torso	<100 bpm	Grimace	Some flexion of extremities	Irregular
2	All pink	≥100 bpm	Sneeze, cough	Active	Regular (crying)

Evaluation and Care of the Normal Neonate

- Chest (cardiac auscultation)
- Abdomen (umbilical site, masses, etc.)
- Genitalia (testicles descended bilaterally)
- Hips
- Neuro (newborn reflexes)

These features are not covered in this book because they are not represented on the shelf. However, a concise reference for all normal exam findings can be found in the Gunner Column.

Normal Developmental Milestones

On the Pediatrics exam, you are guaranteed to get at least three questions on the topic of developmental milestones. These questions first describe the patient's age as well as how well she or he can perform in four developmental categories: gross motor skills, fine motor skills, language, and social cognition. Based on the child's performance of these tasks, you will have to decide if he or she is age-appropriate for each category or if there is one category that lags behind. With milestones for 11 ages to memorize, these questions can be quite challenging. However, don't be discouraged. To master this content, (1) use mnemonics (e.g., 2-year-old uses 2 word phrases and follows 2-step commands), (2) create flashcards and treat milestones as Buzz Words, (3) teach the parents you work with on your rotation (e.g., say what you are looking for to the parents as you examine their 2-month-old infant), and, most importantly, (4) do questions!

Mnemonic for memorizing age of drawing

Table 2.2 shows the milestones you will have to know for the Peds exam (see Table 2.2). You are unlikely to memorize all of them on your first pass. Instead, refer back to this table early and often.

Neonatal Skin Exam

There is a plethora of exam findings for neonates that are harmless but may cause anxiety to the inexperienced. Here

TABLE 2.2 Developmental Milestones to 5 Years of Age

Age	Gross	Fine	Language	Social/Cognitive
2 months	1. Lifts head 45 degrees in prone position	1. Holds placed rattle (palmar grasp = infant grabs anything placed in hand (new-born reflex): Stated in it this way you may confuse it with a 4-mo milestone of holding a rattle 2. Tracks past midline	1. Orients to voice/sound 2. Gurgles/ooo/aah/vocalizes	1. Social smile 2. Regards faces
4 months	1. Sits with trunk support 2. Lifts chest in prone 3. Bears weight on legs	1. Hands mostly open 2. Brings hands to midline and grasps rattle	1. Coos 2. Squeals and laughs	1. Enjoys looking around 2. Self-soothes to sleep 3. Regards own hands
6	1. Pulls to sit 2. Sits tripod, no support 3. Primitive reflexes gone	1. Transfers objects hand to hand 2. Shakes rattle 3. Reaches for objects	1. Looks toward person talking 2. Responds to name 3. Imitates sounds	1. Shows stranger anxiety
9 months	1. Pulls to stand 2. Cruises (walks while holding onto furniture, in need of support), *"cruising with my 9"*	1. **3-finger pincer** grasp 2. Holds cup 3. Bangs two blocks together	1. Understands "no" 2. Says mama and dada (nonspecific) 3. Jabbers	1. Object permanence 2. Plays pat-a-cake
12 months	1. Stands well and walks **first steps** 2. Throws ball	1. **2-finger pincer** grasp 2. **Puts block in cup**	1. **First words** (other than dada and mama, specific)	1. Shows separation anxiety 2. Follows 1-step command 3. Waves bye bye
18 months	1. Runs 2. Stoops and recovers	1. Builds tower of 2–4 cubes 2. Removes clothing	1. 6+ words 2. Identifies body part	1. Pretend play 2. Knows what is "mine"
2 years	1. Kicks ball forward 2. Walks up steps (one foot at a time)	1. Builds 6-cube tower 2. Draws **line** 3. Turns **individual pages**	1. **200** word vocabulary 2. **2-word** phrases 3. **2**/4 (50%) speech intelligible	1. Follows **2-step** command 2. Parallel play 3. Toilet training
3 years	1. Manages stairs with alternating feet 2. Throws ball overhead 3. Jumps 4. Rides **tri**cycle	1. Draws **circle** 2. Uses utensils	1. **3-word** sentences 2. Speech **3**/4 intelligible	1. Knows age/gender 2. Washes/dries hands 3. Can do simple household tasks 4. Puts on t-shirt

Continued

TABLE 2.2 Developmental Milestones to 5 Years of Age—cont'd

Age	Gross	Fine	Language	Social/Cognitive
4 years	1. Hops on 1 foot 2. Jumps over objects	1. Draws a **square** and **cross** 2. Can use **scissors** and crayons	1. Counts to 10 2. Identifies colors 3. Speech 100% intelligible	1. Cooperative play 2. Has imaginary friends 3. Dresses without help
5 years	1. Skips 2. Balances on each foot for 3 seconds	1. Draws a triangle and person with **5+** parts 2. Ties shoelaces 3. Independent dressing/bathing	1. **5**-word sentences	1. Has friends 2. Can do tasks independently (prepares cereal, brushes teeth)

QUICK TIPS

Direct hyperbilirubinemia in a neonate always abnormal.

QUICK TIPS

Jaundice within the first 24 hours is abnormal.

is a high-yield list of commonly tested benign findings, all of which are self-limited and require no further workup:

Physiologic Jaundice: Non-pathologic **indirect** hyperbilirubinemia, seen after day 2 with a total bilirubin level up to 12 mg/dL for term infants. Differentiate from pathologic indirect hyperbilirubinemia where total bilirubin level >20mg/dL.

Breast milk Jaundice: Jaundice in second week of life due to unconjugated bilirubin and glucuronidase in breast milk.

Breastfeeding Jaundice: Jaundice during first week of life due to a lack of breast milk. Characterized by decreased feeding, retained meconium and increased enterohepatic circulation of bilirubin. Treat with increased breast milk intake.

Mongolian spots: Dark-blue macules superior to buttocks (Fig. 2.1). Can actually be anywhere (arms, legs, back), but most common on sacrum and buttocks.

Erythema toxicum: small pustules and papules surrounded by erythematous flare; **eosinophils** found on Wright stain. Easily confused with bacterial infection (Fig. 2.2).

Milia: Whitish papules that are inclusion cysts of the pilosebaceous follicles.

Puberty

Another popular test topic, pubertal development, can be tested in a number of ways. Most importantly, know when puberty is supposed to occur for males and females as well as the first trait of puberty. On the exam, you will only need to distinguish whether the pubertal development is age-appropriate or age-inappropriate. From there, you can begin to delve into the differential diagnosis.

Last, the Tanner Stage of Development is meant to get you familiarized with the terminology. It will not be directly tested on your exam. The best way to think of Tanner

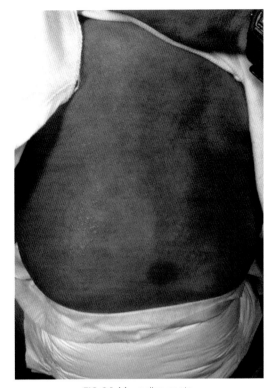

FIG. 2.1 Mongolian spots.

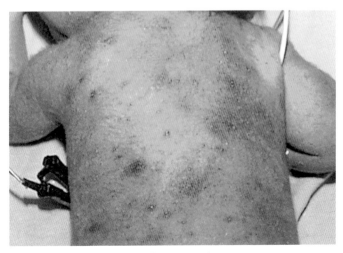

FIG. 2.2 Erythema toxicum.

Staging is as a proxy for puberty; you don't have to know exactly what age correlates with what stage. Instead, know the extremes. For example, a 16-year-old sexually mature male will likely have Tanner stage 4 or 5 development of his genitalia. However, if the exam states Tanner Stage 1 at the same age, you should be suspicious of an underlying endocrine disorder.

Female Puberty

Females begin puberty at a mean of **9.5** years, which is about 2 years younger than the average male. The first organs to mature during puberty are the breasts (thelarche). Thus, whenever you encounter a question about females in the pubertal stage, pay attention to the Tanner Staging of the breasts. If she is 10 years old, Tanner stage 1 or 2 for breast development would be appropriate. If she is 16 years old, however, and still has Tanner stage 1 or 2 breast development, there may be an endocrine dysfunction (Fig. 2.3). Pubic hair development follows after thelarche, and **menarche**, defined as the onset of the first menstrual cycle, will develop last. Typically menarche occurs at 12 or 13 years of age on the exam, or 2 to 3 years after thelarche. Last, it is important to note that the female peak growth spurt occurs during Tanner stage 3 and menarche occurs right after the peak growth spurt is reached.

Male Puberty

Males mature more slowly than females and have a different order of maturation. Instead of breast tissue, the genitalia of males (e.g., testicles) are the first to mature at the age of 11 to 12 (Fig. 2.4). Hair growth (i.e., pubic, facial, axillary) begins a couple years after maturation of the genitalia. Thus, a male patient with Tanner stage 2 development of genitalia and pubic hair at the age of 17 may have an underlying endocrine disorder.

Importantly, 3 out of every 5 males may have normal gynecomastia. The gynecomastia, or enlargement of breast tissue, can be unilateral or bilateral and is a common test question on the Peds exam. Be on the lookout for a 14- to 17-year-old male who comes to his school nurse anxious about "growing breasts." The etiology of normal gynecomastia in teenage boys is unknown and requires **no workup or treatment**.

GUNNER PRACTICE

1. A 4-year-old male is brought to the pediatrician's office by his mother. She is concerned because he is wetting the bed about once a week. He became fully continent 6 months ago, but his nighttime "accidents" have persisted. She explains that he is excelling in his preschool

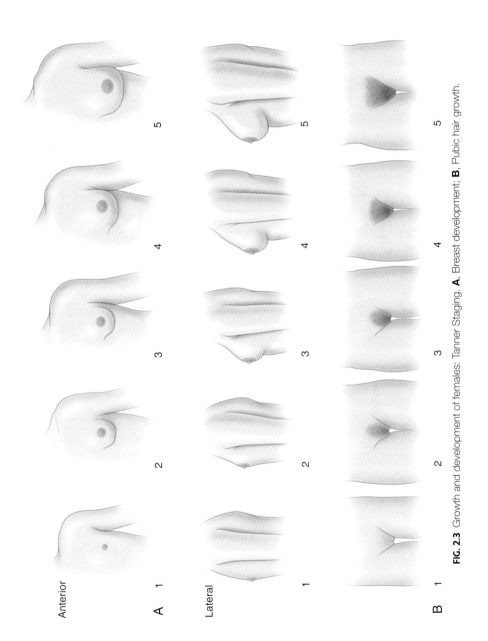

FIG. 2.3 Growth and development of females: Tanner Staging. **A**, Breast development; **B**, Pubic hair growth.

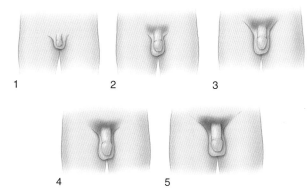

FIG. 2.4 Male genitalia: Tanner Staging.

prep classes and she has no worries about his cognitive development. He has one bowel movement a day and never complains of difficulty or discomfort during his five daily urine voids. His past medical history is significant for mild reactive airway disease and a left fibula fracture at the age of 2. His family history is significant for hypertension in his mother and osteosarcoma in his father. His vital signs are T 98.8°F, HR 102, BP 91/62, RR 18, SpO$_2$ 99% on room air. Examination yields a playful child with a normal gait, no sacral dimple, and normal external genitalia. What is the most likely diagnosis and the most appropriate next step in management?

A. Encopresis; daily laxative administration
B. Nocturnal enuresis; desmopressin administration
C. Child abuse; further investigation
D. Normal development; education and reassurance
E. Occult spinal dysraphism; MRI of the spine

2. A 3-year-old female is brought to the pediatrician's office by her father for a well-child examination. She was born at 35 weeks with no apparent complications. Her medical history is notable for reactive airway disease, recurrent acute otitis media managed with bilateral myringotomy tubes, and a small umbilical hernia. Her length is 13th percentile, her weight is 19th percentile, and her head circumference is 16th percentile for her corrected age. Her father describes her as "happy-go-lucky" and "easygoing." She feeds herself and enjoys playing near other children in preschool. She can balance on one foot for 3 seconds, rides a tricycle at the park, and makes towers with three blocks. She uses about 75 words, 2 at a time in sentences, and is around 50% understandable by strangers. She can draw a circle with crayons and a

person with three parts. She can also state her age and point to different parts of animals. Her physical exam, including hearing testing, is completely normal. What is the most likely diagnosis?

A. Normal development
B. Fine motor developmental delay
C. Gross motor developmental delay
D. Expressive language developmental delay
E. Global developmental delay

3. A 14-year-old male is brought to the pediatrician's office by his father. In private, the boy mentions that he has recently noticed changes in his physical appearance, which have caused him significant distress at school. Specifically, his nipples have protruded from his chest wall, and other students have begun to comment on his "breasts." He is afraid that something is wrong. His past medical history is notable for several episodes of rhinosinusitis, an ulnar fracture at age 9, and moderate eczema, for which he uses petroleum jelly. He denies the use of any other medication, as well as illicit drugs. His height, weight, and body mass index (BMI) are all between the 40th and 60th percentiles. His vital signs are T 98.4°F, HR 82, BP 98/60, RR 16, SpO_2 98% on room air. Examination of his chest reveals approximately 1 cm of subareolar and periareolar rubbery tissue. Examination of his genitalia reveals equal testicular volumes of 7 mL and coarse, dark hair beginning to grow along the penis and scrotum. The remainder of the examination is unremarkable. What is the likely diagnosis and appropriate management?

A. Pseudogynecomastia; education about diet and exercise
B. Drug-induced gynecomastia; cessation of petroleum jelly use
C. Idiopathic pubertal gynecomastia; reassurance
D. Klinefelter syndrome; education
E. Idiopathic pubertal gynecomastia; referral for surgery

ANSWERS: What Would Gunner Jess/Jim Do?

1. WWGJD? A 4-year-old male is brought to the pediatric office by his mother. She is concerned, as he is wetting the bed approximately once per week. He became fully continent around 6 months ago, but his nighttime "accidents" have persisted. She explains that he is excelling in his pre-school preparatory classes, and she has no worries about his cognitive development. He has 1 bowel movement per day and never complains of difficulty or discomfort during his 5 urine voids each day. His past medical history is significant for mild reactive airway disease and a left fibula fracture at the age of 2. His family history is significant for hypertension in his mother and osteosarcoma in his father. His vital signs are T 98.8°F, HR 102, BP 91/62, RR 18, SpO_2 99% on room air. Examination yields a playful child with a normal gait, no sacral dimple, and normal external genitalia. What is the most likely diagnosis and the most appropriate next step in management?

Answer: D, Normal development; education and reassurance

Explanation: This is a 4-year-old child with apparently normal development and isolated, occasional urinary incontinence at night. Up to 16% of 5-year-old children will display "bedwetting," and demonstration of urinary continence at night generally follows after urinary continence during the daytime. As the child has only recently achieved daytime continence and shows no signs of pathology that would cause continued symptoms, the most appropriate response at this time is to continue encouraging and educating the parent and child and await spontaneous resolution.

A. Encopresis; daily laxative administration → Incorrect. Encopresis refers to fecal incontinence. This patient has one bowel movement per day and no complaints about his bowel movements.

B. Nocturnal enuresis; desmopressin administration → Incorrect. Enuresis requires nighttime urinary incontinence in a patient 5 years of age or older. This child is too young for his "accidents" to be termed enuresis. Additionally, desmopressin is not the first-line course of management for isolated enuresis. Of note, it is always important to distinguish primary and secondary incontinence in a child presenting with possible enuresis (see further on). Primary enuresis denotes persistent enuresis with no significant period of "dryness" in the child's lifetime. Secondary enuresis denotes new "bedwetting" after a significant period of nighttime continence.

C. Child abuse; further investigation → Incorrect. There is no evidence in this story or in the physical exam that would support a claim of abuse.

E. Occult spinal dysraphism; MRI of the spine → Incorrect. No sacral dimple or neurologic dysfunction of the lower extremities or gait were noted. There are no coincident complaints of daytime urinary incontinence or fecal incontinence. The most likely explanation remains normal development.

2. WWGJD?

A 3-year-old female is brought to the pediatric office by her father for a well-child examination. She was born at 35 weeks with no apparent complications. Her medical history is notable for reactive airway disease, recurrent acute otitis media managed with bilateral myringotomy tubes, and a small umbilical hernia. Her length is 13th percentile, her weight is 19th percentile, and her head circumference is 16th percentile for her corrected age. Her father describes her as "happy-go-lucky" and "easy-going." She feeds herself and enjoys playing near other children in pre-school. She can balance on one foot for 3 seconds, rides a tricycle at the park, and makes towers with three blocks. She uses about 75 words, 2 at a time in sentences, and is around 50% understandable by strangers. She can draw a circle with crayons and a person with three parts. She can also state her age and point to different parts of animals. Her physical exam, including hearing testing, is completely normal. What is the most likely diagnosis?

Answer: D, Expressive language developmental delay.

Explanation: This is a 3-year-old female who presents for a well-child examination, whose parent has no complaints. Unfortunately, these questions tend to be long and must be read very closely, as they usually assess for developmental milestones, which is a vital topic in pediatrics. This patient has achieved most 3-year-old milestones. REMEMBER that 3-year-olds do a lot of things that involve the number 3, including balance for 3 seconds, build 3-block towers, pedal a 3-wheeled tricycle, draw people with 3 parts, and say that they are 3 years old. Their speech is also expected to be 3/4 (75%) intelligible by strangers, and they use 3-word sentences, which this child does not do. Thus she has an expressive language developmental delay. Note that it is unclear if there is an identifiable cause and if she has an accompanying receptive language delay, but her cognition appears to be within the range of normal. More testing or intervention may be required, but as of now we are convinced only that she has this specific delay of development. Additionally, keep in mind that auditory dysfunction can significantly affect language development in children and will be of particular importance in questions involving language delay or inattention.

A. Normal development → Incorrect. Unlikely normal development because of her delay in speech. She should be 3/4 (75%) intelligible with 3 words at a time in sentences.

B. Fine motor developmental delay → Incorrect. The child draws, feeds herself, and plays with blocks without apparent difficulty for her age.

C. Gross motor developmental delay → Incorrect. The child balances and pedals at the appropriate developmental level.

E. Global developmental delay → Incorrect. This requires a failure to meet milestones of development in several areas. We have, to this point, noted only one area in which this child has a developmental delay.

3. WWGJD?

A 14-year-old male is brought to the pediatrician's office by his father. In private, he mentions that he has recently noticed changes in his physical appearance that have caused significant distress at school. Specifically, his nipples have protruded from his chest wall, and other students have begun to comment on his "breasts." He is afraid that something is wrong. His past medical history is notable for several episodes of rhinosinusitis, an ulnar fracture at the age of 9, and moderate eczema, for which he uses petroleum jelly. He denies any other medication use, as well as illicit drug use. His height, weight, and BMI are all between the 40th and 60th percentiles. His vital signs are T 98.4 °F, HR 82, BP 98/60, RR 16, SpO$_2$ 98% on room air. Examination of his chest reveals approximately 1 cm of sub-areolar and peri-areolar rubbery tissue. Examination of his genitalia reveals equal testicular volumes of 7 mL and coarse, dark hair beginning to grow along the penis and scrotum. The remainder of the examination is unremarkable. What is the likely diagnosis and appropriate management?

Answer: C, Idiopathic pubertal gynecomastia; reassurance
Explanation: This is a 14-year-old male with gynecomastia. The rubbery tissue noted on exam is indeed breast tissue. Gynecomastia, or breast tissue development in males, can be caused by many pathologic conditions and drugs. However, it is also a common occurrence during male puberty. Additionally, idiopathic pubertal gynecomastia resolves spontaneously within 2 years for a majority of patients, especially with areas of tissue less than 2 cm. Thus it is appropriate here to screen for normal pubertal milestones (his testicular volume approximately agrees with the description of his secondary hair development at Tanner stage 3) and pathologic causes and then reassure the patient that this is a common change that will likely go away as he ages. It is also important to help the patient build coping strategies for interactions with his classmates and to monitor the breast tissue over time.

A. Pseudogynecomastia; education about diet and exercise → Incorrect. Pseudogynecomastia refers to fat tissue giving the appearance of breast tissue growth. This patient, per his BMI, is not obese, and physical exam suggests the presence of true breast tissue.

B. Drug-induced gynecomastia; cessation of petroleum jelly use → Incorrect. Petroleum jelly is not associated with gynecomastia.

D. Klinefelter syndrome; education → Incorrect. It is important to think of Klinefelter syndrome in a male with gynecomastia, but he lacks other features of the disorder (hypogonadism, tall stature, etc.), so this is less likely.

E. Idiopathic pubertal gynecomastia; referral for surgery → Incorrect. Especially because this is often a transient physical feature in puberty, it would not be appropriate to refer this patient for surgery at this time.

Immunologic Disorders

Omar Khan, Sila Bal, Peter Capucilli, Hao-Hua Wu,
Leo Wang, and Rebecca Tenney-Soeiro

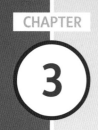

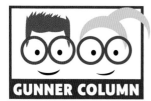

GUNNER COLUMN

The development and maintenance of a robust immune system is essential for a person's survival against microorganisms. As a result, diseases involving impaired immune function have severe clinical manifestations, including anaphylactic reactions, recurrent infections, and chronic diarrhea. For the Pediatrics exam, questions involving congenital abnormalities and allergic reactions are particularly high-yield, as they require comparisons across different physiologic mechanisms. For instance, chronic granulomatous disease (CGD) is the result of defective neutrophil oxidase metabolism. Individuals with this disorder are unable to protect themselves against catalase-positive organisms and are at increased risk of recurrent abscess formation. On the other hand, DiGeorge syndrome (DGS) (aka 22q11.2 deletion syndrome) involves thymic hypoplasia. The resultant T-cell abnormalities lead to an increased risk of viral infections. Do not get bogged down in the details of each mechanism. Understanding enough of the physiology to work out the clinical presentation for each disease is more than sufficient for the exam.

Knowing the cell types involved in the disorder will allow you to further differentiate between various abnormalities. For example, common variable immunodeficiency (CVID) will have a normal number of T cells; however, these cells will be defective. Conversely, severe combined immunodeficiency involves both T and B cells and individuals will have a low T-cell count.

For questions involving hypersensitivity reactions, make sure you are familiar with the expected time course, the antibodies involved, and common clinical presentations, so that you will be able to quickly pick out the important details needed to answer the question.

This chapter is divided into the following sections: (1) disorders associated with immunodeficiency, primarily of humoral immunity; (2) immunologically mediated disorders; (3) adverse effects of drugs on the immune system; (4) infectious disorders; (5) vasculitides; (6) autoimmune disorders; and (7) Gunner Practice.

Immunodeficiency

Disorders associated with immunodeficiency are organized on the US Medical Licensing Examination (USMLE) content by mechanism of disease. Since most of these diseases are congenital or genetic, no prophylactic measures can be implemented. Thus most of the Prophylaxis (PPx) sections will simply say "N/A." Instead, focus your attention on the Buzz Words, Diagnostic Steps (Dx), and Treatment and Management Steps (Tx/Mgmt).

The humoral immune system is comprised of B cells and protects the body against extracellular microbes (e.g., pyogenic bacteria). Examples of disorders of the humoral immune system include CVID, hyper-immunoglobulin (Ig)M syndrome, and Bruton agammaglobulinemia.

Cell-mediated immunity is driven by T cells and protects the body against intracellular microbes (e.g., viruses, fungi). Examples include DGS.

There are instances when diseases can present as a mix of B- and T-cell dysfunction; these diseases include severe combined immunodeficiency disease (SCID) and Wiskott-Aldrich syndrome (WAS).

The complement system defends the body against *Neisseria* organisms. Examples of disorders that arise due to defective complement proteins include terminal complement deficiency and acquired and hereditary angioedema.

Phagocytes and natural killer (NK) cells are part of the innate immune system and help to defend the body against microbes such as bacteria. Examples of disorders that arise due to defective phagocytic or NK cells include Chediak-Higashi syndrome.

Deficiency Primarily of Humoral Immunity

Common Variable Immunodeficiency

Buzz Words: Recurrent pulmonary infections/diarrhea + normal B-cell number + reduced serum IgG/A/M

Clinical Presentation: CVID is a heterogeneous group of diseases that results in defective maturation of B cells into antibody-secreting cells. Genetic lesions can occur in B cells themselves or in T cells and dendritic cells. Although B- and T-cell numbers are often normal, poor B-cell priming and subsequent defects in differentiation result in reduced production of IgG, IgA, and/or IgM. Although most commonly diagnosed in the second or third decade of life, clinical manifestations of CVID can also present in early childhood, with the following:

Recurrent pulmonary infections: Most commonly due to encapsulated bacteria, especially *Streptococcus pneumoniae* and *Haemophilus influenzae.* Patients commonly present with a chronic cough and signs of upper/lower respiratory infection. *Staphylococcus aureus* infections are also common.

Recurrent GI infections: Often caused by *Helicobacter pylori, Giardia lamblia,* or *Campylobacter jejuni.* Results in malabsorption and diarrhea.

Allergic disease: Including asthma, urticaria, eczema, and food allergies.

Autoimmune disease: Autoimmune cytopenias (autoimmune neutropenia, immune thrombocytopenia, hemolytic anemia) are commonly associated with CVID. Patients may also present with rheumatoid arthritis, systemic lupus erythematosus (SLE), or psoriasis.

Malignancy: Children with CVID have an increased risk of malignancy, chiefly B-cell lymphomas.

Failure to thrive: A common finding associated with chronic illness.

PPx: None

Mechanism of Disease (MoD): Multiple possible genetic mutations. Defects in B-cell differentiation/priming → inability to produce secreted antibodies, including IgG, IgA and/or IgM.

Dx:
1. Serum immunoglobulin levels: CVID Dx requires reduced serum levels of IgG in combination with IgA and/or IgM.
2. Antibody function studies: Patients with CVID mount poor responses to vaccines and will therefore have reduced titers against diptheria, tetanus, and *Haemophilus influenzae.*
3. B-cell studies: Will show normal B-cell counts:
   • Absence of B cells **excludes** the Dx of CVID.

Tx/Mgmt:
1. Immune globulin replacement: Can be performed subcutaneously (SCIG) or intravenously (IVIG).
2. Aggressive treatment of infections: Antibiotics may be given prophylactically for refractory infections.
3. Nutritional support.

QUICK TIPS

Live vaccines are contraindicated in patients with CVID.

Hyper-Immunoglobulin M Syndrome

Buzz Words: Recurrent/opportunistic infections + liver disease early in life + increased serum IgM + decreased IgG, IgA, and IgE

Clinical Presentation: Hyper-IgM syndrome (HIGM) is a rare, heterogeneous disease characterized by an increase in serum levels of IgM and a concurrent deficiency in IgG, IgA, and IgE. All types of HIGM involve a defect in the ability of B cells to undergo class-switch recombination, the process through which antibody heavy chains are replaced with other species. The most common cause involves X-linked mutations in CD40L, making the disease more prevalent in males. Clinical manifestations include:

Recurrent pulmonary infections: Patients present with recurrent cases of pneumonia, sinusitis, otitis media.

Opportunistic infections: Most commonly involve *Pneumocystis jirovecii* (resulting in pneumonia), *Cryptosporidium parvum* (resulting in chronic diarrhea), and cytomegalovirus (causing liver disease).

PPx: N/A

MoD: The most common cause of HIGM is a deficiency in CD40L in T cells (X-linked recessive). Mutations in this protein inhibit appropriate B-cell maturation → increase in serum IgM + decrease in IgG, IgA, and IgE.

Dx: Serum immunoglobulin levels: Increase in serum IgM with severe reduction in IgG, IgA, and IgE

Tx/Mgmt:
1. Immune globulin replacement: Can be performed subcutaneously (SCIG) or intravenously (IVIG).
2. Trimethoprim-sulfamethoxazole (TMP/SMX) for PPx against *P. jirovecii* infection.
3. Liver function testing: To detect liver dysfunction.

X-Linked Agammaglobulinemia (Bruton)

Buzz Words: Recurrent bacterial infections very early in life + male child + absence of peripheral B cells + severe reduction in all serum immunoglobulin species

Clinical Presentation: X-linked agammaglobulinemia (XLA) or Bruton agammaglobulinemia is characterized by a significant reduction in B cells secondary to mutations in the signaling molecule Bruton tyrosine kinase (Btk), which plays an important role in B-cell development. As an X-linked disease, XLA is found more commonly in males. Key characteristics of Bruton agammaglobulinemia include:

Age: Patients with XLA, like all newborns, rely on maternal IgG to prevent infections immediately after birth. Patients therefore often present with symptoms after 6 months of age, when the majority of maternal IgGs have been catabolized.

Recurrent bacterial infections: With *Streptococcus pneumoniae, Haemophilus influenzae B, Streptococcus pyogenes.*

Clinical findings: Include absent or small lymph nodes/tonsils.

PPx: N/A

MoD: Mutation in Btk → impaired B-cell development → absence of CD19+ B cells → absence of all antibodies

Dx:

1. Physical exam: Absence of tonsils/lymph nodes.
2. Family history: Incidence of disease in males of family.
3. Serum immunoglobulin levels: Severe reduction in all antibody species.
4. B-cell studies: Show an absence of mature B cells.
5. Genetic studies: Can confirm mutations at the Btk locus.

Tx/Mgmt:

1. Immune globulin replacement: Can be performed subcutaneously (SCIG) or intravenously (IVIG).

Autosomal Recessive Agammaglobulinemia

Buzz Words: Recurrent bacterial infections very early in life of male **OR** female child + absence of peripheral B cells + severe reduction in all serum immunoglobulin species

Clinical Presentation: Many genetic lesions can result in autosomal recessive agammaglobulinemia (ARA). Patients with this disease will present in exactly the same way as those with XLA and are also treated similarly. Differentiating between XLA and ARA requires a compatible family history (i.e., incidence of disease in females within the family) or exclusion of mutations in Btk.

PPx: N/A

MoD: See XLA

Dx: As XLA, but with autosomal recessive inheritance pattern

Tx/Mgmt: See XLA

Selective Immunoglobulin A Deficiency

Buzz Words: Recurrent infections/autoimmune disease or anaphylactic reaction after transfusion + isolated reduction in serum IgA

Clinical Presentation: IgA deficiency is the most common antibody defect in humans and occurs in 1:100 to 1000 children of non-Asian descent (in Asians, the incidence is slightly lower). The vast majority of patients with IgA deficiency are asymptomatic, with fewer than 30% presenting with the following symptoms:

Recurrent pulmonary infections: Recurrent episodes of otitis media, sinusitis, and pneumonia secondary to infection with *S. pneumoniae* or *H. influenzae*.

Gastrointestinal manifestations: Patients with IgA deficiency have an increased susceptibility to *G. lamblia* infection. Noninfectious GI manifestations include celiac disease and inflammatory bowel disease.

Autoimmune disease: Can be found in up to 30% of patients. The most common autoimmune diseases include systemic lupus erythematosus (SLE), Graves disease, rheumatoid arthritis (RA), type 1 diabetes (T1D), and vitiligo.

Atopy: Risk of food and respiratory allergies is increased in patients with IgA deficiency. Asthma, eczema, and urticaria are also commonly associated with this disease.

Transfusion reactions: A minority of patients can develop anaphylactic reactions to blood or plasma products that contain IgA. This generally occurs only in patients with undetectable levels of serum IgA. This clinical pearl, however, may be highlighted in board questions.

PPx: N/A

MoD: IgA deficiency can occur secondary to many different defects in B and/or T cells. Although B cells expressing surface IgA are still present, secretion of IgA is impaired → severe reduction in serum IgA.

Dx:
1. Serum immunoglobulin levels: less than 7 mg/dL serum IgA with normal levels of IgG and IgM

Tx/Mgmt:
1. Primarily focuses on managing infections and other complications:
   - IVIG/SCIG is not indicated in this case because secreted IgA dimers cannot be replaced. In fact, IVIG and SCIG contain only small amounts of IgA.
   - Moreover, if patients with undetectable levels of IgA are given exogenous immunoglobulins, they may be at risk for an anaphylactic reaction (due to preformed antibodies against IgA).

Selective Immunoglobulin M Deficiency

Buzz Words: Recurrent infections and/or atopy in child + isolated reduction in IgM

Clinical Presentation: An exceedingly rare selective immunodeficiency characterized by an isolated reduction in serum IgM and normal levels of IgG and IgA. Although many patients remain asymptomatic, some may present with serious, recurrent infections and atopy:

QUICK TIPS

Atopy: Patients have increased incidence of asthma, allergic rhinitis, and eczema.

Recurrent bacterial/viral infections: Patients most commonly present with recurrent cases of otitis media, bronchitis, pneumonia, or chronic rhinosinusitis. Sepsis has also been documented in some patients.

PPx: N/A

MoD: Cause is unknown, but most likely due to multiple different mechanisms that effect B and T cells. Although most patients have normal surface levels of IgM, B- and/or T-cell dysfunction results in severe reductions in secreted IgM.

Dx:

1. Serum immunoglobulin levels: less than 10–15 mg/dL serum IgM with normal levels of IgG and IgA

Tx/Mgmt:

1. Management of atopic disease: Aggressive treatment of asthma and allergic rhinitis may reduce risk of pulmonary infections.
2. Immune globulin replacement and prophylactic antibiotics: In patients with recurrent infections.

Immunoglobulin G Subclass Deficiency

Buzz Words: Recurrent sinopulmonary infections + normal total IgG levels → IgG2/3/4 deficiency. IgG1 deficiency generally results in hypogammaglobulinemia.

Clinical Presentation: Clinical presentation is variable, characterized by a significant decrease in the serum levels of one or more IgG subclasses (IgG1, IgG2, IgG3, IgG4). The majority of IgG-deficient patients remain asymptomatic. In fact, upward of 20% of healthy individuals have a deficiency in at least one IgG subclass. Therefore IgG deficiency is relevant in patients who present with recurrent infections or have poor responses to vaccines. Characteristics of this disease include:

Age/gender: IgG subclass deficiencies are 3 times more common in male children, but this gender distribution flips in adulthood, as the disease is primarily seen in women after age 16.

Recurrent sinopulmonary infections: All subclass deficiencies increase the risk of recurrent infection. Patients generally present with recurrent bronchitis, sinusitis, and/or otitis. Specific characteristics of individual subclass deficiencies are as follows:

IgG1 deficiency: Occurs mostly in adults. Patients commonly have hypogammaglobulinemia (as IgG1 is the primary IgG species in serum).

IgG2 deficiency: Is more prevalent in children. Patients have an increased risk of infection with *S. penumoniae, H. influenzae B*, and *Neisseria meningitidis*.

IgG3 deficiency: Is more common in adults. This sub-class deficiency is associated with an increased risk of infection with *Moraxella catarrhalis* and *Streptococcus pyogenes*.

IgG4 deficiency: Is relatively common. Most patients with isolated IgG4 deficiency remain asymptomatic but can present with recurrent infections, as with the other subclass deficiencies.

PPx: N/A

MoD: Subclass deficiencies can be caused by numerous different mechanisms, including genetic mutations and dysregulation of cytokine responses.

Dx:
1. Serum immunoglobulin levels: With the exception of IgG1 deficiency, patients with other subclass defi-ciencies have normal levels of total IgG. Dx is made by the measurement of serum levels of specific IgG species.
2. Vaccine challenge: Patients with clinically relevant IgG subclass deficiency have poor responses to vaccina-tion. This is measured by analyzing antibody titers prior to and after the administration of a vaccine.

Tx/Mgmt: As with other selective immunodeficiencies, aggressive management of sinopulmonary infections, vaccination, prophylactic antibiotics, and IVIG are main-stays of management.

Selective Immunoglobulin E Deficiency

Buzz Words: Recurrent sinopulmonary infections and/or nonallergic reactive airway disease + isolated, signifi-cant decrease in serum IgE

Clinical Presentation: Selective IgE deficiency is largely a laboratory finding and is not always associated with a clinically relevant disease.

Recurrent sinopulmonary infections and nonallergic reac-tive airway disease (including congestion, rhinorrhea, cough, and wheezing) can occur in patients with selec-tive IgE deficiency.

PPx: N/A

MoD: Largely unknown

Dx: Serum immunoglobulin levels: Dx can be made when serum IgE levels fall below 2.5 U/mL with normal levels of IgG and IgA.

Tx/Mgmt:
1. IVIG is not indicated, as serum IgE replacement is currently not available. Management of associated infections and conditions remains the primary form of care.

Cell Mediated

Cell-mediated immunity is driven by T cells. As stated in Table 3.1, defects in cell-mediated immunity lead to largely intracellular pathogens and fungi. Use infectious etiology to differentiate defects in cell-mediated and humoral immunity.

Severe Combined Immunodeficiency Disease

Buzz Words: Recurrent infections + common gamma chain mutation + B- and T-cell defect

Clinical Presentation: The term *SCID* covers a heterogeneous group of diseases that results in significant dysfunction of both B and T cells as well as natural killer cells ("combined"). These diseases are termed "severe" as they often lead to death within the first year of life secondary to uncontrolled infection unless patients reach medical care. Given severity, efforts in recent years have focused on newborn screening for SCID, early recognition, and treatment.

Infections early in life: Due to significant loss in adaptive immunity. This results in susceptibility to common viruses (including but not limited to rotavirus, norovirus, cytomegalovirus, Epstein–Barr virus), opportunistic pathogens (*P. jirovecii*), and poor responses to vaccination. Mucocutaneous candidiasis early in life is often one of the first indications of SCID. Other key presenting histories include failure to thrive and chronic diarrhea.

PPx: N/A

MoD: (1) X-linked SCID: Most common form of SCID. Genetic lesion in the IL-2 receptor common gamma chain → loss of functional receptors for interleukins 2, 4, 7, 9, 15, and 21. (2) Autosomal recessive SCID: The most common autosomal cause for SCID, due to adenosine deaminase deficiency (ADA).

TABLE 3.1 Type of Immunologic Deficiency Versus Types of Infections

Immunological Deficiency	Types of Susceptible Infections
B-cell deficiency	Pyogenic bacteria, parasites, enteric bacteria, and viruses (largely extracellular)
T-cell deficiency	Viruses, atypical mycobacteria, fungi, bacteria within the cell (largely intracellular)
Terminal complement deficiency	*Neisseria meningitides* and *Neisseria gonorrhoeae*

TABLE 3.2 Types of Hypersensitivity Reactions: Mechanisms and Examples

Hypersensitivity	Mediated by	Mechanism of Action	Example
Type 1	IgE	Allergen binds and cross-links 2 IgE molecules attached to mast cells	Atopy/ urticaria/ anaphylaxis
Type 2	Antibodies	Antibody attack antigen	ABO blood type incompatibility + Rh hemolytic disease
Type 3	Immune complex–mediated	IgG or IgM antibodies form immune complexes → nonspecifically activates inflammatory process	Serum sickness syndrome (mediated by antibody-containing blood) Arthus reaction Serum sickness–like reaction (mediated by drug)
Type 4	Cell-mediated (T-cell)	Prior exposure to allergen before developing reaction; reexposure activates cell-mediated response	**Allergic contact dermatitis** from poison ivy, oak, or sumac

Ig, Immunoglobulin.

- Several other mutations may also result in severe combined immunodeficiency. SCID may result from defects in T cells + B cells or T cells alone (T cells play an important role stimulating B cells to produce antibodies, therefore T-cell defects can substantially dampen humoral responses).

Dx:

1. Complete blood count (CBC) to look for lymphopenia: Absolute lymphocytes counts generally fall below 2500/mL.
2. Flow cytometry to measure abnormality in T-cell subsets.

3. Poor T-cell function: T cells from patients with SCID are poorly proliferative in response to mitogens.
4. Hypogammaglobulinemia: Is generally found but may be complicated by maternal IgGs, especially early in life.
5. Chest radiograph: Will commonly show the absence of a thymic "shadow"; this finding is not specific for SCID.

Tx/Mgmt:
1. Protection from infection: Children with SCID are incredibly susceptible to infection, therefore early and expedient protective measures are an important part of management.
2. Patients should be kept in isolation, must receive irradiated blood products (if necessary), and should not be given live vaccines.
3. IVIG: To replenish and maintain serum globulin levels.
4. Prophylactic antibiotics and antivirals: Trimethoprim-sulfamethoxazole (for *P. jirovecii*). Consider palivizumab during the winter to protect from respiratory syncytial virus (RSV) in those less than 2 years old.
5. Hematopoietic stem cell transplant: May be curative in SCID.

DiGeorge Syndrome (Old Name; Now Part of 22q11.2 Deletion Syndrome)

Buzz Words: Cardiac defects + abnormal facies + thymic hypoplasia + cleft palate + hypocalcemia → DGS

Clinical Presentation: DiGeorge is now part of the 22q11.2 deletion syndrome. However, since the National Board of Medical Examiners (NBME) sometimes recycles old questions, the term *DiGeorge syndrome* may come up. Clinical findings in patients with DGS stem from defects in the development of the pharyngeal pouch system.

Cardiac defects: Most patients present with conotruncal/outflow tract defects including interrupted aortic arch, truncus arteriosus, tetralogy of Fallot, septal defects, or vascular rings.

Abnormal facies: May include ear and ocular defects, but these findings are not specific for DGS.

Thymic hypoplasia: The thymus can also be completely absent in DGS patients. The severity of the hypoplasia determines the degree of immunodeficiency. Patients can present with recurrent infections or symptoms of SCID.

Cleft palate

Hypocalcemia: Due to poor parathyroid development. Hypocalcemia in DGS patients can therefore be paired with low levels of parathyroid hormone. Patients may present with seizures due to the hypocalcemia.

PPx: N/A

MoD: Microdeletions on chromosome 22q11.2 lead to the loss of several genes that play an important role in the sequence of pharyngeal development → CATCH-22 clinical presentation.

Dx:

1. T-cell enumeration: less than 500/mm^3 CD3+ T cells.
2. Conotruncal defect: Such as interrupted aortic arch, truncus arteriosus, tetralogy of Fallot (ToF).
3. Persistent hypocalcemia.
4. Detection of chromosome 22q11.2 deletion: Performed using fluorescence in situ hybridization (FISH).

Tx/Mgmt:

1. Cardiothoracic surgery: Cardiac emergencies may necessitate surgical correction of conotruncal abnormalities.
2. Calcium supplementation: With intravenous calcium gluconate or calcium chloride.
3. Immune symptoms: For patients with partial DGS, and therefore some immune function, vaccination and PPx against recurrent sinopulmonary infections are important.
4. Correction of palate defects:
   - Patients with complete DGS should be treated like those with SCID.
   - Thymic transplants are the preferred curative therapy, but the procedure is not widely available.
   - Bone marrow transplant does not completely restore the T-cell repertoire but improves immune function adequately and should be performed as soon as possible.
   - Bottom line: Treatment of DiGeorge usually requires a multidisciplinary team approach with specialists from various fields. Specialized clinics are largely found in the nation's children's hospitals.

Wiskott–Aldrich Syndrome

Buzz Words: Clotting deficiency immediately at birth + recurrent infections + malignancy + family history of similar disease in males

Clinical Presentation: X-linked congenital disorder caused by mutation in the *WAS* gene, which plays an important role in linking T-cell receptor signaling pathways to cytoskeletal rearrangement. Although patients initially have normal serum lymphocyte levels, both T- and B-cell counts decrease over time, therefore increasing infection susceptibility with age.

Recurrent infections: Increase in frequency as the patient ages. Typical pathogens include *S. pneumoniae, N. meningitidis*, and *H. influenzae.*

Thrombocytopenia: Is found in the vast majority of *WAS* patients. Manifestations can be observed immediately after birth (prolonged bleeding of umbilical cord). Platelet defect can be life-threatening in the case of gastrointestinal or intracranial bleeding.

Eczema: Is common within the first year of life. (This is often used as a clue to board questions.)

Malignancies: Are found with increasing incidence as patient ages. B-cell lymphoma and leukemia are most common.

PPx: N/A

MoD: Mutation in X chromosome *WAS* gene → defective cytoskeletal remodeling and subsequent poor T- and B-cell function → increased susceptibility to infection and thrombocytopenia

Dx:
1. **Congenital thrombocytopenia:** As observed from complete blood count. Small platelets are also seen in WAS.
2. Detection of mutation in *WAS* gene.
3. Compatible family history: Evidence of *WAS* in maternal male cousins, uncles, or nephews.
4. Poor antibody response to polysaccharides/ polysaccharide vaccines, which include protection against the encapsulated bacteria *N. meningitidis, S. pneumoniae,* and *H. influenzae* B.
5. T-cell studies: Lymphocyte counts are generally normal early in life, but levels fall over time. T cells may also exhibit poor proliferative responses to mitogen. Abnormal antibody distribution: Patients generally have normal levels of IgG but lower levels of IgM and higher levels of IgA and IgE.

Tx/Mgmt:
1. Hematopoietic cell transplantation (HCT): Patients generally respond well to this, the only curative therapy currently available.
2. Immune globulin replacement: IVIG is recommended for patients with antibody deficiencies.
3. Splenectomy: Resolves thrombocytopenia in the majority of patients. After the procedure, patients must receive IVIG and prophylactic antibiotics for life.

Deficiencies of the Innate Immune System

Chediak–Higashi Syndrome

Buzz Words: Azurophilic granules in neutrophils + recurrent pyogenic infections + streaked blond hair + neutropenia + toddler → Chediak–Higashi syndrome

Clinical Presentation: This is an extremely rare autosomal recessive disorder that stems from a defect in lysosomal trafficking. Patients who survive the severe and recurrent infections early in life often go through a period of accelerating disease, when the following symptoms drastically worsen:

Oculocutaneous albinism: Defect in melanosome transfer to keratinocytes/epithelial cells result in speckled hypo/hyperpigmentation and characteristic streaks of blond hair (which also have a metallic appearance).

Recurrent pyogenic infections: Defect in neutrophil and cytolytic T-cell function results in frequent and severe pyogenic infections. Cutaneous and respiratory infections are common and are generally caused by *S. aureus, S. pyogenes,* and *Pneumococcus.*

Neutropenia: Is a common finding. Moreover, neutrophil function is also severely hampered.

Platelet abnormalities: Mild coagulation defects are common.

Neurologic manifestations: Large granules can be found in Schwann cells. Diffuse atrophy of the brain and spinal cord may be present during the accelerated phase of disease. Patients can experience difficulty walking, poor balance, and reduction in cognitive function.

PPx: N/A

MoD: Congenital defect in lysosomal trafficking (*CHS1/LYST* gene) → poor melanosome delivery, poor cytotoxicity/cytolytic granule release, reduction in platelet-dense bodies → clinical symptoms

Dx:
1. Peripheral blood smear: Will show giant azurophilic granules within neutrophils and other granulocytes.

Tx/Mgmt:
1. HCT is the therapy of choice to correct immune deficiency. Importantly, this does not correct neurologic symptoms/damage or albinism.
2. Aggressive treatment of infections, once they occur, and prophylaxis for patients with recurrent infections.

MNEMONIC
Wiskott–Aldrich mnemonic: walT for ME. Immunodeficiency, Thrombocytopenia, Malignancy, Eczema.

Chronic Granulomatous Disease

Buzz Words: Severe/recurrent infection with catalase-positive bacteria/*Aspergillus* + nicotinamide adenine dinucleotide phosphate (NADPH) oxidase deficiency

Clinical Presentation: High yield for exams. CGD is a genetically heterogeneous disease (with both X-linked and autosomal recessive forms) that stems from mutations in the NADPH oxidase system. Defects in NADPH oxidase result in the defective production of the reactive oxygen species (ROS) required for robust immune function. Specifically, CGD results in poorly functional granulocytes, which therefore increases the susceptibility of patients to bacterial infection. As the X-linked form of CGD is more common, this is primarily a disease of males.

Recurrent and severe infections: Pneumonia is the most prevalent type of infection, but abscesses, suppurative adenitis, osteomyelitis, and skin infections are also common. Typical bacterial organisms include *S. aureus, Pseudomonas, Serratia,* and *Nocardia* species. *Aspergillus* infection is also common in CGD patients.

PPx: N/A

MoD: Defect in NADPH oxidase system → poor granulocyte respiratory burst → defective clearance of catalase-positive bacteria and *Aspergillus*

Dx:
1. Neutrophil function testing to identify deficiencies in superoxide production; the DHT (dihydrorhodamine 123) and NBT (nitroblue tetrazolium) tests are commonly used.

Tx/Mgmt:
1. Infection PPx: TMP-SMX (antibacterial) + itraconazole (antifungal) administration drastically increase patient's life span.
2. Prophylactic immunomodulation with administration of interferon gamma (IFN-gamma).
3. Infection management: Patients must be treated aggressively with antibiotics and abscess drainage as necessary.
4. HCT can be curative for patients with CGD.

Schwachman-Diamond Syndrome

Buzz Words: Neutropenia + steatorrhea + skeletal abnormalities + recurrent infections in a young child

Clinical Presentation: Schwachman-Diamond syndrome (SDS) is an autosomal recessive disease that involves mutations in the *SBDS* gene in the majority of patients. *SBDS* has multiple enzymatic functions, including the regulation of neutrophil chemotaxis.

Neutropenia: Absolute neutrophil count (ANC) of less than 1500/μL

Recurrent infections: Pneumonia, otitis media, and abscesses

Exocrine pancreatic dysfunction: SDS is a major cause of exocrine pancreatic dysfunction, with many patients presenting with steatorrhea.

Skeletal abnormalities: Also common in SDS patients, with many having short stature.

Hepatic dysfunction: Elevated transaminases and hepatomegaly are common.

PPx: N/A

MoD: Autosomal recessive with 90% having mutation in the *SBDS* gene, although the function of the protein is unknown.

Dx: Based on clinical findings of pancreatic dysfunction and neutropenia. Dx can be confirmed by genetic testing.

Tx/Mgmt:

1. HCT is curative for the immune defects seen in SDS but does not improve pancreatic function.
2. For neutropenia + fever in SDS, tx with broad-spectrum antibiotics with blood cultures ordered immediately.
3. Supplementation for pancreatic dysfunction: Oral pancreatic enzymes and fat-soluble vitamins administered as needed.

Leukocyte Adhesion Deficiency

Buzz Words: Recurrent infections + delayed umbilical cord separation + impaired leukocyte trafficking

Clinical Presentation: High yield on exams. The migration of leukocytes from the bloodstream to the site of infection or injury is critical for efficient wound healing and immunity. Upon receiving a specific stimulus (such as inflammatory cytokine signals), leukocytes loosely bind to endothelial cells, roll, arrest, and extravasate into the tissue. Each of these steps is crucial for leukocyte migration and requires the function of several different adhesion molecules.

There are three described leukocyte adhesion deficiency (LAD) syndromes: LAD1, LAD2, and LAD3. As LAD2/3 are exceedingly rare, only LAD1 is discussed here. LAD1 is an autosomal recessive disorder. The clinical presentation of LAD1 results from mutations in CD18, the common beta chain of the beta 2 integrin family. This results in deficiencies in the expression of LFA-1 and Mac-1.

Stems from impaired leukocyte trafficking. Classic clinical findings include:

Recurrent bacterial infection: Omphalitis (infection of umbilical stump) and delayed umbilical cord separation. Patients frequently present with cutaneous, respiratory, and perirectal infections. *S. aureus* is a primary infectious organism.

Leukocytosis: An increase in blood leukocyte levels due to poor extravasation.

Severe gingivitis: More common later in life.

PPx: N/A

MoD: Mutation in CD18 → impaired extravasation of leukocytes from the bloodstream → leukocytosis and poor responses to infection and wound healing

Dx:

1. Primarily based on clinical findings, particularly leukocytosis + recurrent infections in an infant.
2. CD18/CD11a flow cytometry can confirm Dx.

Tx/Mgmt:

1. Aggressive management of active infections.
2. For severe cases of LAD1, patients may receive HCT, which is curative.

Complement Deficiency

C1 Esterase Inhibitory Deficiency

Buzz Words: Increased bradykinin + recurrent angioedema + laryngeal angioedema + strong family history of similar symptoms + chronic reduction in C4 levels

Clinical Presentation: C1 esterase inhibitor (C1INH) is a serine protease inhibitor (serpin) that limits the activity of several plasma proteases including C1r/C1s (classical complement pathway), MASP1/2 (MBL complement pathway), coagulation factors XI/XII, plasma kallikrein, and plasmin. C1INH plays an important role in limiting the catalytic product of factor XII and kallikrein: bradykinin, a potent vasodilator and enhancer of vascular permeability.

Both C1INH deficiency (defect in protein production) and C1INH dysfunction (normal levels of a defective protein) can result in hereditary angioedema (HAE). Inability to limit bradykinin production can result in significant swelling of the skin, gastrointestinal tract, and respiratory tract.

HAE is inherited in an autosomal dominant fashion; 25% of cases develop due to spontaneous mutation.

Age: Many patients show symptoms before the age of 5. Frequency of symptoms increases after puberty.

Recurrent angioedema, which resolves spontaneously and occurs without urticaria or pruritus. Can manifest cutaneously, in the GI tract (leading to abdominal pain), or in the respiratory tract.

Laryngeal edema, which can result in asphyxiation if not immediately treated.

MoD: Dysfunction/deficiency in C1 esterase inhibitor → increased bradykinin → increased vasodilation and vascular permeability → recurrent episodes of angioedema

Dx:

1. Clinical findings: Recurrent angioedema, especially in a patient with a family history of HAE, is highly suspicious for the disease.
2. Low C4 levels: C1r/C1s function to cleave C4 in the complement cascade.
3. Deficiency/dysfunction of C1INH results in chronically low levels of C4 in patients.

Tx/Mgmt:

1. C1 Inhibitor concentrate: Is the most commonly used therapy for acute angioedema attacks.
2. Angioedema PPx: Antifibrinolytics or androgens can help control symptoms in many patients.
3. Avoidance of exacerbating factors: Including estrogen (certain contraceptives) and angiotensin-converting enzyme (ACE) inhibitors.

Immunologically Mediated Disorders

In contrast to the "disorders associated with immunodeficiency," where the immune system is too weak to mount an adequate immune response, the "immunologically mediated disorders" can be thought of as involving an overactive immune response.

Multisystem Infectious Disorders

Lyme Disease (*Borrelia burgdorferi*)

Buzz Words: Bilateral Bell palsy + no other signs of peripheral neuropathy → Lyme disease (be sure to differentiate from Guillain-Barré syndrome, which can present with bilateral Bell palsy associated with ascending paralysis.

Hiking in tall grass + ECG shows third-degree AV block + joint pain (arthritis) + facial nerve palsy → Lyme disease

Clinical Presentation: This is the most high-yield bacterial infection to know for the exam because it affects multiple organ systems and can present in a variety of ways. Lyme disease is caused by *B. burgdorferi* via the *Ixodes* deer tick. Lyme presents in multiple stages, spreading from local to multisystem:

Stage 1 (early): Erythema migrans (targetoid lesion)

Stage 2: Third-degree AV block, facial nerve palsy (Bell), migratory arthritis and myalgias

Stage 3 (late): Encephalopathy and chronic arthritis

QUICK TIPS
Definition of serum sickness syndrome: immune complex–mediated hypersensitivity to nonhuman proteins.

QUICK TIPS
Fever + urticarial rash + polyarthralgia + lymphadenopathy (LAD) + viral infection + use of penicillin + amoxicillin + cefaclor → serum sickness-like reaction. Although serum sickness–like reaction is drug-induced, it does not represent a true drug allergy since it is an immune complex–mediated (type 3) reaction. Treat by withdrawing offending agent.

QUICK TIPS
Patient returned from trip to woods + itching/burning/oozing lesions of skin → allergic contact dermatitis due to poison ivy → type IV (cell-mediated) hypersensitivity.

AR

Lyme disease patient presentation

Typically patients on the exam will present with either stage 1 or 2 symptoms, although be wary of stage 3 in considering the differential for encephalopathies. Also keep a keen eye out for exposure to tall grass and hiking in the northeastern US.

Be sure to differentiate Lyme from *Babesia microtii*, which is also transmitted by *Ixodes* ticks but will present with hemolytic anemia instead (Fig. 3.1).

PPx:

1. Avoid skin exposure while hiking in tall grass in the northeastern US.

MoD: *Ixodes* deer tick → *B. burgdorferi* bacterium transmitted through bite → Lyme disease

Dx:

1. Diagnosis of lyme disease is generally made exclusively from clinical presentation. Importantly, patients may not present with a classic EM lesion (absence cannot rule out lyme disease).
2. Serological testing (ELISA) for IgM/IgG antibodies against B. burgdorferi should only be used as an adjunct to clinical diagnosis. In fact, early in disease, patients will be seronegative.

Tx/Mgmt:

1. If patient is over 9 years old, doxycycline (on medicine, all question-stem patients will be adults, so doxycycline is the default answer for treatment. For your pediatrics

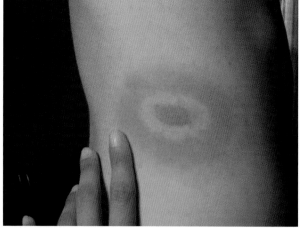

FIG. 3.1 Erythema migrans (characteristic "bull's-eye" or targetoid lesion). (From Wikipedia: https://en.wikipedia.org/wiki/Erythema_chronicum_migrans#/media/File:Bullseye_Lyme_Disease_Rash.jpghttps://en.wikipedia.org/wiki/Erythema_chronicum_migrans - /media/File:Bullseye_Lyme_Disease_Rash.jpg; https://en.wikipedia.org/wiki/Erythema_chronicum_migrans - /media/File:Bullseye_Lyme_Disease_Rash.jpg)

exam, however, keep in mind that Lyme disease in kids younger than 9 is treated with amoxicillin).
2. If disseminated (e.g., stage 3) and doxycycline is not an answer choice, ceftriaxone.

Toxic Shock Syndrome

Buzz Words: History of recent tampon use OR nasal packing + septic shock + scalded skin syndrome + no other plausible explanation → toxic shock syndrome due to bacterial toxin

Male or female + septic shock + diffuse maculopapular rash + desquamation of palms/soles (scalded skin syndrome) + strawberry tongue (indicative of *Streptococcus pyogenes* infection) → toxic shock syndrome (can also present without clear source of infection)

Clinical Presentation: *Toxic shock syndrome* refers to the devastating sequelae of infection by *S. aureus* or *S. pyogenes* through an intramucosal nidus (e.g., tampon or nasal packing) and toxin-mediated overactivation of the immune system. Learn the Buzz Words as well as the workup/management of these types of patients, which will touch upon how one manages a patient in septic shock.

PPx: (1) Avoid prolonged use of same tampon or nasal packing. (2) Avoid food poisoning.

MoD: Caused by **toxins** released by *S. aureus* or *S. pyogenes*. Toxic shock syndrome toxin (TSST-1) or exotoxin A (*S. pyogenes*) binds to MHC II and T-cell receptor → activation of T-cell (cell-mediated immunity) → release of pyrogenic cytokines such as IL-1, IL-2, and TNF-alpha → symptoms such as shock.

Dx:
1. CBC
2. Comprehensive metabolic panel (CMP)
3. Liver panel (decreased aspartate aminotransferase [AST], alanine aminotransferase [ALT], bilirubin)
4. Blood cultures

Tx/Mgmt:
1. ABCs (e.g., fluids to stabilize pressure)
2. Antibiotics (broad-spectrum or with penicillin + clindamycin once inciting agent is known)
3. Admission, often to an intensive care unit (ICU)

Rickettsiosis (Rocky Mountain Spotted Fever)

Buzz Words: Headache + fever + rash that starts in the wrists and spreads proximally/distally + rash of palms and soles + pancytopenia + hyponatremia → RMSF

QUICK TIPS

Rash of the palms or soles of foot → only 3 diseases should be on your differential: hand-foot-mouth disease caused by Coxsackie A virus, syphilis (secondary), and RMSF.

Clinical Presentation: Rocky Mountain spotted fever (RMSF) is a disease commonly seen on the East Coast. On the exam, it can present in both kids (Pediatrics shelf) and adults (Medicine shelf). RMSF rash starts at the wrists and spreads to the palms and soles. Most patients went hiking or camping in the southeastern United States, NOT the Rocky Mountains. Patients are treated with doxycycline.

PPx: Long sleeves and pants when hiking

MoD: (1) *Rickettsia rickettsiae* is carried by and transmitted by *Dermacentor variabilis* (dog or wood) tick.

Dx: Clinical; BMP often shows hyponatremia

Tx/Mgmt: Doxycycline; no age restriction due to severity of RMSF

Viral

Multisystem viral infections are the second most high-yielding because of Epstein-Barr virus (EBV) and CM5.

Infectious Mononucleosis (aka "Mono")

Buzz Words: Young adult + posterior cervical lymphadenopathy + fever/fatigue + hepatosplenomegaly + exudative pharyngitis + cold autoimmune hemolytic anemia (e.g., painful extremities w/ hemolytic anemia) + heterophile antibodies → infectious mononucleosis

Young adult + persistent abdominal pain after trauma (e.g., physical contact during sports) to left upper quadrant + shock + recent history of fever/sickness that had "resolved" → rupture of the spleen due to splenomegaly from mononucleosis infection

Fever/fatigue + polymorphous maculopapular rash status post-amoxicillin → Indicative of infection with EBV (rash seems to occur when amoxicillin is given in setting of EBV infection; not considered a drug allergy and mechanism unknown)

Burkitt lymphoma + nasopharyngeal carcinoma → EBV infection

Tonsillar exudates + fever + anterior lymphadenopathy → GA strep pharyngitis (vs. mono, which has posterior LAD) (Fig. 3.2)

Fever + fatigue + exudative pharyngitis + diffuse, posterior cervical LAD + splenomegaly (and hepatomegaly) → infectious mononucleosis

Clinical Presentation: Mono is the highest-yielding multisystemic viral infection because it is commonly seen and affects many different organ systems (e.g., upper respiratory tract, liver, spleen). Furthermore, EBV, the infectious agent, has been implicated in a couple of well-known cancers (e.g., Burkitt lymphoma and nasopharyngeal carcinoma).

QUICK TIPS

Complications of EBV-mediated mono: (1) increased risk for splenic rupture, (2) rash if exposed to penicillin (PCN), (3) can remain dormant in B cells → increases risk of recurrence and lymphoma (pathoma)

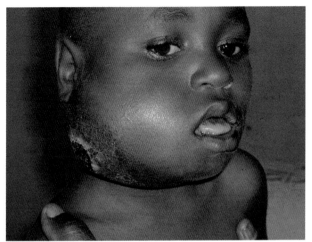

FIG. 3.2 Burkitt lymphoma, jaw swelling. (From Wikipedia: https://en.wikipedia.org/wiki/Burkitt%27s_lymphoma#/media/File:Large_facial_Burkitt%27s_Lymphoma.JPG)

PPx: (1) Avoid kissing someone with mono (or anyone with a fever who is clearly sick). (2) If infected, avoid sports for at least 3 weeks to prevent splenic rupture.

MoD: Caused by EBV (aka HHV-4) transmitted through saliva (kissing) → infects B cells through CD21

Dx:

1. Monospot
2. Positive heterophile antibody test (will show antibodies detected by agglutination of animal red blood cells)

Of note, monospot can be negative in an EBV+ child, so important to perform heterophile antibody test if there is high suspicion.

Tx/Mgmt:

1. Supportive care
2. Steroids

Vasculitides

Henoch-Schönlein Purpura (HSP)

Buzz Words: Palpable purpura + joint pain + IgA immune complex deposition in kidney **and** skin/GI tract + normal-elevated platelets + hematuria + GI bleed/pain + recent upper respiratory tract infection → HSP

Clinical Presentation: Henoch-Schönlein purpura (HSP) is a small-cell vasculitis associated with palpable purpura, IgA immune complex deposition in both the kidney and organs outside the kidney (e.g., skin or GI tract), and normal-elevated platelets. Often presents after an upper respiratory tract infection.

If IgA deposition is found only in kidney, the disease is likely IgA nephropathy. If platelets are low in a patient with palpable purpura, suspect thrombotic thrombocytopenic purpura (TTP). Given its penchant for affecting multiple organ systems and mimicking pathology, HSP is frequently tested on the Medicine and Pediatrics exams.

Other disorders that mimic HSP include:

- Pupura fulminans: Associated with *N. meningitidis*, *S. pneumoniae*; presents with hypotension and disseminated intravascular coagulopathy (DIC)
- Leukemia: Bone marrow infiltration → purpura → elevated WBCs and decreased platelet count
- Viral exanthems
- Vesicular/macular/maculopapular rather than purpuric
- Rocky Mountain spotted fever + atypical measles; can progress to purpura but has **fever** as well
- Von Willebrand factor (vWF) deficiency
- Hemophilia A/B

PPx: Unknown

MoD:

1. Inflammation of small vessels such as arterioles, venules, and capillaries of unknown cause
2. Palpable purpura due to bleeding from IgA immune complex–mediated inflammation
3. Hematuria due to IgA immune complex deposition in the mesangium of the glomerulus

Dx:

1. CBC (normal platelets)
2. Coags (normal coags)
3. BMP (Nl to mildly elevated Cr)
4. UA (hematuria + red cell casts + mild proteinuria)
5. Skin exam to look for palpable purpura
6. Renal biopsy → immunofluorescence microscopy → IgA IC deposition in the kidney, mesangial deposition of IgA

Tx/Mgmt:

1. Supportive management (hydration/pain control with NSAIDs)
2. Hospitalization indicated for severe abdominal pain + renal insufficiency + AMS + poor PO
3. Glucocorticoids (e.g., steroids) in patients with severe abdominal pain unresponsive to NSAIDs

Kawasaki Disease

Buzz Words: Red eyes + rash on body + arthritis + strawberry tongue + skin peeling off hands + fever for 5 days or more

---

MNEMONIC

CRASH and Burn
Conjunctivitis
Rash
Arthritis
Strawberry tongue
Hands with skin peeling
BURN (high fever ≥5 days): http://kawasakidiseaseawareness.blogspot.com/2009/05/crash-and-burn.html, Accessed 25.05.17

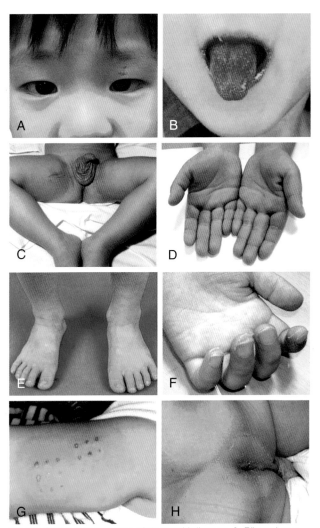

FIG. 3.3 Clinical presentation of Kawasaki disease. **A,** Bilateral, non-exudative conjunctival injection; **B,** strawberry tongue; **C,** perineal rash; **D,** erythema of palm; **E,** erythema of soles; **F,** desquamation of fingers; **G,** erythema at site of previous BCG vaccination; **H,** perianal desquamation. (From Kim D.S., Kawasaki Disease, Yonsei Medical Journal, Vol. 47, No. 6, pp. 759-772, 2006.)

Clinical Presentation: Kawasaki disease is a medium-vessel vasculitis that affects children (e.g., more common on Pediatrics shelf). Includes coronary artery aneurysms, myocardial infarction (MI), and myocarditis. Classically, Kawasaki is associated with a child presenting with a fever lasting 5 or more days plus a strawberry tongue and desquamation of the hands/feet (Fig. 3.3).

PPx: (1) Monitor with echocardiography to avoid cardiovascular sequelae (such as coronary vessel thrombosis/aneurysm)

QUICK TIPS

Scarlet fever, a toxin-mediated illness caused by group A beta hemolytic strep; can also present with strawberry tongue and desquamation. However, unlike Kawasaki, can resolve with PCN.

QUICK TIPS

Adenoviruses, like Kawasaki, can also cause conjunctivitis. However, unlike Kawasaki, adenovirus has discharge.

MoD: (1) Inflammation of medium vessels, such as arteries lined with smooth muscle, of unknown cause

Dx:
1. PEx to look for limbic-sparing conjunctivitis, erythema/fissured lips, and **strawberry tongue**
2. C-reactive protein (CRP) and erythrocyte sedimentation rate (ESR) (both elevated)
3. CBC → leukocytosis with neutrophilia, anemia, thrombocytosis (late finding)
4. UA → sterile pyuria on UA due to urethritis
5. Echo → perform at time of diagnosis and repeat at 6 to 8 weeks to look for changes/monitor coronary artery aneurysm

Tx/Mgmt: (Start within 10 days of fever onset.)
1. To prevent coagulopathy/reduce CVD → aspirin (prevents coronary thrombosis)
2. Can substitute with clopidogrel if there is flu or varicella infection
3. To treat autoimmune reaction/reduce CVD → IVIG
4. Usually will self-resolve in 12 days but treat to prevent cardiac complications

Autoimmune Disorders

Autoimmune disorders are characterized by damaged tissues from aberrant attacks from the patient's own immune system. These typically affect multiple organ systems. In addition, many of these autoimmune disorders, such as SLE, are known as great imitators and should be on the differential for most chief complaints. In studying autoimmune disorders, keep two organizing principles in mind: First, there is typically an environmental trigger that sets off the immune system to attack the patient's own cells. For instance, in lupus, ultraviolet rays from the sun can damage exposed skin and release intranuclear contents into the bloodstream, whereby they are recognized and attacked by the humoral immune system. Second, disease activity of autoimmune disorders can wax and wane. Treatment aims to reduce disease activity during flares and prevent future flares from occurring.

Systemic Lupus Erythematosus (aka Lupus)

Buzz Words: RPR- and VDRL-positive + elevated PTT + recurrent abortions + malar rash → antiphospholipid antibody in s/o SLE

Presents with recurrent pregnancy loss, stroke, and venous thrombosis. Treat with anticoagulation. Can be a primary disorder or associated with SLE.

gg AR

Aspirin is typically contraindicated as a treatment for children because it may cause **Reye syndrome** (acute live failure with characteristic microvesicular fatty infiltration). Treatment of Kawasaki disease is the one exception.

QUICK TIPS

Antiphospholipid antibodies include (1) lupus anticoagulant (elevates PTT), (2) anticardiolipin (false-positive VDRL and RPR), (3) anti–beta$_2$ glycoprotein

QUICK TIPS

Antiphospholipid disorder characterized by hypercoagulable state due to antiphospholipid antibodies

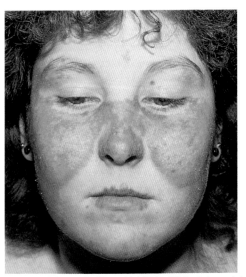

FIG. 3.4 Malar rash. (From Habif TP: Clinical dermatology: a color guide to diagnosis and therapy, ed. 3, St. Louis, 1996, Mosby.)

Antihistone antibody + malar rash + new drug/medication → drug-induced lupus

IgG + malar rash + discoid rash + ANA + mucositis (mouth ulcers) + neurologic dysfunction + serositis (pleuritis/pericarditis) + hematologic disorder (pancytopenia) + arthritis + renal disorder (wire loops) + photosensitivity + psychosis → SLE

Clinical Presentation: SLE is an autoimmune disorder that can present like almost any chief complaint and is thus often kept somewhere on the differential. It is therefore very easy to get lost in thinking about SLE. Here are two organizing principles to guide your study:

First, be clear on how SLE presents on the shelf. Although, SLE is the "great imitator," there are only a handful of Buzz Words or clinical vignettes that can be used to describe SLE. First, be on the lookout for a (most likely) female patient with a malar (e.g., "butterfly") rash over the bridge of her nose who presents with constitutional symptoms, such as fatigue, fever, and night sweats (Fig. 3.4).

On the exam, these patients typically have recently been exposed to sun (e.g., beach trip) or perhaps forgot to put on sunscreen.

PPx: (1) Sunscreen (avoid sun exposure)

MoD: (1) Mostly considered type 3 hypersensitivity because damage is mediated by antigen-antibody immune complexes. Sun damage → apoptotic debris → activation

99 AR

Oral ulcers in SLE

99 AR

Lupus presentation video

and production of antibodies that target antigens from patient's cell nuclei → immune complex formed → immune complex deposited in body tissues, upregulates immune responses (using up complement proteins and leading to deficient C1, C2, and C4). (2) In pregnancy, **lupus anticoagulant** leads to thrombus development within the placenta → spontaneous abortion/pregnancy loss. (3) Pancytopenia in SLE mediated by direct antibody attack on RBCs, WBCs, and platelets (type 2 hypersensitivity).

Dx:
1. CBC/BMP
2. ANA
3. Anti-Smith and anti-dsDNA antibodies (specific/gold standard for diagnosis)
4. Complement levels (may show decrease C1, C3, C4)

Tx/Mgmt:
1. NSAIDs
2. Steroids
3. Anticoagulation (e.g., warfarin, heparin) if antiphospholipid antibody syndrome
4. Discontinue drug if drug-induced lupus
5. Disease-modifying antirheumatic drugs (DMARDs: e.g., methotrexate)
6. Biologics (e.g., TNF-alpha inhibitors)
7. Renal transplant if kidney failure

GUNNER PRACTICE

1. A 6-year-old girl with a history of seasonal allergies is brought to the pediatrician's office owing to a pruritic rash. She has a family history of asthma and eczema. Her mother is concerned that she is suffering from an allergic reaction. She denies any recent change in laundry detergent, lotion, or jewelry. On exam, the child has a linear, vesicular rash extending across her chest. She has a similar rash on her right arm. Physical exam is otherwise unremarkable. What type of hypersensitivity reaction is responsible for this rash?
   A. Type I
   B. Type II
   C. Type III
   D. Type IV
   E. This is not the result of a hypersensitivity reaction

2. A 14-year-old girl presents to your clinic with a rash on her cheeks. She has a history of joint pain and complains that her fingers turn white and are extremely painful when it is cold. You notice a red rash on her

cheeks. The rash on her cheeks gets worse in the sun. On exam, her vitals are HR 82, BP 114/78, T 37, RR 18, SaO2 98% on room air. Exam is otherwise unremarkable. Laboratory results have not yet returned. Which of the following complement levels would be associated with her diagnosis?

A. Low level of early complement factors (C1, C2, C4)
B. Low level of late complement factors (C5, C6, C8)
C. Deficiency of C1 esterase inhibitor
D. Increased total serum complement levels (CH50)

3. A 15-year-old boy presents to the trauma bay following a severe motor vehicle accident. His vitals on admission are HR 110, BP 90/70, T 37, RR 24, SaO2 98% on room air. He is confused and disoriented as to time and place. His abdomen is distended and diffusely tender to palpation. He has severe ecchymoses and abrasions across his chest, arms, and face. Your team decides to transfuse him with one unit of packed red blood cells. During the transfusion, his vitals are HR 125, BP 80/65, T 39, RR 35, SaO2 90% on room air. He is noticeably shaking and has an audible wheeze. Which of the following would you most likely see in this patient?

A. Lack of mature B cells
B. Defective neutrophil oxidase
C. Thymic hypoplasia
D. Low IgA levels
E. Low B- and T-cell levels

ANSWERS: What Would Gunner Jess/Jim Do?

1. WWGJD? A 6-year-old girl with a history of seasonal allergies is brought to the pediatrician's office due to a pruritic rash. She has a family history of asthma and eczema. Her mother is concerned that she is suffering from an allergic reaction. She denies any recent change in laundry detergent, lotion, or jewelry. On exam, she has a linear, vesicular rash extending across her chest. She has a similar rash on her right arm. Physical exam is otherwise unremarkable. What type of hypersensitivity reaction is responsible for this rash?

Answer: D, Type IV hypersensitivity

Explanation: The linear, vesicular rash in a child is a classic presentation for poison ivy. She has the rash in more than one location. This is actually rather common as children scratch and transfer the oils from one location to another. Contact dermatitis, as is the case for poison ivy, is a delayed (type IV) hypersensitivity reaction. There is no humoral component and the cell types involved include T cells and macrophages. Other common examples of type IV hypersensitivity reactions include the tuberculin skin test.

A. Type I → Incorrect. These IgE-mediated reactions are dominated by basophils and mast cells. A common example is anaphylaxis or an allergic reaction such as rhinosinusitis. Although this patient has a history of allergies, the rash in this vignette is nearly pathognomonic for poison ivy.

B. Type II → Incorrect. These IgG-mediated reactions are dominated by eosinophils, neutrophils, and macrophages. Common clinical presentations include autoimmune hemolytic anemia and Goodpasture disease.

C. Type III → Incorrect. These immune complex–mediated reactions are dominated by neutrophils. Examples include serum sickness and lupus nephritis.

E. This is not a hypersensitivity reaction → Incorrect.

2. WWGJD?

A 14-year-old-girl presents to your clinic with a rash on her cheeks. She has a history of joint pain and complains that her fingers turn white and are extremely painful when it is cold. The rash on her cheeks gets worse in the sun. On exam, HR 82 BP 114/78 T 37 RR 18 SaO2 98% on room air. You notice a red rash on her cheeks. Exam is otherwise unremarkable. Laboratory results have not yet returned. Which of the following complement levels would be associated with her diagnosis?

Answer: A, Low level of early complement factors (C1, C2, C4).

Explanation: This patient is presenting with a malar rash, which is classically seen in lupus. She additionally has clinical findings consistent with lupus, including joint pain and the Raynaud phenomenon. Deficiencies of the classic complement pathway are associated with autoimmune disorders such as lupus.

B. Low level of late complement factors (C5, C6, C8) → Incorrect. Deficiencies of these complement factors would commonly result in recurrent infections, particularly meningococcal and gonococcal.

C. Deficiency of C1 esterase inhibitor → Incorrect. A deficiency of C1 esterase inhibitor would result in hereditary angioedema and is not associated with autoimmune disease.

D. Increased total serum complement levels → Incorrect. Lupus patients have a decreased total complement level, specifically the early complement factors.

3. WWGJD?

A 15-year-old boy presents to the trauma bay following a severe motor vehicle accident. His vitals on admission are: HR 110, BP 90/70, T 37, RR 24, PO_2 98% on room air. He is confused and disoriented to time and place. His abdomen is distended and diffusely tender to palpation. He has severe ecchymoses and abrasions across his chest, arms, and face. Your team decides to transfuse his with one unit of packed red blood cells. During the transfusion, his vitals are: HR 125 BP 80/65, T 39, RR 35, PO_2 90% on room air. He is noticeably shaking and has an audible wheeze. Which of the following would you most likely see in this patient?

Answer: D. Low IgA levels.

Explanation: This patient is likely losing a significant amount of blood in his abdomen. The most common sources in trauma such as this include the spleen and the liver. However, you are not being asked to answer this. Instead, you should focus on what is taking place during the transfusion. The patient has become considerably more hypotensive and has developed a fever with a new wheeze.

Hypotension could be due to blood loss in this case, but you should also consider hypotension due to leaky vessels secondary to anaphylaxis as a reaction to the transfusion. In any patient developing posttransfusion hypotension or other symptoms of anaphylaxis, you must consider IgA deficiency as a possible cause. Remember, anaphylaxis does not always result in shock! Two systems must be involved to raise concern: CNS, respiratory, GI, circulatory, skin. Therefore, in this case, if the patient developed wheeze and vomiting following transfusion but had normal blood pressure, that would also be consistent with the diagnosis.

A. Lack of mature B-cells → Incorrect. X-linked agammaglobulinemia often presents with recurrent infections and is not associated with transfusion reactions.

B. Defective neutrophil oxidase → Incorrect. CGD results in recurrent infections from catalase-positive bacteria and fungi and is commonly associated with repeated abscess formation.

C. Thymic hypoplasia → Incorrect. Thymic hypoplasia is associated with DiGeorge syndrome and results in defective/low T cells. Patients often present with viral infections. Furthermore, these patients will have cardiac abnormalities, abnormal facies, cleft palate, and hypocalcemia.

E. Low B- and T-cell levels → Incorrect. This would be seen in severe combined immunodeficiency. These patients present with infection in the first few months of life, with failure to thrive and chronic diarrhea. Blood products require irradiation to prevent infection. However, it is not associated with anaphylaxis.

Diseases of the Blood and Blood-Forming Organs

Sila Bal, Hao-Hua Wu, Susan McClory, Leo Wang, and Rebecca Tenney-Soeiro

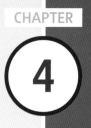

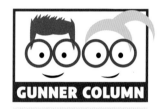

GUNNER COLUMN

Introduction

Blood sustains life through a myriad of mechanisms, ranging from gas exchange to immune function and coagulation. Consequently, diseases of the blood have a wide scope of clinical manifestations including disorders affecting hemoglobin and subsequent delivery of oxygen to tissue, infection in the setting of poor bone marrow function and neutropenia, and bleeding secondary to thrombocytopenia or platelet dysfunction. For the Pediatrics exam, questions about anemia, hemoglobinopathies, leukemia, and inherited blood disorders are particularly high-yield as they are common general pediatric presentations and may have overlapping clinical features that require considerable insight to decipher.

There are several organizing principles for this chapter. First, set up a framework to work within each hematologic abnormality. For example, given a patient with anemia, first decide whether the anemia is an isolated abnormality or is associated with thrombocytopenia or leukopenia. If anemia is isolated, decide whether the anemia is microcytic, macrocytic, or normocytic. Refer to your differential for each category and use hints from the clinical picture to come to a conclusion.

It is important to recognize basic pediatric lab values, in particular the complete blood count (CBC), as it may not always be provided in a question stem. Be sure you are familiar with the clinical presentations associated with each abnormality. For example, patients with moderate/severe thrombocytopenia will generally present with symptoms of bleeding, particularly mucosal bleeds. Likewise, question stems may provide you with alternative laboratory findings or tests. Become familiar with the types of tests AND the expected results for common pathologies. This will allow you to quickly work through the question stems without getting bogged down in the details.

This chapter is divided into five sections: (1) Immunologic and Inflammatory Disorders of the Blood; (2) Neoplasms; (3) Anemia, Cytopenias, and Polycythemia; (4) Coagulation Disorders; and (5) Traumatic, Mechanical, and Vascular Disorders.

Health Maintenance and Screening

All pregnant females are screened for potential inherited hemoglobinopathies. Patients with increased risk factors have the option of obtaining a hemoglobin analysis prenatally, and every child receives a newborn screen at 24–48 hours of life. Since the high-oxygen-affinity fetal hemoglobin (HbF) stays elevated until approximately 6 months of age, clinical symptoms may not appear until that time and are discovered through hemoglobin electrophoresis (Figs. 4.1 and 4.2).

All infants should have an iron-deficiency anemia risk assessment at 4 months for factors including low birth weight, premature birth, or diet deficient in iron. Universal hemoglobin levels should be evaluated at 12 months with annual repeat in high-risk populations.

Immunologic and Inflammatory Disorders of the Blood

Immune Thrombocytopenic Purpura

Buzz Words: Petechiae + isolated thrombocytopenia + s/p viral infx/immunization

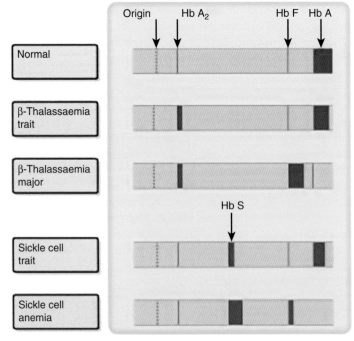

FIG. 4.1 Hemoglobin electrophoresis results by disease.

Clinical Presentation: Mucosal bleeding, purpura, petechiae, and isolated thrombocytopenia. Should NOT see evidence of hemarthrosis or other deep bleed; if so, consider alternative diagnosis. Prothrombin time (PT)/partial thromboplastin time (PTT) will be normal, **only bleeding time will be elevated.**

   Age: Varies

   Gender: No predilection

   Site of care: Generally outpatient

   Chief complaint: Mucosal bleeding

   PMH/PSuH/PFH/PSoH: History of urinary tract infection (URI) or other viral infection

Prophylaxis (PPx): N/A

Mechanism of Disease (MoD): Immune-mediated isolated thrombocytopenia (<100 K). Due to idiopathic, drug, or virally induced formation of antiplatelet antibodies. Neonatal immune thrombocytopenic purpura (ITP) includes both passive (mother with ITP passes the antibodies) and isoimmune (normal platelets in mother, who forms antibodies against fetal platelets only).

Diagnostic Steps (Dx):

1. CBC
2. H&P

Treatment and Management Steps (Tx/Mgmt): Generally self-limited, especially in pediatric populations. A subset of patients will go on to develop chronic disease. If platelet

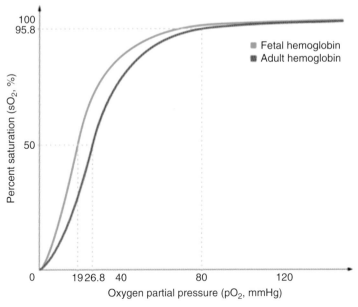

FIG. 4.2 Comparison of fetal and adult hemoglobin curve.

count drops below 10 K, treat with intravenous immunoglobulin (IVIG). Steroids are also used in therapy.
Transfusion is reserved for severe cases.

Thrombotic Thrombocytopenic Purpura

Buzz Words: Severe hemolytic anemia and thrombocytopenia

Clinical Presentation: Pentad: microangiopathic hemolytic
anemia w/ elevated lactate dehydrogenase (LDH); thrombocytopenia; neurologic symptoms such as headache,
stroke, seizure, confusion (CNS involvement cause of
mortality); fever; renal dysfunction.

Age: Acquired TTP is more common in adults than
children.

Gender: No predilection

Site of care: Inpatient

Chief complaint: Fatigue, dizziness, vomiting,
petechiae/purpura

PMH/PSuH/PFH/PSoH: N/A

PPx: N/A

MoD: Deficient ADAMTS13 (protease that cleaves von
Willebrand factor [vWF]) → vWF buildup provides a site
for platelet aggregation and accumulation.

Dx:

1. Clinical picture
2. CBC
3. Coagulation studies
4. ADAMTS13 activity and inhibitor testing (treatment
   should not be delayed for confirmatory testing)

Tx/Mgmt:

1. Plasma electrophoresis
2. Glucocorticoids

Hemolytic Uremic Syndrome

Buzz Words: Hemolytic anemia + thrombocytopenia + renal
dysfunction

Clinical Presentation: Triad of hemolytic anemia, thrombocytopenia, and renal dysfunction. Purpura usually not
seen despite the thrombocytopenia. May have history
of recent infection with abdominal pain, diarrhea (usually bloody), and low urine output or pallor.

Age: Most commonly seen in children

Gender: No predilection

Site of care: Outpatient unless severe

Chief complaint: Pallor, abdominal pain, diarrhea, and
low urine output

PMH/PSuH/PFH/PSoH: N/A

PPx: N/A

QUICK TIPS

In TTP, both PTT and PT are normal (as opposed to disseminated
intravascular coagulation).

MoD: Shiga toxin binds to glomerular vascular endothelium, most commonly due to *Escherichia coli* (EHEC 0157:H7), but also seen following *Shigella* infection.

Dx:
1. Clinical picture
2. Urinalysis
3. CBC
4. May culture for bacterial infection, though not always present at the time of presentation

Tx/Mgmt: DO NOT give antibiotics as they may increase the shiga toxin and cause worsening renal dysfunction. Supportive care only.

Neoplasms

Acute (Precursor Cell) Leukemia (White Blood Cell Disease)

Buzz Words: Greater than 20% blasts or greater than 20% immature myeloid cells

Clinical Presentation: Acute onset of nonspecific symptoms that include fever, lymphadenopathy, bone pain, anemia, thrombocytopenia with bleeding, or neutropenia with infections. Some less common presentations include unilateral testicular enlargement or mediastinal masses.

> Age: The peak incidence of acute lymphoblastic leukemia (ALL) is between 2 and 5 years. Conversely, acute myeloid leukemia (AML) is seen in older adults with average age of 50–60.
>
> Gender: In ALL, boys > girls
>
> Site of care: Inpatient and outpatient
>
> Chief complaint: Varies (see Clinical Presentation above)
>
> PMH/PSuH/PFH/PSoH: N/A

PPx: N/A

MoD: Genetic transformation of immature blasts (or myeloid) cells causes accumulation of precursor cells. These immature cells will overtake normal hematopoiesis, resulting in anemia, thrombocytopenia, and neutropenia. The overpopulating immature cells will then enter the bloodstream, resulting in leukocytosis.

Dx: Bone marrow aspirate for phenotype, cytology, and immunogenetics. Patients with acute leukemias will have greater than 20% blasts or myeloid in their bone marrow.

Tx/Mgmt:
1. ALL has excellent response to chemotherapy.
2. AML treatment varies based on cytogenic abnormalities.

QUICK TIPS

8ur14itt's (8:14 translocation)

Burkitt Lymphoma

Buzz Words: Epstein–Barr virus (EBV) + **Rapidly growing extranodal mass** + "starry-sky" appearance on hematoxylin and eosin (H&E)

Clinical Presentation: Very rapidly growing extranodal mass with tumor lysis and associated laboratory findings of elevated LDH and uric acid. African form involves jaw.

Age: Child or young adult

Gender: No predilection

Site of care: Varies

Chief complaint: Rapidly growing mass

PMH/PSuH/PFH/PSoH: There is an association between immunodeficiency and Burkitt lymphoma; ask about human immunodeficiency virus (HIV) risk factors. History of EBV infection.

PPx: N/A

MoD: Proliferation of intermediate B cells, associated with **constitutively active** c-Myc proto-oncogene. Often associated with EBV infection. Will see starry sky appearance on H&E.

Dx: Tissue biopsy of the mass

Tx/Mgmt:

1. Chemotherapy
2. Management of tumor lysis syndrome with hydration and electrolyte repletion

Non-Hodgkin Lymphoma

Buzz Words: Painless lymphadenopathy

Clinical Presentation: Varies: Some cases rapid, others with waxing and waning painless lymphadenopathy. Symptoms of fever, chills, night sweats, weight loss. May see compressive symptoms such as facial plethora, respiratory distress, or asymmetric tonsils.

Age: Any age

Gender: No predilection

Site of care: Varies

Chief complaint: Rapidly growing, painless mass

PMH/PSuH/PFH/PSoH: May be associated with a history of prior cancer therapy, HIV, EBV infection, primary immune deficiency, and autoimmune disorders.

PPx: N/A

MoD: Proliferation of lymphoid cells including T cells, B cells, or natural killer cells. More common than Hodgkin lymphoma. Often with extranodal involvement. Pediatric cases are high grade and rapidly progressive.

Dx: Excisional lymph node biopsy

Tx/Mgmt: Depending on the type and location, may require chemotherapy, radiation, or a combination of the two. Surgical intervention generally limited to diagnostic excisional biopsy.

Tumor Lysis Syndrome

Buzz Words: Recent cancer diagnosis + started therapy + N/V + lethargy + hematuria

Clinical Presentation: Metabolite abnormalities (see later). Nausea, vomiting, lethargy, hematuria, seizures, cardiac abnormalities, flank pain, and possible death.

Age: Varies

Gender: No predilection

Site of care: Inpatient

Chief complaint: Varies

PMH/PSuH/PFH/PSoH: Recent chemotherapy

PPx: (1) Hydration for all patients. (2) High-risk populations may receive allopurinol to decrease uric acid production.

MoD: Most often seen after initiation of cytotoxic therapy in patients with high-grade lymphomas such as Burkitt lymphoma. Tumor cell lysis releases large amounts of potassium, uric acid, and phosphate into circulation. May lead to acute kidney injury, cardiac abnormalities, and/or seizures.

Dx: Laboratory findings of hyperuricemia, hyperphosphatemia, hyperkalemia, or hypocalcemia up to 7 days after initiating chemotherapy.

Tx/Mgmt:
1. Supportive care with cardiac monitoring
2. Treat electrolyte abnormalities
3. Loop diuretics
4. Hydration to flush out uric acid

Tx/Mgmt:
1. Vitamin K is used for reversal
2. For acute reversal, FFP may also be used

Anemia, Cytopenias, and Polycythemia (Fig. 4.3)

Decreased Production

Iron-Deficiency Anemia

Buzz Words: Fatigue + dizziness + pallor + microcytic anemia + **low ferritin** + low reticulocyte count + increased total iron-binding capacity (TIBC) → Iron-deficiency anemia

Pica + koilonychias (concave nails) + cheilosis + glossitis → severe iron-deficiency anemia

	Serum Fe	TIBC	% Sat	Ferritin
Fe Deficiency	↓↓	↑↑	↓↓ <10	↓
Chronic Disease	↓	NI or ↓	↓ >15	NI or ↑
Sideroblastic	↑↑	NI or ↓	↑↑	↑↑
Thalassemia others	NI	NI	NI	NI

FIG. 4.3 Results of iron study labs by disease type. *TIBC*, Total iron-binding capacity.

Clinical Presentation: Iron deficiency is the most common cause of anemia and more likely to be found in females (especially those who are pregnant), infants, and the elderly. Suspect in female patients who present with a chief complaint of fatigue. In elderly patients, suspect occult blood loss until otherwise proven (e.g., melena or peptic ulcer disease).

PPx: (1) No screening recommended by the USPSTF. (2) Counseling about foods that contain iron.

MoD: Variable but can be most commonly due to insufficient intake and blood loss. Can also be due to increased iron requirement (e.g., infants, pregnancy) or decreased iron absorption (e.g., celiac disease, gastrectomy).

Dx:
1. CBC
2. Peripheral blood smear
3. Iron studies (iron, TIBC, ferritin, transferrin, reticulocyte count, red cell distribution width)

Tx/Mgmt:
1. Oral supplemental iron
2. Parenteral iron

Anemia of Chronic Disease

Buzz Words: Microcytic or normocytic anemia + elevated ferritin + decreased Fe/TIBC + any chronic illness

Clinical Presentation: Microcytic/normocytic anemia with elevated ferritin (storage form of iron) but decreased serum iron levels. TIBC decreased. Can be seen in the setting of malignancy and autoimmune conditions or other chronic illness. Associated with autoimmune disorders, endocarditis, malignancy, any chronic illness

99 AR

The most current USPSTF guidelines state that pregnant women and children between the age of 6-24 months do NOT have to be screened. This is a departure from their old guidelines, which did recommend screening. Keep this in mind as there may be texts that are out of date.

including malnutrition, irritable bowel disease (IBD), or chronic infection.

PPx: N/A

MoD: Chronic disease state → elevated acute-phase reactants (hepcidin) → hepcidin pushes iron into storage form in order to prevent bacterial access to iron → decreased free iron causes decreased hemoglobin production → anemia

Dx:

1. CBC
2. Iron studies
3. Acute-phase reactants

Tx/Mgmt:

1. Treat underlying cause; otherwise no treatment for asymptomatic anemia
2. EPO if symptomatic
3. Transfusion if severely decreased hemoglobin

Hemolysis (Increased Breakdown)

Autoimmune Hemolytic Anemia

Buzz Words: Hemolytic anemia + prior viral infection + pallor/jaundice

Clinical Presentation: Hemolytic anemia with fatigue, weakness, pallor, jaundice, and/or dark urine.

Age: Infancy to adolescence

Gender: No predilection

Site of care: Outpatient unless severe anemia

Chief complaint: See presentation

PMH/PSuH/PFH/PSoH: Generally unrevealing, but look for family history of immune disorders or recent systemic illness, especially viral prodrome.

PPx: N/A

MoD: Autoantibodies against erythrocytes lead to premature destruction and subsequent anemia. May be primary or secondary. Often categorized based on thermal reactivity of antibodies: Warm (immunoglobulin [Ig]G, more common) or cold (IgM, postinfectious). Pediatric cases are most often secondary, with causes including autoimmune conditions such as lupus, infections such as mycoplasma or EBV, immunodeficiency, malignancy such as lymphomas or leukemias, or drugs, especially antibiotics.

Dx:

1. Laboratory findings of hemolytic anemia, anemia, high indirect bilirubin, high LDH, low haptoglobin)
2. Direct antiglobulin test (formerly known as Coombs)

QUICK TIPS

Hemolysis laboratory findings: Increased indirect bilirubin, increased lactate dehydrogenase, reduced haptoglobin, may also see reticulocytosis

Direct Coombs test / Direct antiglobulin test

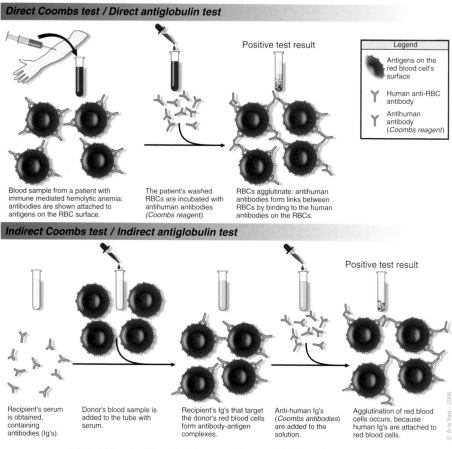

Positive test result

Legend

Antigens on the red blood cell's surface

Human anti-RBC antibody

Antihuman antibody (*Coombs reagent*)

Blood sample from a patient with immune mediated hemolytic anemia: antibodies are shown attached to antigens on the RBC surface.

The patient's washed RBCs are incubated with antihuman antibodies (*Coombs reagent*).

RBCs agglutinate: antihuman antibodies form links between RBCs by binding to the human antibodies on the RBCs.

Indirect Coombs test / Indirect antiglobulin test

Positive test result

Recipient's serum is obtained, containing antibodies (Ig's).

Donor's blood sample is added to the tube with serum.

Recipient's Ig's that target the donor's red blood cells form antibody-antigen complexes.

Anti-human Ig's (*Coombs antibodies*) are added to the solution.

Agglutination of red blood cells occurs, because human Ig's are attached to red blood cells.

© Aria Rad - 2006

FIG. 4.4 How to differentiate between direct and indirect Coombs tests.

Tx/Mgmt:

1. Warm autoimmune hemolytic anemia: Steroids
2. Cold autoimmune hemolytic anemia: Frequently self limited, but may try steroids

Glucose-6-Phosphate Dehydrogenase Deficiency

Buzz Words: Male, less commonly female, with dark urine following exposure to oxidative stressor (fava beans, sulfa drugs, dapsone, antimalarials such as primaquine, infection)

Clinical Presentation: Usually asymptomatic; hemoglobinuria, back pain, fever, jaundice, pallor. Neonates with unexplained hyperbilirubinemia.

Age: All ages

Gender: Male > female (females must be homozygous)

Site of care: Varies

Chief complaint: Dark urine or severe fatigue following infection or other oxidative stressor

PMH/PSuH/PFH/PSoH: Family history of G6PD

PPx: Avoidance of oxidative stressors (see earlier)

MoD: Most common enzymatic disorder of RBCs: X-linked recessive deficiency in G6PD. G6PD is necessary for glutathione regeneration, with decreased G6PD cells become vulnerable to oxidative stress, resulting in intravascular hemolysis of the damaged RBCs.

Dx:

1. Suggested by newborn screen.
2. Peripheral smear with precipitated hemoglobin as Heinz body, which is then removed by the spleen, forming bite cells.
3. Enzyme activity: Assays may yield false-negative result if performed during acute attack, as all affected cells would be hemolyzed. Repeat enzyme studies weeks after episode.

Tx/Mgmt: Generally self-limited. May require transfusion in extreme cases.

Pyruvate Kinase Deficiency

Buzz Words: Low pyruvate kinase activity + hemolytic anemia + autosomal recessive

Clinical Presentation: Varies: May present as life-threatening hemolytic anemia in utero or at birth. Otherwise, signs of hemolytic anemia, including pallor, icterus, splenomegaly.

Age: Varies

Gender: No predilection

Site of care: Outpatient

Chief complaint: Fatigue and pallor

PMH/PSuH/PFH/PSoH: Family history

PPx: Daily folic acid supplementation

MoD: Autosomal recessive deficiency in erythrocyte pyruvate kinase. Mechanism behind source of hemolysis is unclear. Thought that decreased ATP production as a result of defective glucose metabolism may have a role.

Dx:

1. Enzyme studies for low pyruvate kinase activity
2. Genetic testing
3. Lab findings of hemolysis

Tx/Mgmt: For severe hyperbilirubinemia in neonates, phototherapy is required. In most cases transfusions will be required and splenectomy or hematopoietic cell transplantation for refractory cases. As with all patients requiring repeated transfusions, iron chelation may be necessary.

Disorders of Hemoglobin, Heme, or RBC Membrane
Hereditary Spherocytosis/Elliptocytosis

Buzz Words: Spherocytes + osmotic fragility test + anemia with pigmented gallstones + spectrin defect + parvovirus B19 infection

Clinical Presentation: Jaundice in the neonatal period. Otherwise, mild jaundice, splenomegaly, anemia. Mean cell hemoglobin concentration (MCHC) increases due to smaller cell size. RBC distribution width (RDW) is also increased due to varying time for individual membrane dysfunction and thus varying RBC sizes. Patients at increased risk of pigmented bilirubin stones and **aplastic crisis following parvovirus B19 infection.**

Age: Varies

Gender: No predilection

Site of care: Generally outpatient

Chief complaint: Anemia

MH/PSuH/PFH/PSoH: Family history of hereditary spherocytosis

PPx: N/A

MoD: Inherited defect of **RBC cytoskeletal proteins** → loss of membrane integrity → formation of spherocyte (or elliptocyte)-shaped RBC → hemolytic anemia secondary to extravascular hemolysis of the spleen

Dx:
1. Evidence of hemolysis
2. Spherocytes on peripheral smear
3. Increased spherocyte fragility on **osmotic fragility test**
4. **Abnormal eosin-5-maleimide binding test**

Tx/Mgmt:
1. Transfusion for symptomatic anemia
2. Folic acid supplementation for moderate/severe anemia
3. Splenectomy after age 6 in cases of moderate/severe anemia

Paroxysmal Nocturnal Hemoglobinuria

Buzz Words: Coombs-negative hemolytic anemia

Clinical Presentation: Anemia symptoms such as fatigue, dyspnea, dark urine (hemoglobinuria); does NOT have to be nocturnal only. Most common cause of death is thrombosis of the hepatic, portal, and cerebral veins.

Age: All ages

Gender: X-linked gene defect (PIGA, see later); however, **equal distribution in males and females,** since it is a somatic disorder and only requires one X chromosome.

Site of care: Outpatient

Chief complaint: Anemia symptoms

PMH/PSuH/PFH/PSoH: Family history of paroxysmal nocturnal hemoglobinuria (PNH)

PPx: N/A

MoD: Mutation in the PIGA gene of hematopoietic stem cells → **decreased anchoring proteins** on the surface of RBCs (absent glycosylphosphatidylinositol [GPI])→ loss of complement protection → complement-mediated intravascular hemolysis. Some patients will present with thrombosis secondary to increased free hemoglobin, causing systemic response.

Dx: Flow cytometry for patients presenting with Coombs-negative hemolytic anemia. Will see laboratory findings of hemolytic anemia (high indirect bilirubin, high LDH, low haptoglobin).

Tx/Mgmt:

1. Eculizumab (complement inhibitor) + iron supplement + folic acid
2. Allogeneic hematopoetic stem cell transplantation

Methemoglobinemia, Acquired and Congenital

Buzz Words: Cyanosis + normal pulse oximetry reading

Clinical Presentation: Blue or gray skin, lips, nails. Light-headedness, headache, fatigue, tachycardia. In severe cases may lead to coma, shock, respiratory depression, and death. Congenital methemoglobinemia patients have lifelong cyanosis but are otherwise asymptomatic.

Age: Infants and premature neonates

Gender: No predilection

Site of care: Inpatient

Chief complaint: See earlier

PMH/PSuH/PFH/PSoH: Recent use of dapsone or topical analgesic

PPx: N/A

MoD: Iron in hemoglobin oxidized to methemoglobin → impaired oxygen delivery to tissues:

- Acquired: Increased production of methemoglobin causes **acute** impairment in oxygen delivery to tissues that does not allow sufficient time for compensatory changes:
  - Most commonly associated with sepsis, antibiotics (trimethoprim, dapsone), nitrates in drinking water and topical anesthetic agents such as lidocaine. Infants and premature infants are particularly susceptible to the development of methemoglobinemia because of decreased enzymatic activity in erythrocytes.
- Congenital: Decreased enzymatic reduction of methemoglobin

Dx:
1. Chocolate- or dark-colored blood
2. Methemoglobin detected by the co-oximeter; pulse oximetry is inaccurate

Tx/Mgmt:
1. Methylene blue
2. Severe cases may need adjuvant transfusion or hyperbaric oxygen treatment.

Sickle Cell Disease

Buzz Words: Schistocytes + splenic infarct + vaso-occlusion + **salmonella osteomyelitis** + pigment stones + **HgbS**

Clinical Presentation: First symptoms of vaso-occlusion are **dactylitis in infants** with swollen extremities, followed by **autosplenectomy** with risk of encapsulated infection, especially *Streptococcus pneumoniae*, as well as increased risk of *Salmonella* osteomyelitis. Vaso-occlusion in the musculoskeletal system can cause repeat episodes of significant bone pain. Vaso-occlusion in the pulmonary circulation precipitated by pneumonia results in acute chest syndrome. In renal circulation, results in **renal papillary necrosis**. Evidence of extramedullary hematopoiesis includes chipmunk facies from facial bone involvement or crewcut appearance of skull on x-ray. Hemolysis, both intra- and extravascular, is common. Children are at increased risk of avascular necrosis of the femoral head.

Age: Congenital

Gender: No predilection

Site of care: Varies

Chief complaint: Varies

PMH/PSuH/PFH/PSoH: History of sickle cell or trait

PPx: (1) Penicillin prophylaxis against *S. pneumoniae*. (2) Pneumococcal and meningococcal vaccine by age 2. (3) Magnetic resonance angiogram (MRA) or ultrasound at age 2 to screen for stroke.

MoD: Autosomal recessive point mutation of beta globin gene results in a valine substitution for glutamic acid → stressors such as dehydration, acidosis, or hypoxia cause this abnormal hemoglobin protein to stack within the RBC membrane → sickling of RBC → Sickled RBC leads to hemolysis, extramedullary hematopoiesis, and vaso-occlusive crises.

Dx: Often diagnosed on newborn electrophoresis, as symptoms will not present until approximately 6 months when HbF levels begin to decrease.

Tx/Mgmt:
1. Hydroxyurea to increase HbF levels
2. Folic acid supplementation
3. Stem cell transplant
4. Chronic transfusion therapy

Sideroblastic Anemia

Buzz Words: Microcytic anemia without evidence of thalassemia or iron deficiency

Clinical Presentation: Most commonly seen in a young boy with severe microcytic anemia without a positive family history. Serum iron is often elevated, as the excess iron in the mitochondria spills out of the cell. Ferritin levels also subsequently increase as excess iron is taken up. TIBC is decreased.

Age: Varies
Gender: Male > female
Site of care: Varies
Chief complaint: General symptoms of anemia including malaise, fatigue, and dyspnea on exertion
PMH/PSuH/PFH/PSoH: N/A

PPx: N/A

MoD: Acquired or congenital defect in protoporphyrin synthesis. Heme is composed of protoporphyrin and iron in erythrocyte mitochondria. When there is a protoporphyrin deficiency, iron remains trapped inside the mitochondria, forming ringed **sideroblasts** (mitochondria forming a ring around the nucleus). The congenital defect is most commonly due to X-linked ALAS deficiency. Acquired causes include alcoholism, vitamin B6 deficiency due to isoniazid treatment (B6 is a cofactor for ALAS), and lead poisoning.

Dx: Ringed sideroblasts on bone marrow aspirate

Tx/Mgmt: Varies based on cause. Splenectomy is generally avoided.

Thalassemias

Buzz Words: Target cells + Mediterranean descent → beta thalassemia; **HbA2** + HbBarts/HbH + Southeast Asian → alpha thalassemia

Clinical Presentation: Microcytic anemia of varying severity (see MoD, further on). In severe cases may see signs of extramedullary hematopoiesis with crewcut appearance of skull on x-ray, chipmunk facies due to facial bone involvement, and hepatosplenomegaly.

Age: Generally presents a few months after birth, as HbF is protective.

Gender: No predilection

Site of care: Varies

Chief complaint: Often asymptomatic

PMH/PSuH/PFH/PSoH: Family history of thalassemia

PPx: Prenatal genetic testing

MoD: The major hemoglobin found in adults is hemoglobin A, composed of 2 alpha and 2 beta chains. Thalassemia is an inherited mutation in the alpha or beta globin chain of hemoglobin, resulting in decreased hemoglobin synthesis. Both forms lead to increased hemolysis and extramedullary hematopoiesis, with resultant enlarged bones.

- **Alpha thalassemia** is more commonly seen in Southeast Asian populations with four variations:
  - One to two gene deletions result in normal or mild anemia.
  - Three gene deletions result in Barts (HgH) disease: Severe anemia with a chain that binds strongly to oxygen, similar to fetal Hb.
  - Four gene deletions are incommensurate with life, resulting in hydrops fetalis.
- **Beta thalassemia** is more commonly seen in Mediterranean populations:
  - Heterozygotes will have beta thalassemia minor and present with mild microcytic anemia.
  - Homozygotes will have **Cooley anemia**, with hepatosplenomegaly, bone marrow hyperplasia, and thalassemia facies. These patients may require lifelong transfusions, resulting in **secondary hemochromatosis (iron overload)**.

Dx:

1. Hemoglobin electrophoresis with **HbA2 or HbF and little/no HbA**.
2. Peripheral smear shows microcytic, hypochromic RBCs as well as target cells.

Tx/Mgmt: For minor cases, no treatment is necessary. Patients with beta thalassemia minor do not require iron supplementation. For severe cases, lifelong exchange transfusions.

Other Causes of Anemia

Blood Loss, Acute and Chronic

Buzz Words: Normocytic anemia

Clinical Presentation: Normocytic anemia **most common cause of anemia overall.** May see spoon-shaped nails or diminished attention.

Age: Varies

Gender: Varies

Site of care: Varies

Chief complaint: Varies

PMH/PSuH/PFH/PSoH: Varies, look for recent trauma or surgery. Bleeding into the retroperitoneal space or the thigh is often missed. **Infants with exposure to cow's milk** prior to age 1 may have occult GI blood loss.

PPx: N/A

MoD: Blood loss → increased reticulocyte formation + decrease in iron levels necessary to produce new RBCs → iron deficiency → worsening anemia. Blood loss may be secondary to cow's milk, peptic ulcer disease (PUD), IBD, or Meckel diverticulum.

Dx:

1. CBC
2. Iron studies
3. Source of bleed

Tx/Mgmt:

1. Management of the source
2. Iron supplementation for several months if there was evidence of iron deficiency on iron studies
3. Transfusion if Hb <7 with symptoms (dyspnea, dizziness, severe fatigue)

Platelet Disorders

Glanzmann Thrombasthenia and Bernard–Soulier Syndrome

Buzz Words: Congenital thrombocytopenia

Clinical Presentation: mucocutaneous bleeding.

Age: Varies

Gender: No predilection

Site of care: Varies

Chief complaint: Bleeding

PMH/PSuH/PFH/PSoH: N/A

PPx: N/A

MoD: Both are autosomal recessive disorders of platelet function. In Glanzmann thrombasthenia, platelets are unable to attach due to defective IIa/IIIb. In Bernard–Soulier syndrome, it is a result of platelet glycoprotein abnormalities resulting in defective platelet adhesion.

Dx: Platelet morphology on peripheral smear followed by specific platelet testing

Tx/Mgmt: Varies but include factor VIIa, desmopressin, and platelet transfusions.

Thrombocytopenia/Absent Radius

Buzz Words: No radius bone in forearm + low platelets + newborn (Fig. 4.5)

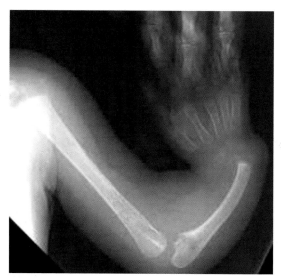

FIG. 4.5 Radiographic example of thrombocytopenia absent radius.

Clinical Presentation: Severe thrombocytopenia. Absent radii, thumbs present. Often associated with congenital cardiac abnormalities. High mortality in early infancy due to intracranial hemorrhage.
    Age: Birth to within the first few weeks of life
    Gender: No predilection
    Site of care: Varies
    Chief complaint: N/A
    PMH/PSuH/PFH/PSoH: N/A
PPx: N/A
MoD: Autosomal recessive disorder with severe thrombocytopenia and bilateral absent radii, though thumbs are always present.
Dx: Clinical and severe thrombocytopenia in neonate
Tx/Mgmt: Platelet transfusions as needed

Cytopenias

Aplastic Anemia
Buzz Words: Pancytopenia with **low reticulocyte count**
Clinical Presentation: Varies based on severity. Common manifestations include fatigue, bleeding, and infection.
    Age: Varies
    Gender: No predilection
    Site of care: Varies
    Chief complaint: Varies
    PMH/PSuH/PFH/PSoH: History of chemotherapy; recent viral illness, especially parvovirus B19 infection; use of certain medications (sulfonamides); exposure to certain chemicals (benzenes)

PPx: N/A
MoD: Injury to hematopoietic stem cells caused by infection, autoimmune damage, inherited disorders, or drugs → pancytopenia
Dx:
1. Bone marrow aspirate shows hypocellular marrow.
2. Low reticulocyte count.
Tx/Mgmt:
1. Remove causative agents
2. Marrow-stimulating factors including granulocyte colony stimulating factor (GM-CSF), granulocyte-macrophage colony stimulating factor (G-CSF), and erythropoietin (EPO) may be used.
3. Transfusion if severe

Lymphopenia

Buzz Words: Isolated decrease in lymphocytes
Clinical Presentation: Varies depending on the cause.
   Age: Varies
   Gender: No predilection
   Site of care: Varies
   Chief complaint: Varies
   PMH/PSuH/PFH/PSoH: History of radiation or recent infection
PPx: N/A
MoD: Most common following a viral infection, especially aviral URI. Also seen in immunodeficiency states such as HIV and DiGeorge syndrome, systemic diseases such as SLE, Cushing syndrome, high-cortisol states, and following whole-body radiation or chemotherapy.
Dx: CBC with manual differential of WBC count
Tx/Mgmt:
1. Treat underlying cause
2. Remove inciting agent

Neutropenia

Buzz Words: Infection with endogenous bacteria
Clinical Presentation: Infection of the bloodstream (especially gram-negative bacteremia), oral mucosa, skin, or mucous membranes, generally due to endogenous pyogenic bacteria (*Staphylococcus aureus*), fungi, or gram-negative organisms of the GI/GU tract. Not viral or parasitic.
   Age: Varies
   Gender: Varies
   Site of care: Varies
   Chief complaint: Infections
   PMH/PSuH/PFH/PSoH: Varies

PPx: Be sure to cover with broad-spectrum antibiotics in neutropenic patient with fever. Gram-negative are the most common and will need coverage to include *Pseudomonas* (i.e., cefepime). May also consider vancomycin if concern for gram-positive organisms. If fever does not resolve in 3 days or patient is severely ill, consider adding fungal coverage.

MoD: Absolute neutrophil count <1500 due to:

- Increased destruction: Following infection, autoimmune antineutrophil antibodies (seen in systemic lupus erythematosus [SLE], juvenile rheumatoid arthritis [JRA], or isoimmune from mother to fetus), hypersplenism, or drugs.
- Decreased production: Due to viral > bacterial infection:
  - Viral agents include HIV, cytomegalovirus (CMV), Hep A/B, parvovirus, influenza
  - Others: Malaria, typhus, Rocky Mountain spotted fever
  - Malnutrition: Folic acid deficiency may result in neutropenia
- Sequestration (movement into tissues): Due to severe gram-negative sepsis.
- Congenital:
  - In children younger than 4 years old, **chronic benign neutropenia of childhood** is a common inherited abnormality with isolated noncyclic neutropenia and mild infections.
  - **Cyclic neutropenia is an autosomal dominant disorder** causing regular episodes of neutropenia approximately every 21 days. May see symptoms of fever, oral ulcers, and stomatitis during these repeat episodes.
  - Other congenital causes include Chediak-Higashi syndrome and Schwachman-Diamond syndrome (see page 93).

Dx:

1. CBC with manual differentiation
2. Peripheral smear with decreased neutrophils
3. Most of the body's neutrophils are found in the bone marrow; therefore an aspirate is better than peripheral blood.

Tx/Mgmt:

1. For isolated mild neutropenia, serial monitoring of blood counts every 8 weeks is sufficient.
2. GM-CSF or G-CSF may also be used to stimulate bone marrow.

Congenital Agranulocytosis (Kostmann Syndrome)

Buzz Words: Pyogenic bacterial infections in infancy

Clinical Presentation: Infants with life-threatening oropharyngeal, respiratory, or skin infections secondary to *S. pneumoniae* or *S. aureus.* Otitis media also commonly seen. Will see oral ulcers and painful gingivitis. Absolute neutrophil count (ANC) often less than 200.

Age: Infancy
Gender: No predilection
Site of care: Inpatient
Chief complaint: Pyogenic infection
PMH/PSuH/PFH/PSoH: N/A

PPx: Prophylactic antibiotics (abx) no longer used. G-CSF may cause osteopenia; therefore, if used, close monitoring needed of bone density and vitamin D.

MoD: Form of severe congenital neutropenia; autosomal recessive inheritance

Dx: Bone marrow aspirate and genetic analysis

Tx/Mgmt: G-CSF or hematopoietic cell transplantation

Polycythemia

Polycythemia Vera/Secondary Polycythemia

Buzz Words: Elevated hematocrit + itching after bathing + flushed face + blurry vision

Clinical Presentation: Cyanosis of the tongue and mucosa (central cyanosis), ruddy complexion, fatigue, headache, blurry vision. Elevated RBC count, hematocrit greater than 60% or Hb concentration.

Age: Varies
Gender: No predilection
Site of care: Outpatient
Chief complaint: Ruddy facial complexion, central cyanosis
PMH/PSuH/PFH/PSoH: Assess for cardiac/pulmonary disease; polycythemia seen in infants born small for gestational age (SGA), infants of diabetic mothers or smokers, or delayed clamping of umbilical cord.

PPx: N/A

MoD: Increased number of RBCs. Polycythemia vera, or primary polycythemia, is uncommon in pediatric populations and is a malignancy of RBCs associated with JAK2 kinase mutation. Secondary polycythemia is more common in pediatrics and can be due to appropriate or inappropriate EPO production. Appropriate erythropoietin responses include congenital cardiac/pulmonary anomalies, high altitude, or other causes of hypoxemia.

Peripartum hypertension can also result in neonatal polycythemia. Inappropriate causes include malignancy, renal dysfunction, and inappropriate hormone production:

- Relative polycythemia secondary to contraction is seen in dehydration; RBC mass will be normal.
- Itching while bathing due to histamine release.

Dx:
1. CBC
2. Clinical exam to determine the cause
3. EPO level will be decreased in polycythemia vera

Tx/Mgmt: Treat the underlying cause:
1. In cases of volume overload or symptomatic hyperviscosity, phlebotomy may be used.
2. Hydroxyurea

Coagulation Disorders

Hypocoagulable
Disseminated Intravascular Coagulation
Buzz Words: Bleeding and thrombosis

Clinical Presentation: May be acute or chronic: In acute cases, bleeding is the more common manifestation, which includes petechiae and oozing from wound/IV. In chronic cases, thrombosis is more common and leads to thromboembolism.

Age: Varies

Gender: no predilection

Site of care: Inpatient

Chief complaint: Varies

PMH/PSuH/PFH/PSoH: History of malignancy, bacterial sepsis, preeclampsia, trauma, recent blood transfusion

PPx: Check for ABO compatibility prior to transfusions

MoD: An inciting event such as pregnancy, sepsis, malignancy → thrombin generation and fibrin deposition in the microcirculation → unregulated stimulation of coagulation consumes platelets and clotting factors → secondary bleeding.

Dx:
1. Coagulation studies (PT/PTT elevated, D-dimer elevated, decreased fibrinogen)

Tx/Mgmt:
1. If the patient is bleeding, fresh frozen plasma to replete clotting factors.
2. If the patient has clot-related complications, use heparin.

Hemophilia
Buzz Words: Hemarthrosis or deep hematoma, especially in child

Clinical Presentation: In newborns with severe disease, initial bleed may present as cephalohematoma or uncontrolled bleeding after circumcision. In infants, musculoskeletal bleeding, bleeding joints, or "goose egg" hematomas on the head may be seen.

Age: In severe cases presents younger than 1 year old; however, in mild cases may not present until adulthood or when patient is subjected to trauma or surgery.

Gender: Males, although heterozygous female carriers may display mild disease.

Site of care: Outpatient unless acute complication

Chief complaint: N/A

PMH/PSuH/PFH/PSoH: Relative with coagulation disorder (one-third of patients have a negative family history), history of deep hematomas

PPx: (1) Factor replacement. (2) Prophylactic therapy = current standard of care.

MoD: Both hemophilias are X-linked recessive and result in elevated PTT (not bleeding time because platelets not affected). Defined as:

- Severe: Spontaneous bleeding with less than 1% of normal factor activity
- Moderate: Bleeding with trauma and 1%–5% normal factor activity
- Mild: Bleeding with surgery and 5%–40% normal factor activity

Dx: Platelets and PT should be normal. **Only PTT will be elevated** and should resolve with mixing study as there is a factor deficiency rather than a factor inhibitor present. Be sure to test for vWF antigen in cases of suspected hemophilia A. Carriers may get genetic testing.

Tx/Mgmt:

1. Factor replacement is preferred both for acute and chronic treatment.
2. Desmopressin increases VIII and vWF, used for hemophilia A.

Von Willebrand Disease

Buzz Words: Uncontrolled bleeding + no binding with ristocetin

Clinical Presentation: The most common inherited bleeding disorder. Easy bruising, bleeding gums/mucosal surfaces, uncontrolled epistaxis, uncontrolled bleeding post–dental procedure, heavy menses.

Age: Varies

Gender: No predilection

Site of care: Outpatient

Chief complaint: Bleeding

PMH/PSuH/PFH/PSoH: Family history of von Willebrand disease (vWD), or undiagnosed symptoms of bleeding (ask about transfusions after childbirth, heavy menstruation).

PPx: N/A

MoD: Autosomal dominant inheritance of decreased or defective vWF → decreased platelet adherence to vessel wall:

- vWF synthesized by endothelial cells, binds to GP Ib-IX receptors on platelets to mediate platelet aggregation/adhesion to subendothelial collagen.

Dx:
1. **Ristocetin cofactor activity** for vWF activity
2. Plasma vWF antigen
3. Factor VIII activity
4. **Prolonged bleeding time and PTT**, unlike hemophilia A, in which bleeding time is normal.

Tx/Mgmt:
1. Desmopressin acetate (DDAVP) increases circulating vWF in patients with decreased vWF; however, it is ineffective in patients who have defective vWF.
2. Replacement of vWF (Humate or other available blood products).
3. Tranexamic acid or aminocaproic acid for acute bleeding.

Hypercoagulable

Heparin-Induced Thrombocytopenia

Buzz Words: Thrombocytopenia following heparin initiation

Clinical Presentation: Thrombocytopenia in a patient 5–10 days after initiation of heparin treatment. Paradoxical thrombosis; bleeding is less common. Thrombotic sequelae include skin necrosis at the injection site, limb gangrene, and organ ischemia.

Age: Varies

Gender: Female > males

Site of care: Inpatient

Chief complaint: Varies

PMH/PSuH/PFH/PSoH: Exposure to unfractionated heparin > low-molecular-weight heparin (LMWH)

PPx: None

MoD: Autoantibody formation against the heparin-platelet complex

Dx:
1. 4T score: Thrombocytopenia (<20,000); timing (5–10 days). Thrombosis. Other causes for thrombocytopenia ruled out.
2. ELISA for antibodies

Tx/Mgmt:
1. Discontinue ALL heparin (including heparin carriers in central lines and IV)
2. Alternative methods of anticoagulation; warfarin; direct thrombin inhibitors

Antithrombin III Deficiency

Buzz Words: Renal vein thrombosis

Clinical Presentation: Venous thromboembolism (VTE). Think of this when a patient presents with **renal vein thrombosis**, but may cause other venous thrombotic events too

Age: Varies, mean age of presentation is 10–15

Gender: No predilection

Site of care: Varies

Chief complaint: N/A

PMH/PSuH/PFH/PSoH: VTE

PPx: Anticoagulation during pregnancy or preoperatively

MoD: Autosomal dominant condition with variable penetrance causing deficiency of antithrombin III, which, as the name would suggest, acts as a thrombin inhibitor.

Dx: AT-heparin cofactor assay measures antithrombin activity

Tx/Mgmt:
1. Anticoagulation in cases of VTE development
2. Antithrombin concentrate available for severe cases

Protein C/Protein S Deficiency

Buzz Words: VTE in pediatric patient without a central line or known underlying predisposing disorder

Clinical Presentation: Homozygous protein C deficiency will present with neonatal purpura fulminans, rapidly progressive intravascular thrombosis, and hemorrhagic infarction of the skin leading to intravascular collapse and disseminated intravascular coagulation (DIC). Heterozygotes may present with VTE. Adults may present with warfarin-induced skin necrosis.

Age: Varies

Gender: Varies

Site of care: Varies

Chief complaint: Recurrent VTE

PMH/PSuH/PFH/PSoH: Family history of recurrent VTE

PPx: Lifelong anticoagulation for patients with unprovoked VTE

MoD: Autosomal dominant inheritance of decreased protein C, a vitamin K–dependent anticoagulant that inhibits factors V and V3. Vitamin K deficiency, meningococcal infection, liver disease, and DIC may also lead to secondary protein C deficiency.

Dx: Protein C (or S) levels <50% of normal

Tx/Mgmt: For warfarin-induced skin necrosis, immediately discontinue the warfarin, administer vitamin K and protein C (or S) concentrate or fresh frozen plasma (FFP), then start heparin.

Factor V Leiden

Buzz Words: VTE

Clinical Presentation: VTE generally presents as deep venous thrombosis (DVT) or pulmonary embolism. Female patients may present with repeat early fetal loss.
Age: Varies
Gender: Varies
Site of care: Outpatient
Chief complaint: VTE
PMH/PSuH/PFH/PSoH: Family history of thrombotic events

PPx: Generally not recommended even in homozygous individuals unless they are in a high-risk situation (i.e., surgery or pregnancy).

MoD: Most common thrombophilia in Caucasians. Point mutation that eliminates a cleavage site in factor V, resulting in **resistance to inactivation by protein C.**

Dx: Genetic testing for all five inherited thrombophilias at once (antithrombin deficiency, protein C/S deficiency, prothrombin mutation, FVL)

Tx/Mgmt: Manage the acute thrombotic event with anticoagulation

Antiphospholipid Antibodies (Anticardiolipin Antibodies, Lupus Anticoagulant)

Buzz Words: Autoimmune disease (e.g., SLE) + isolated DVT or other VTE + stroke/transient ischemic attack (TIA)

Clinical Presentation: Both arterial and venous thromboses. Repeat VTE especially in young patients or unexplained thrombocytopenia. Livedo reticularis, valvular heart disease, and neurologic findings such as cognitive deficits and white matter lesions. History of autoimmune disease, especially SLE. Arterial events include stroke and TIA. Repeat pregnancy complications including premature labor and preterm loss are the hallmark.
Age: Varies
Gender: Female > male
Site of care: Outpatient
Chief complaint: Varies

PMH/PSuH/PFH/PSoH: Repeat pregnancy loss, history of rheumatologic condition, repeat VTE

PPx: Aspirin prophylaxis for patients with SLE and no previous thrombotic event

MoD: Susceptible individuals are exposed to a second hit, such as infection or rheumatic disease that leads to overexpression of antiphospholipids. Antiphospholipids are procoagulants and influence the action of protein C as well as increasing vascular tone.

Dx:
1. Antiphospholipid antibody testing
2. Evaluation for SLE and other rheumatologic conditions

Tx/Mgmt:
1. Treat the underlying rheumatologic condition
2. Lifelong anticoagulation with warfarin or heparin following first thrombotic event

> **QUICK TIPS**
> Antiphospholipid antibodies may cause false elevation in PTT or false +RPR.

Prothrombin G20210A Mutation

Buzz Words: VTE + elevated PT levels

Clinical Presentation: Three to four times increased risk of VTE in heterozygotes, even higher in homozygotes. Thrombotic events include DVT, pulmonary embolism (PE), and sites of atypical thrombosis including the portal, hepatic, and cerebral veins.

Age: Varies

Gender: Varies

Site of care: Varies

Chief complaint: VTE

PMH/PSuH/PFH/PSoH: Recurrent VTE or VTE at young age, family history

PPx: Anticoagulation only if there is a strong family history of VTE or patient has recurrent VTE

MoD: Point mutation results in substitution of adenine for guanine → higher plasma prothrombin levels → increased risk of VTE.

Dx: Genetic testing for the point mutation, NOT plasma levels

Tx/Mgmt: Anticoagulation for thrombotic events. Avoid contraceptives

Reactions to Blood Components

ABO Incompatibility

Buzz Words: Group O recipient with fever and flank pain following blood transfusion

Clinical Presentation: Classic triad of fever, flank pain, and red/brown urine. May progress to DIC with blood oozing from venipuncture sites. Neonatal ABO incompatibility with a group O mother presents less severe than Rh disease; these neonates generally have only mild anemia that resolves with phototherapy.

Age: Varies

Gender: No predilection

Site of care: Inpatient

Chief complaint: Fever

PMH/PSuH/PFH/PSoH: Recent transfusion, blood group O

PPx: Strict protocols to prevent errors

MoD: Acute hemolytic reaction due to the presence of **preformed antibodies** in the recipient. Generally a group O recipient receives A or B blood by medical error. The recipient's IgM anti-A or anti-B fixes complement and causes destruction of erythrocytes.

Dx: Repeat typing and cross-matching of the transfused blood

Tx/Mgmt:
1. Immediately discontinue the transfusion and start intravenous fluid (IVF) with normal saline.
2. Supportive care with care to maintain hemodynamic stability.

Rh Incompatibility

Buzz Words: Rh-negative mother with one or more previous pregnancies

Clinical Presentation: Ranges from mild anemia with signs of hyperbilirubinemia in the first 24 hours of life and tachycardia/lethargy to severe hydrops fetalis with edema, effusions, and ascites.

Age: Maternal/fetal

Gender: No predilection

Site of care: Inpatient

Chief complaint: N/A

PMH/PSuH/PFH/PSoH: Rh-negative mother with previous pregnancy

PPx: (1) Rh type and screen at first prenatal visit. (2) Repeat screen at 28 weeks and delivery in Rh-negative mother. (3) Administer anti-D immunoglobulin (RhoGAM) to all Rh-negative mothers at 28 weeks, within 72 hours of delivery of Rh positive fetus, and any time there is increased risk of fetomaternal hemorrhage.

MoD: Alloimmunization when Rh-negative mother is exposed to Rh-positive RBCs either from previous pregnancy, transfusions, or exposure to the fetal blood during the current pregnancy.

Dx: Detection of anti-Rh antibody in maternal serum

Tx/Mgmt:

1. Pregnancies affected by hemolysis may receive intrauterine transfusions and early delivery
2. Severe hemolytic anemia will require blood transfusions
3. Phototherapy to manage hyperbilirubinemia
4. Supportive care

Hemolysis, Delayed

Buzz Words: Hemolysis 3–30 days posttransfusion

Clinical Presentation: Fever, falling hematocrit, signs of anemia, increased unconjugated bilirubin.

Age: Varies

Gender: No predilection

Site of care: Outpatient

Chief complaint: Fever

PMH/PSuH/PFH/PSoH: Increased risk with multiple transfusions or chronic transfusion therapy

PPx: N/A

MoD: Reexposure to a previously encountered foreign RBC antigen during pregnancy, transfusion, or transplant triggers antibody formation with extravascular hemolysis occurring 3–30 days posttransfusion. These antibodies are undetectable pretransfusion and increase in number following the second exposure to antigen.

Dx:

1. New positive antibody screen by blood bank
2. Falling hematocrit

Tx/Mgmt: Generally self-limited. Patient will need to avoid the inciting antigen in the future.

Febrile Nonhemolytic Transfusion Reaction

Buzz Words: Fever + chills within a few hours of transfusion

Clinical Presentation: Most common transfusion reaction. **Fever with chills** (distinguishes from acute hemolytic reaction) 1–6 hours posttransfusion. Patients may also experience mild to moderate dyspnea.

Age: Varies

Gender: No predilection

Site of care: Inpatient to monitor for hemolytic reaction

Chief complaint: Fever with chills

PMH/PSuH/PFH/PSoH: Recent transfusion

PPx: Leukoreduction of blood products, no evidence to support the value of premedicating with acetaminophen or antihistamines

MoD: **Cytokine-mediated** stimulation of the immune system following transfusion

> **MNEMONIC**
>
> ABCDs of RhoGAM: Within 72 hours of:
> **A**mniocentesis/ **A**bruptio placenta
> **B**aby RhD-positive delivered
> **C**VS (Chorionic Villus Sampling)
> **D**&E

Dx:

1. Clinical; rule out hemolytic reaction.

Tx/Mgmt:

1. Hold transfusion until hemolytic reaction is ruled out.
2. Antipyretics and supportive care.

Infection Related to Blood Product Transfusion

Buzz Words: N/A

Clinical Presentation: Fever with hypotension, tachycardia, rigors following transfusion.

Age: Varies

Gender: No predilection

Site of care: Inpatient

Chief complaint: Fever

PMH/PSuH/PFH/PSoH: N/A

PPx: (1) Donor selection protocol. (2) Sterile collection.

MoD: Donor blood in the United States is screened for a number of infections, including HIV, hepatitis B and C viruses, human T-cell leukemia virus, West Nile virus, *Trypanosoma cruzi*, and *Treponema pallidum*. However, bacterial contamination, either due to donor infection or contamination of the blood products, is much more common than viral infection. Platelets carry higher risk due to storage at room temperature:
- Gram-negative rods contaminate RBC products
- Gram -positive bacteria contaminate plasma products

Dx:

1. Culture transfused and patient's blood
2. Screen for hemolytic reaction as clinical picture is similar

Tx/Mgmt:

1. Broad-spectrum antibiotics (vancomycin and beta-lactam) if high suspicion for bacterial infection with fever and hypotension/rigors.
2. As always, discontinue the transfusion.
3. Send blood for antibody screen and bacterial culture.

Transfusion-Related Acute Lung Injury

Buzz Words: Respiratory distress within 6 hours of transfusion

Clinical Presentation: Onset of hypoxemic respiratory failure with in 6 hours of transfusion. Cyanosis, hypotension, pink frothy sputum, and fever are seen. Leading cause of transfusion-related mortality.

Age: Varies

Gender: No predilection

Site of care: Inpatient/ICU

Chief complaint: Respiratory distress

PMH/PSuH/PFH/PSoH: N/A

PPx: Avoid plasma products from multiparous women as they have the highest rate of antileukocyte antibodies (see further on).

MoD: Current belief is that two hits are required. Susceptible neutrophils in the recipient are activated by preformed antileukocyte antibodies in the transfused product. As such, plasma products pose the highest risk.

Dx: Clinical diagnosis

Tx/Mgmt:
1. Immediately discontinue blood products
2. Supplemental oxygen and respiratory support as needed
3. CXR

Anaphylactoid Reaction (Immunoglobulin A Deficiency)

Buzz Words: Urticaria that may progress to symptoms of anaphylaxis during or following blood product transfusion

Clinical Presentation: Urticaria, angioedema, respiratory distress with wheezing, vomiting, and even shock within minutes of blood product transfusion.

Age: Varies

Gender: No predilection

Site of care: Inpatient/ICU

Chief complaint: Rash

PMH/PSuH/PFH/PSoH: History of IgA deficiency

PPx: In patients with IgA deficiency, use only IgA-deficient blood products or products that have been washed 3 times.

MoD: Presence of IgG anti-IgA antibodies in patients who are IgA-deficient

Dx: Clinical diagnosis based on physical exam; if present, shock/hemodynamic instability. IgA deficiency diagnosis.

Tx/Mgmt:
1. Immediately discontinue the blood products
2. Epinephrine
3. Supportive care (albuterol, antihistamines, steroids)

Traumatic, Mechanical, and Vascular Disorders

Mechanical Injury to Erythrocytes

Buzz Words: RBC fragmentation + hx of cardiac valve replacement

Clinical Presentation: Anemia with increased fatigue, pallor, etc. Evidence of hemolysis (premature breakdown of RBCs). Increased indirect bilirubin, increased LDH, decreased haptoglobin. Most often intravascular hemolysis as hemoglobin is released from the RBCs into circulation; patients may present with increased free plasma Hb and/or hemoglobinuria.

Age: Varies
Gender: No predilection
Site of care: Varies
Chief complaint: Anemia-related fatigue and pallor
PMH/PSuH/PFH/PSoH: History of cardiac hardware
PPx: Varies
MoD: Intravascular RBC shearing due to malfunctioning heart valve or vascular access device (VAD), platelet microthrombi in thrombotic thrombocytopenic purpura (TTP), or fibrin shearing across vessels, as seen in DIC
Dx: Peripheral smear with fragmented RBCs
Tx/Mgmt:
1. Treat underlying defect
2. In the case of prosthetic valve damage, replace the valve
3. Folic acid or iron supplementation to optimize RBC production

Kasabach–Merritt Syndrome (Fig. 4.6)

Buzz Words: Hemangioma + anemia/thrombocytopenia
Clinical Presentation: Rapidly enlarging vascular lesion, usually on the extremities or trunk, associated with cytopenia.
Age: Within the first year of life
Gender: No predilection
Site of care: Varies
Chief complaint: Rapidly enlarging lesion
PMH/PSuH/PFH/PSoH: N/A
PPx: N/A
MoD: Large hemangioma causes microangiopathic hemolytic anemia and thrombocytopenia due to platelet trapping and consumption of fibrinogen.

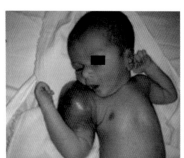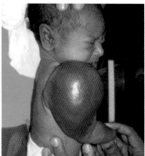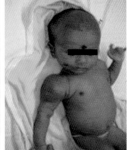

FIG. 4.6 Patient with clinical presentation of Kasabach-Merritt syndrome.

Dx: Biopsy
Tx/Mgmt: Supportive care. For smaller lesions, surgical removal is indicated. If too large for surgery, steroids and vincristine may be used.

Disorders of the Spleen

Splenic Rupture/Laceration
Buzz Words: Pain radiating to the left shoulder (Kehr sign), hypotension and signs of blood loss without an obvious source following blunt trauma to the chest
Clinical Presentation: Left upper quadrant (LUQ) pain ± radiation to left shoulder, splenomegaly, abdominal bruising.
Age: Varies
Gender: No predilection
Site of care: Inpatient
Chief complaint: LUQ pain
PMH/PSuH/PFH/PSoH: History of malaria, recent trauma, recent mononucleosis infection with subsequent sports injury
PPx: Varies
MoD: Direct blow to the upper trunk (handlebars) or high-speed motor vehicle accident. Malaria is the most common cause of nontraumatic splenic rupture.
Dx:
1. If hemodynamically stable, get CT abdomen with contrast if possible.
2. If not stable, will need peritoneal lavage and surgery.
Tx/Mgmt: Hemodynamically stable patients can be treated nonoperatively. Patients may require transfusions.

Splenic Infarct
Buzz Words: Fibrotic spleen in sickle cell patient
Clinical Presentation: Acute onset, severe, left-sided abdominal pain. Often accompanied by fever, nausea/vomiting, leukocytosis, and splenomegaly.
Age: Varies, during childhood for sickle cell patients
Gender: No predilection
Site of care: Inpatient
Chief complaint: LUQ pain
PMH/PSuH/PFH/PSoH: History of Gaucher disease (marked splenomegaly), sickle cell disease, hypercoagulability, embolic disease
PPx: N/A
MoD: Occlusion of one or more branches of the splenic artery results in infarction of splenic tissue.

Dx: CT abdomen with contrast or ultrasound in some cases

Tx/Mgmt: Varies based on severity:

1. Pain management
2. If rupture or abscess formation, may require surgical intervention.

Splenic Abscess

Buzz Words: N/A

Clinical Presentation: Persistent fever despite antibiotics, LUQ pain, splenomegaly. May also be accompanied by left pleural effusions or splenic infarcts due to septic emboli.

Age: Varies

Gender: No predilection

Site of care: Inpatient

Chief complaint: LUQ pain and fever

PMH/PSuH/PFH/PSoH: History of endocarditis, recent infection with antibiotic treatment

PPx: N/A

MoD: Splenic infection secondary to septic emboli, most commonly from endocarditis.

Dx: CT abdomen

Tx/Mgmt: Antibiotics therapy; usually requires splenectomy.

Effects/Complications of Splenectomy (e.g., Sepsis Due to Encapsulated Bacteria)

Buzz Words: Sepsis secondary to encapsulated organisms

Clinical Presentation: Patients with recent splenectomy OR sickle cells patients who have infarcted their spleen, making them functionally asplenic.

Age: Varies

Gender: No predilection

Site of care: Varies

Chief complaint: Varies

PMH/PSuH/PFH/PSoH:

PPx: (1) Pneumococcal, meningococcal, and *H. influenzae* type b vaccines. (2) Must go to emergency room for all fevers for antibiotics and evaluation.

MoD: The spleen plays an important role in humoral immunity and bacterial clearance. As such, asplenia results in increased risk of severe bacterial sepsis secondary to encapsulated organisms, most notably *S. pneumoniae*, *H. influenzae*, and *N. meningitidis*.

Dx: High suspicion for encapsulated bacteria. With onset of fever, obtain blood cultures.

Tx/Mgmt: For any febrile patient, immediate broad coverage with ceftriaxone and transfer to nearest hospital.

Hypersplenism

Buzz Words: N/A

Clinical Presentation: Anemia, thrombocytopenia with splenomegaly. May be painful.

Age: Varies

Gender: No predilection

Site of care: Inpatient

Chief complaint: Varies

PMH/PSuH/PFH/PSoH: Sickle cell patient with acute drop
in hemoglobin; portal hypertension, liver failure

PPx: Varies

MoD: The spleen normally sequesters 30% of the circulating platelets. With splenomegaly, this may double or
triple, resulting in thrombocytopenia. Also see anemia
and neutropenia. Splenic sequestration crisis is seen in
pediatric sickle cell patients who have not yet infarcted
their spleen. Splenomegaly in these patients causes
severe drop in hemoglobin.

Dx: Splenomegaly with anemia, thrombocytopenia, and/or
neutropenia

Tx/Mgmt:

1. Supportive care
2. In sickle cell disease, IV fluids may help marginalize
   RBC and platelets
3. Transfusion may be required in cases of sequestration
   crisis
4. May require splenectomy

GUNNER PRACTICE

1. A 9-month-old male is brought to the pediatrician's
   office due to sudden swelling and pain in his hands. The
   child was born at home and had poor prenatal care. His
   diet consists solely of breast milk. His mother is concerned, as he suffered from a runny nose for the week
   prior to this incident. He had an episode of diarrhea 2
   weeks earlier, which has since resolved. You draw a
   hemoglobin level and find that the patient has an MCV
   of 88. Which of the following would likely be seen on
   hemoglobin electrophoresis?
   A. Hemoglobin A2 and hemoglobin A
   B. Nearly 100% hemoglobin F with some hemoglobin A2
   C. Hemoglobin S
   D. Hemoglobin S and hemoglobin A
   E. Hemoglobin A

2. An 18-month-old female presents with chronic diarrhea, failure to thrive, and recurrent pyogenic soft tissue
   infections. Family history is significant for asthma and

eczema. She has a dog and two cats in the home. She is nonverbal. Abdomen is tender to palpation. You are awaiting laboratory results. Which of the following are associated with this syndrome?

A. Parvovirus
B. Pancreatic insufficiency
C. Albinism
D. Autosomal dominant inheritance
E. Smooth red tongue

3. A 7-year-old male with a history of asthma and seasonal allergies is brought to the emergency room due to prolonged bleeding following a dental procedure. According to his mother, he has a history of easy bruising since infancy. Upon further questioning, you find that his uncle also has a history of easy bleeding. Physical exam is remarkable for watery eyes and several ecchymoses. Laboratory results show hemoglobin 13.3, platelets 300,000, WBCs 7, elevated PTT, and prolonged bleeding time. Which of the following findings will most likely lead to the diagnosis?

A. Ristocetin cofactor assay
B. Factor IX activity
C. Factor VIII activity
D. Elevated D-dimer

Notes

ANSWER: What Would Gunner Jess/Jim Do?

1. WWGJD? A 9-month-old male is brought to the pediatrician's office due **to sudden swelling and pain in his hands.** The child was born at home and had poor prenatal care. His diet consists solely of breast milk. His mother is concerned as he suffered from a runny nose for the past week prior to this incident. He had an episode of diarrhea 2 weeks ago, which has since resolved. You decide to draw a hemoglobin level and find that the patient has an **MCV of 88.** Which of the following would likely be seen on **hemoglobin electrophoresis**?

Answer: C, Hemoglobin S

Explanation: This question requires multiple steps. First, determine the type of anemia: Macrocytic anemia. Next, make a diagnosis: The painful swelling following a viral illness points to acute dactylitis in a child with previously undiagnosed sickle cell disease. The poor prenatal care and home birth make newborn electrophoresis unlikely. Children with sickle cell disease often do not present with an acute crisis until after 6 months of age, as fetal hemoglobin drops. Finally, determine which hemoglobin electrophoresis findings are found in sickle cell disease.

A. Hemoglobin A2 and hemoglobin A → Incorrect. This is the finding of beta-thalassemia minor, a microcytic anemia. Remember that hemoglobin A is the normal hemoglobin found in adults. Patients with beta thalassemia minor will have very mild anemia.

B. Nearly 100% hemoglobin F → Incorrect. This is the finding of beta thalassemia major, a microcytic anemia. These patients have no normal hemoglobin (hemoglobin A) and present with severe anemia and evidence of extramedullary hematopoiesis.

D. Hemoglobin S and hemoglobin A → Incorrect. This is the finding of sickle cell trait, a macrocytic anemia. This is the likely hemoglobin electrophoresis of this boy's parents, as sickle cell disease is autosomal recessive.

E. Hemoglobin A → Incorrect. This would be a normal finding and would not explain the MCV of 110 and symptoms of this child.

2. WWGJD? An 18-month-old female presents with **chronic diarrhea, failure to thrive, and recurrent pyogenic soft tissue infections.** Family history is significant for asthma and eczema. She has a dog and two

cats in the home. She is nonverbal. Abdomen is tender to palpation. You are awaiting laboratory results. Which of the following are associated with this syndrome?

Answer: B, Pancreatic insufficiency

Explanation: First, determine the abnormality. This is tricky, given the vague symptoms. However, recurrent pyogenic soft tissue infections should not occur in a healthy 18-month-old child and should make you think of neutropenias. Next, determine the source of her neutropenia. The important clues here are her failure to thrive and chronic diarrhea. Schwachman-Diamond is an autosomal recessive disorder associated with pancreatic insufficiency and neutropenia. Remember that pancreatic insufficiency will result in malabsorption, leading to chronic diarrhea and failure to thrive. Another approach to this question is to check the answer choices and decide what the association of each answer is. You may then use the diagnoses to match the clinical scenario described.

A. Parvovirus → Incorrect. Viral infections are the leading cause of neutropenia in childhood. However, this is unlikely to be the source in this patient, who is presenting with chronic rather than acute diarrhea.

C. Albinism → Incorrect. Albinism is associated with Chediak-Higashi, an autosomal recessive disorder of protein trafficking associated with neutropenia, thrombocytopenia, and neurologic abnormalities.

D. Autosomal dominant inheritance → Incorrect. Cyclic neutropenia has an autosomal dominant inheritance. This is unlikely to be the cause in this child, as there was no mention of recurring neutropenia in 21-day cycles. Both Chediak-Higashi and Schwachman-Diamond are autosomal recessive disorders.

E. Smooth, red tongue → Incorrect. Glossitis would be expected in B12 deficiency. Folic acid deficiency, not B12 deficiency, may be associated with diarrhea and neutropenia. Clues to this would be a diet deficient in folic acid or classically consisting of only goat's milk.

3. WWGJD? A 7-year-old male with a history of asthma and seasonal allergies reports to the emergency room due to prolonged bleeding following a dental procedure. According to his mother, he has a history of easy bruising since infancy. Upon further questioning, you find

out that his uncle also has a history of easy bleeding. Physical exam is remarkable for watery eyes and several ecchymoses. Laboratory results show hemoglobin 13.3, platelets 300,000, WBC 7, elevated PTT, and prolonged bleeding time. Which of the following findings will most likely lead to the diagnosis?

Answer: A, Ristocetin cofactor assay

Explanation: First, determine the type of coagulation disorder in this child with bleeding. This patient has a normal platelet count, elevated PTT, and prolonged bleeding time, effectively ruling out thrombocytopenia as a cause of the bleed. The prolonged bleeding time suggests platelet dysfunction, while the elevated PTT points to intrinsic pathway dysfunction. Next, determine the most likely diagnosis. vWD is the most common inherited coagulopathy and would present both with platelet and intrinsic pathway dysfunction. Finally, what diagnostic test would be used for vWD?

B. Factor IX assay → Incorrect. This would be useful if we believed the patient had hemophilia B. This is a mild bleed, and hemophilias generally present with hemarthrosis or more severe bleeding. Both hemophilias feature the loss of clotting factors in the intrinsic pathway only and would have an elevated PTT, not bleeding time.

C. Factor XIII assay → Incorrect. Factor XIII deficiency is associated with hemophilia A. Although hemophilia XIII and vWD can both be treated with DDVAP, hemophilia A is generally more severe and will not have prolonged bleeding time (see previous, hemophilia B).

D. Elevated D-dimer → Incorrect. Elevated D-dimer in a bleeding patient should make you think of DIC. This patient, however, is asymptomatic other than the bleed and does not have any other risk factors (pregnancy, malignancy, sepsis). DIC is highly unlikely in this case.

Mental Disorders

Leo Wang, George Dalembert, Hao-Hua Wu, and Rebecca Tenney-Soeiro

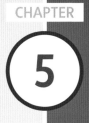

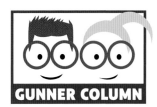

Mental disorders encompass abnormal mental processes in children and are traditionally thought of as pediatric psychiatry. This chapter is organized into several subsections: adjustment disorders, eating disorders, incontinence, learning disorders, disruptive disorders, pervasive developmental disorders, genetic disorders, and infectious diseases. Only a basic understanding of most of these conditions will be tested, as there are only 1 to 5 such questions on the Pediatrics exam. As usual, focus on the **Buzz Words**, which will clue you in to recognizing the disorder from the vignette. On recognizing a disorder from the Buzz Words, the most important steps in most instances are diagnosis, treatment, and management. Prophylaxis rarely exists for many of these and will be presented when relevant. Mechanisms are even less well understood and, as such, are infrequently tested. In many cases, you will notice that parents are heavily involved in various aspects of each disorder. This is because parents play a **major** role in many of these conditions, and fixing the disorder in the child often requires treating or managing both the child and the parents.

Adjustment Disorders in Children

Adjustment disorders comprise symptoms that children can feel after a stressful life event because adequate coping mechanisms have yet to develop. These include reactive attachment disorder, posttraumatic stress disorder (PTSD), acute stress disorder, and separation anxiety. Major depressive disorder (MDD) is also included because it is on the differential of patients who are anxious or irritable, especially in the pediatric population. Understand everything from the Buzz Words to the treatment/management for these disease processes.

Reactive Attachment Disorder of Infancy/Early Childhood

Buzz Words: Limited response to caregivers and others + limited positive affect + repeated changes in primary caregivers + **>9 months** + **<5 years** + episodes of irritability

Clinical Presentation: There are two types of reactive attachment disorder. Although it is unlikely that you will be asked the difference between types I and II, the defining characteristics are here:

Both types I and II:

- Cruelty to animals, siblings, or other children
- Weak crying response
- No reciprocal smile response
- Often malnourished
- Tactile defensiveness

Type I = inhibitory:

- Does not respond in developmentally appropriate fashion to social interactions
- Is hypervigilant, ambivalent, contradictory

Type II = disinhibited:

- Has varied, indiscriminate attachments

Prophylaxis (PPx): Ensure that the patient has a safe and stable living situation and positive interactions with caregivers.

Mechanism of Disease (MoD): Pathogenic care due to one of the following:

- Persistent disregard of child's basic emotional needs
- Disregard of physical needs
- Repeated changes of primary caregiver
- Neglect (sensory deprivation) leading to brain abnormalities

Diagnostic Steps (Dx):

1. Rule out autism, depression, intellectual disability, adjustment disorder
2. Thorough psychiatric evaluation with assessment of episodes

Treatment and Management Steps (Tx/Mgmt):

1. Individual and family counseling

Posttraumatic Stress Disorder in Children

Buzz Words: Major life stressor + separation anxiety + decreased sociability + avoidance/arousal symptoms occurring months/years after event + bed wetting + increased muscle tone/startle response + **for greater than 1 month**

Clinical Presentation: Children can develop PTSD just as adults can. In these situations, assess for the symptoms of PTSD, which include avoidance and arousal symptoms occurring for longer than 1 month. Recognize that these symptoms, when occurring for less than 1 month, are actually known as acute stress disorder.

PPx: N/A, although severity depends on patient responses to trauma

TABLE 5.1 Avoidance Versus Arousal Symptoms in Posttraumatic Stress Disorder

Avoidance Symptoms	Arousal Symptoms
Efforts to avoid thoughts, feelings related to event	Difficulty falling/staying asleep
Inability to recall events	Irritability or outburst of anger
Markedly diminished interest	
Feeling detached or estranged	Hypervigilance
Restricted range of affect	Exaggerated startle
Sense of foreshortened future	response

MoD: Increased catecholamine activity caused by dysregulation of the hypothalamic-pituitary axis; prolonged sympathetic response with loss of self-regulation

Dx:
1. Psychiatric evaluation
2. Assess for presence of ≥3 avoidance symptoms and ≥2 arousal symptoms (Table 5.1)

Tx/Mgmt:
1. Cognitive behavioral therapy (CBT)
2. Psychological first aid (PFA) to teach problem-solving skills and calming
3. Eye movement desensitization and reprocessing (EMDR) therapy
4. Play therapy

Acute Stress Disorder in Children

Buzz Words: Exposure to traumatic event + reexperiencing of event + numbing/detachment or depersonalization + amnesia + reduced awareness + **2 days to 4 weeks**

Clinical Presentation: Acute stress disorder in children is the early equivalent of PTSD, taking place for less than 4 weeks. Children will often present with symptoms similar to those of adults, which includes reexperiencing of the event with numbing and detachment.

PPx: Parental response to trauma affects severity

MoD: Thought to be precursor to PTSD

Dx: Assess exposure to event in setting of avoidance and arousal symptoms for more than 2 days and less than 1 month

Tx/Mgmt: Cognitive behavioral therapy (CBT):
1. Overcome denial/avoidance, teach coping
2. Selective serotonin receptor inhibitor (SSRI)
3. Anticonvulsant
4. Problem-focused coping to control stressor
5. Emotion-focused coping

QUICK TIPS

Some 80% of child burn victims will get this.

QUICK TIPS

PTSD >1 month; acute stress disorder <1 month

Separation Anxiety Disorder

Buzz Words: Abdominal pain during school days or excessive fear of going to school + no physical symptoms during the weekends/summers when child is with caregiver + refuses to sleep alone + >4 weeks

Clinical Presentation: Separation anxiety disorder is high-yield on the Pediatric shelf. This behavior is normal for patients who are 7 to 11 months old. Most patients diagnosed are between the ages of 7 and 11 years. About 5% of patients between 7 and 11 years of age will get this disorder. Parents are likely to have anxiety disorder.

PPx: Overprotective parents can precipitate separation anxiety; counseling for parents is suggested

MoD: Often develops as coping mechanism to major life stressor

Dx: Thorough psychiatric and medical evaluation

Tx/Mgmt:
1. CBT
2. SSRIs

> **QUICK TIPS**
> Associated with panic disorder, depression, and agoraphobia as an adult.

Major Depressive Disorder (>2 Weeks)

Buzz Words: SIGECAPS (anhedonia + depressed or "down" mood + suicidal ideation + sleep troubles + trouble concentrating + psychomotor retardation [moving slower than usual] + low energy + lack of appetite) + 2 or more weeks

Clinical Presentation: MDD is high-yield. The chief complaint on the Pediatrics shelf depends on age. Teenagers can articulate feeling down or depressed. Prepubertal patients may present with vague individual somatic symptoms as already noted (e.g., trouble sleeping, low energy, trouble concentrating, weight loss, lack of appetite). The parents may provide previous personal history of mood disorders or a family history of mood disorders. Most importantly, look for symptoms that last at least 2 weeks and impair the patient's ability to participate in normal activity (e.g., school).

PPx: None

MoD: Unknown, but decreased serotonin in cerebrospinal fluid (CSF) and possibly decreased norepinephrine and dopamine

Dx:
1. Urine drug screen (UDS) to r/o substance use.
2. Clinical diagnosis, satisfying 5/9 SIGECAPS criteria for greater than 2 weeks continuously (see criteria).

Tx/Mgmt:
1. **SSRIs**
2. Tricyclic antidepressants (TCAs)

> **QUICK TIPS**
> SIGECAPS = sleep interest guilt energy concentration anxiety psychomotor agitation suicidal ideation

> **QUICK TIPS**
> Psychiatric disorders cannot be diagnosed in the setting of substance use. Thus, if patients exhibit symptoms of a mood disorder, always make sure first that their urine tox or drug screen is negative. This is a high-yield point for both the exam and clinics.

3. Monoamine oxidase inhibitors (MAOIs)
4. Various forms of therapy (supportive, CBT, interpersonal) can be used in conjunction with medication.

Eating Disorders in Children

Eating disorders in children are characterized by a persistent failure to eat, decreased weight, and symptoms lasting for longer than 1 month. An important point for the physician is always to rule out food insecurity. Anorexia and bulimia nervosa are high-yield eating disorders seen in adolescents and frequently tested on the exam.

Pica

Buzz Words: Patient eats nonnutritive substances + 1 month or more

Clinical Presentation: Pica is present in 10% to 30% children between the ages of 1 and 6 and in 25% of children with intellectual disability. It is equally prevalent in boys and girls, usually begins at age 1 or 2, and remits by adolescence in most cases. Some major complications of pica include poisoning, anemia, intestinal obstruction, and parasites.

PPx: N/A

MoD: Thought to be due to nutritional insufficiency

Dx:
1. Rule out anemia and other medical causes:
   a. Schizophrenia
   b. Iron deficiency
   c. Zinc deficiency
   d. Kleine-Levin (aka "Sleeping Beauty") syndrome (sleeps for weeks and wake up ravenously hungry)
2. Test for iron deficiency, check hemoglobin levels, iron, and zinc

Tx/Mgmt:
1. CBT
2. SSRIs

Rumination Disorder

Buzz Words: Repeated food regurgitation that is pleasurable, tension-relieving, or attention-getting + failure to thrive + pain/nausea + bad breath + chapped lips + >1 month

Clinical Presentation: Rumination disorder is rare; it is most common in children from 3 months to 1 year, particularly in those with intellectual disability. It is slightly more common in males and occurs in nervous and anxious individuals. Side effects include esophagitis, recurrent dental problems, excessive salivation, anemia, and social ostracism.

PPx: N/A

MoD: Thought to arise from physical illness or severe stress in setting of parental neglect; may also be an attention-seeking behavior in a child.

Dx:

1. Rule out medical causes, including gastroesophageal reflux disease (GERD) and pyloric stenosis (projectile vomiting).
2. Review eating habits, observe infants during feeding.

Tx/Mgmt:

1. Behavioral changes:
   a. Postural adjustments
   b. Reduce feeding distractions
   c. Encourage parental attention
2. Psychotherapy

Anorexia Nervosa

Buzz Words: Young female with excessive dieting, exercise, or binging and purging + body mass index (**BMI**) **below 18.5**

Clinical Presentation: Usually seen in young females with an intense fear of gaining weight and a distorted body image. Associated symptoms include severe weight loss, lanugo, decreased bone density (osteopenia), anemia, metatarsal stress fractures, amenorrhea (from loss of pulsatile GnRH) and electrolyte imbalances. Two subtypes:

- Restricting type (excessive dieting)
- Binge-eating/purging type (excessive dieting with episodes of eating large quantities of food, followed by purging, which may consist of laxatives/diuretics, vomiting, etc.)

PPx: N/A

MoD: Unknown; however, genetic (first-degree relative with anorexia increases risk) and psychosocial factors (societal pressures to be slender, more common in adolescents) have some implication.

Dx:

1. Patient history

Tx/Mgmt:

1. Nutritional rehabilitation (most common complication is refeeding syndrome—increased insulin leads to hypophosphatemia, causing cardiac complications)
2. Psychotherapy (family therapy/group therapy)

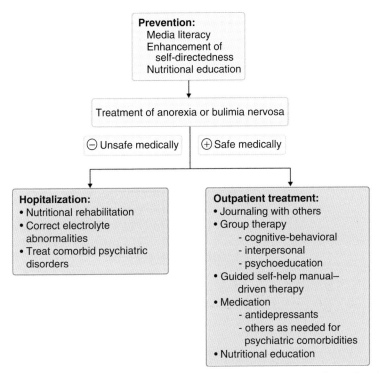

FIG. 5.1 Cleveland clinic comprehensive plan for the treatment of eating disorders. (Reproduced with permission of the Cleveland Clinic Center for Continuing Education. Franco KN, Sieke EH, Dickstein L, Falcone T. Eating Disorders. Disease management project (http://www.clevelandclinicmeded.com/medicalpubs/diseasemanagement/psychiatry-psychology/eating-disorders/). © 2000-2015 The Cleveland Clinic Foundation. All rights reserved.)

Bulimia Nervosa

Buzz Words: Parotitis + enamel erosion + electrolyte imbalances + alkalosis + Russell sign (calluses on dorsal hand) + normal BMI

Clinical Presentation: Usually occurs in young females who practice binge eating with inappropriate compensatory behaviors (vomiting, laxative/diuretic use, fasting, or excessive exercise). It must occur weekly for at least 3 months. Additionally, it typically coexists with overvaluation of body image. Importantly, patients with bulimia nervosa maintain a normal BMI. The two subtypes are the purging and the nonpurging types.

PPx: N/A

MoD: Unknown

Dx:

1. Patient history

Tx/Mgmt:

1. Nutritional rehabilitation
2. Psychotherapy (cognitive and behavioral)
3. Antidepressants (SSRIs, fluoxetine)
4. Group counseling (Fig. 5.1)

Cleveland Clinic Comprehensive plan for treatment of eating disorders

Incontinence in Children

Encopresis

Buzz Words: Involuntary or intentional passage of feces in inappropriate places + occurs once/month for more than 3 months + **4 years of age or older**

Clinical Presentation: These children defecate in inappropriate places and at least once a month for 3 or more months. Often they are constipated and, as a result, defecate at inappropriate intervals. This is why stool softeners are great treatments for these patients. As a rule, encopresis must be diagnosed **after** age 4.

PPx: Regular toileting habits

MoD: Often caused by child not defecating for several days due to constipation, followed by passage of stool at inappropriate times.

Dx:
1. Check for fecal retention
2. Thorough medical and psychiatric evaluation

Tx/Mgmt:
1. Psychotherapy = behavioral modification that only rewards defecation
2. Stool softeners
3. Bowel catharsis

Enuresis

Buzz Words: Urinating into bed or clothes + occurs 2x/week for 3 months + **5 years old or more** + causes marked impairment → enuresis

Urinating into bed or clothes + occurs 2x/week for 3 months + **less than 5 years old** + causes marked impairment → **normal**

Clinical Presentation: Patients with enuresis void at inappropriate times or locations. There are two subtypes: primary enuresis occurs in patients who were never previously continent; secondary enuresis occurs in patients who were previously continent. This must occur in patients after the age of 5 and must occur at least twice a week for 3 months. Enuresis can further be classified by when it occurs; nocturnal enuresis occurs at night and diurnal enuresis occurs in the day. Remember, this process can be voluntary or involuntary.

If a patient presents with enuresis-like symptoms before the age of 5, he or she cannot be diagnosed yet, by definition! This is a common question on the shelf (<5 year old vs. ≥5 year old).

PPx: N/A

MoD: Caused by combination of anxiety, genetics, sleep apnea, structural abnormalities

Dx:

1. Urinalysis and urine culture
2. Rule out diuretic use
3. Rule out medical causes:
   a. Diabetes mellitus
   b. Seizures
   c. Urethritis

Tx/Mgmt:

1. Behavioral training (shock, bell, alarm and pad)
2. Imipramine (TCAs)
3. DDAVP (watch out for H_2O intoxication):
   a. **Headaches** = main side effect
   b. Nausea
   c. Hyponatremia

Learning Disorders

Learning disorders include a group of disorders in which young children have difficulty understanding and responding to information. The most commonly tested learning disorder is attention deficit disorder (ADD)/attention deficit hyperactivity disorder (ADHD). For this, know everything from the Buzz Words to the treatment/management. The single most important thing you can do for a patient with a learning disorder is to test his or her hearing and vision; this concept is important both in real life and on the Pediatrics exam.

Attention Deficit Hyperactivity Disorder

Buzz Words: Temper tantrum in preschool + difficulty with peers in elementary school + sense of restlessness as an adolescent + chronic disorganization as an adult + inattention and hyperactivity (easily distracted, careless mistakes, forgetful, difficulty listening, reluctance to put forth effort) + occurs in both school and at home + present for less than 6 months + presentation before 7 years of age

Clinical Presentation: ADHD is the most high-yield topic in this chapter and guaranteed to be on your test. It is 67% comorbid with conduct and oppositional defiant disorder (ODD), and these patients have a 25% chance of developing antisocial personality. This is a disorder where genetics probably plays a key role, and remember, these kids may have low self-esteem. In 20%, these symptoms last into adulthood.

QUICK TIPS

Some 20% continue to have symptoms in adulthood.

QUICK TIPS

Associated with low birth weight

PPx: Prevent alcohol exposure, tobacco exposure

MoD: Likely dysregulation of norepinephrine and dopamine (both lower than normal); no dopamine in frontal lobe means all gas and no brakes.

Dx:

1. Rule out hearing/vision problems
2. Complete medical history
3. Assess for six symptoms of attentiveness, hyperactivity, or both that persist >beyond 6 months and present before age 7 and that occur in two settings (e.g., home + school).
4. Inattentiveness symptoms:
   a. Careless mistakes
   b. Difficulty with attention
   c. Difficulty listening
   d. No instructions
   e. Lack of organization
   f. Reluctance to put forth effort
   g. Loses things easily
   h. Forgetful, easily distracted
5. Hyperactivity/impulsivity symptoms:
   a. Restlessness
   b. Difficulty remaining quiet
   c. Driven by a motor
   d. Excessive talking
   e. Blurts out answers (impulsive)
   f. Does not wait turn (impulsive)

Tx/Mgmt:

1. Methylphenidate (Ritalin, Concerta, Metadate, Focalin):
   a. Blocks dopamine (DA) reuptake
   b. Upregulates DA
   c. Side effects are those of stimulants
   d. Can still be used if tics already there
2. Dextroamphetamine (Dexedrine, Dextrostat)
3. Amphetamine salts (Adderall):
   a. Blocks DA **and** norepinephrine (NE) reuptake **and** stimulates release
   b. Upregulates DA and NE
   c. Side effects are those of stimulants
4. **Pemoline** = stimulant drug
5. Atomoxetine:
   a. **Nonstimulant**, so it will NOT cause tics
   b. NE reuptake inhibitor, so upregulates NE
   c. Side effects include dry mouth, insomnia, decreased appetite

   Indications:
   • ADHD w/substance abuse
   • ADHD with tics

6. Reboxetine:
   a. Nonstimulant
   b. NE reuptake inhibitor
   c. Side effects include dry mouth, insomnia, decreased appetite
7. SSRIs
8. If stimulants do not work, can try alpha$_2$ agonists like clonidine or guanfacine:
   a. Cause sedation
9. Psychotherapy
10. Parental counseling
11. Group therapy
12. Additional help through an individualized educational plan should be available in a public school setting; some children attend **therapeutic day schools** if not working out in regular classroom

Learning Disorders, Not Otherwise Specified

Buzz Words: Does not meet expected achievement for age, education, intelligence + no organic cause

Clinical Presentation: Learning disorder not otherwise specified (NOS) was recently renamed "specific learning disorder," which is a catch-all term that now includes problems like dyslexia, dyscalculia, and more. Dyslexia is trouble with reading despite normal intelligence. Dyscalculia is trouble with math despite normal intelligence. Dysgraphia is trouble with writing despite normal intelligence. A rarer learning disorder is language processing disorder, which is a condition in which children have trouble attaching meaning to the sounds that they hear.

PPx: None

MoD: None

Dx:
1. Rule out vision/hearing problems
2. Full medical exam including ruling out dyspraxia (difficulty in motor control)

Tx/Mgmt: Specific to type of learning disorder and is not commonly tested.

QUICK TIPS
Dyspraxia is comorbid with many learning disorders.

Selective Mutism

Buzz Words: Child refuses to speak in certain situations only but has normal language development; lasts more than 1 month.

Clinical Presentation: Selective mutism is typically thought of as an extension of social anxiety. This can also be present in adults. Patients with selective mutism refuse to speak in certain situations where speech would be expected, although they fully understand speech and are able to speak. Selective mutism is often perceived as shyness.

PPx: N/A

MoD: Inherited predisposition to anxiety with increased function in amygdala

Dx:

1. Test language and speech.
2. Rule out other problems affecting communication (autism, schizophrenia, ADHD).
3. Ensure symptoms occur only in specific setting, is present for more than 1 month, and affects function.

Tx/Mgmt:

1. Psychotherapy
2. Behavioral therapy
3. Anxiety management
4. SSRIs

QUICK TIPS

Selective mutism, if left untreated, can cause chronic depression and anxiety.

Tourette Syndrome

Buzz Words: Repetitive blinking, throat-clearing or licking + clearing throat or other vocal tic occurring many times a day + every day + lasting longer than 1 year + in child below 18 years of age

Clinical Presentation: This is a disorder with motor and verbal tics in children below 18 years of age. Tourette occurs more often in boys and will usually begin at about age 7.

PPx: Avoid stimulants

MoD: Too much dopamine and too little GABA in the caudate; 50% concordance in monozygotic twins, suggesting genetic predisposition.

Dx:

1. Test for OCD and ADHD
2. Assess for:
   a. Greater than or equal to 2 motor tics, greater than or equal to 1 vocal tic that occurs many times a day, almost every day, for more than 1 year; **onset prior to age 18.** It must cause distress or impairment in social/occupational functioning.

Tx/Mgmt:

1. Pimozide (DA receptor antagonist):
   a. Causes QT prolongation
2. Haloperidol
3. Clonidine (activates presynaptic autoreceptors in locus ceruleus to decrease NE)
4. Guanfacine (activates presynaptic alpha$_2$ adrenergic receptor to decrease NE)

Intellectual Disability

Buzz Words: Impairment in self-care, learning, mobility, receptive/expressive language + patient below age 18 years

Clinical Presentation: Intellectual disability is infrequently tested on the Pediatrics exam and is a complicated umbrella term for many different pathologies. As such, the ability to recognize etiologies of intellectual disability is typically sufficient.

PPx: N/A

MoD:

1. Organic/idiopathic:
   - No discernible pathologic basis
   - Comorbidities include:
     - Epilepsy
     - Cerebral palsy
     - Autism
     - Fetal alcohol
     - Trisomy 21
   - Men > women
   - Higher among nonwhites
2. Prenatal (genetic):
   - **Fragile X** → 30%–50%
   - Trisomy 21
   - **TORCH** infections
   - Prader-Willi (50%–70% paternal deletion)
   - Chromosomal basis
3. Perinatal or postnatal (problems by 2 years):
   - Alcohol-related
   - Anoxia
   - Lead
   - Mercury
   - Associated with maternal smoking

Dx:

1. Evaluate hearing/vision
2. Thorough medical exam
3. IQ test
4. Assess for disability in two areas, such as self-care, learning, mobility, receptive/expressive language, etc. (Table 5.2)

Tx/Mgmt: Not tested

Disruptive Disorders in Pediatric Populations

Oppositional Defiant Disorder

Buzz Words: Hostile and defiant behavior + temper tantrums + arguments + deliberately annoying/trolling + blaming others + no violation of laws + occurring for at least 6 months

> **QUICK TIPS**
>
> In individuals with moderate to profound disability as well as limited means of communication, it is important to remember that medical conditions causing pain can result in aggressive or self-destructive behavior.

TABLE 5.2 Severity of Intellectual Disability

Severity	IQ	Characteristics	Function
Mild	50–70	Not detected until child is in school; child will complete elementary education	Can live/work independently, requires modest level of support
Moderate	35–50	Social isolation in elementary school	Requires high level of support but can work in some capacity independently
Severe	20–35	Minimal speech, poor motor development	Requires extensive supervision
Profound	<20	Absent speech, absent motor skills	Constant supervision with nursing throughout life

Clinical Presentation: ODD is a disorder in which children are generally defiant toward authority but importantly do not actually break any rules or laws. ODD is usually diagnosed at 3 to 8 years of age and is highly associated with ADHD (50%). ODD can occasionally lead to conduct disorder and is estimated to affect 5% of children.

PPx: Precipitated from parent and family environment; prevent violent discipline by parents

MoD: Thought to occur through a combination of genetics and parenting environment including violent disciplinary actions.

Dx:
1. Complete medical evaluation
2. Assess for frequency and intensity of hostile and aggressive behaviors occurring for at least 6 months

Tx/Mgmt:
1. Psychotherapy (behavioral training)
2. Parenting skills training
3. Parent–child interaction therapy
4. Social skills training

Conduct Disorder

Buzz Words: Violation of social norms (destruction of property, theft) + significant impairment + less than 18 years old + occurring for more than 6 months

Clinical Presentation: Conduct disorder is the big brother of ODD and in some sense is more of an exaggerated version, where hostile and defiant behavior has evolved into actual violation of rules and laws. Some 40% of these patients will be diagnosed with antisocial personality disorder. Conduct disorder is also highly comorbid with ADHD and substance abuse. Of note, children with conduct disorder can feel remorse about their actions; however, children with conduct disorder who do not feel remorse will often later be diagnosed with antisocial personality disorder.

PPx: Precipitated from parent and family environment

MoD: Thought to occur through a combination of genetics and parenting environment, including violent disciplinary action; patients have serotonin dysfunction or **decreased 5-HIAA** in CSF.

Dx:
1. Complete medical evaluation
2. Assess for frequency and intensity of hostile and aggressive behaviors occurring for more than 6 months with violation of social norms and rules, causing significant impairment

Tx/Mgmt:
1. Multimodal:
   a. Firm rules, consistency
   b. Psychotherapy
2. Antipsychotics and lithium for aggression
3. SSRI for impulsivity and aggression
4. Some patients enjoy **psychodynamic therapy**

> **QUICK TIPS**
> Subtypes are child-onset conduct disorder (<10 yo) and adolescent-onset conduct disorder (10-17 yo.)

Pervasive Developmental Disorders

Pervasive developmental disorders include a spectrum of diseases that impair all aspects of development. On the exam, you will be expected to recognize and differentiate between the pervasive developmental disorders and to work these patients up thoroughly. This includes medical, lab, psychological, physical testing, and speech and language evaluation. The most commonly tested developmental disorder is autism.

Autism Spectrum Disorder

Buzz Words: Social impairment + lack of interest + poor eye contact + stereotyped use of language or language delay + repetitive motor movements + preoccupation with objects

Clinical Presentation: ASD is an umbrella term encompassing a lack of social function and communication, with restricted behavior and interests. The term *Asperger syndrome* used to describe children with purely motor delays but without delays in speech and development. However, this is now categorized simply as a disorder that falls within the spectrum. Seventy percent of patients on the autism spectrum have comorbid intellectual disability.

PPx: 18-month screening for autism

MoD: Unknown

Dx:

1. R/O medical causes:
   a. Vision and hearing test
   b. Acquire maternal age, health, alcohol use, smoking
   c. Acquire gestational age, perinatal complications, stay in neonatal intensive care unit (NICU)
   d. Look for presence of infection, maternal diabetes, jaundice, birth defects
   e. Look for neurologic problems
   f. Look for cardiac problems
2. Lab testing should include:
   a. **Lead** levels → pica, ASD
   b. Chromosomal analyses
   c. Molecular/genetic analysis
3. Psychological evaluation:
   a. Developmental progression
   b. Intelligence
   c. Behavioral observation scales
4. Physical evaluation:
   a. Somatic growth/height
   b. Weight
   c. Head circumference
5. Speech and language evaluation

Tx/Mgmt:

1. Behavioral and family interventions
2. Speech, occupational, and physical therapy
3. Community support, parent training

Criteria for diagnosis of autism:

1. Assess for 6+ total symptoms, from social interaction impairment, social communication problems, and restrictive behavior/interests
2. Social Interaction impairment (2 or more):
   a. Impairment of nonverbal behavior such as **poor eye contact**
   b. Failure to develop peer relationships
   c. Lack of spontaneous seeking of shared enjoyment

3. Social communication problem (1 or more):
   a. Stereotyped use of language
   b. Language delay (if no language delay or cognitive delay, question suggests Asperger syndrome)
   c. Lack of varied or spontaneous play
4. Restrictive behavior/interests (1 or more):
   a. Intense preoccupation with objects
   b. Inflexible adherence to rules
   c. Repetitive motor movements

Rett Disorder

Buzz Words: Decreased head circumference **growth rate** during 5 to 48 months + loss of previously acquired hand skills + loss of social interaction + impaired language, psychomotor development + stereotyped hand movements + cyanosis + seizures + gastrointestinal (GI) problems + occurring at 5 months only in females

Clinical Presentation: Rett disorder is caused by an abnormality on the X-chromosome and is associated with the MECP-2 gene. It is affects only girls. The most common findings include small head, hands, feet, and repetitive hand movements. Rett was recently removed from the *Diagnostic and Statistical Manual* (DSM) and is now more often categorized as a neurologic disorder.

PPx: Screen females who were normal for the first 5 months of life and then started deteriorating.

MoD: Associated with MECP2 gene on X chromosome

Dx: Same workup as ASD

Tx/Mgmt:
1. Physical therapy/hydrotherapy
2. Occupational therapy
3. Speech-language therapy
4. Feeding assistance
5. Medications for seizures, cardiac abnormalities

Childhood Disintegrative Disorder (Heller Syndrome)

Buzz Words: Loss of language and social skills (bladder/bowel control, ability to play) + impaired social interactions + stereotyped behaviors or stereotyped interests + typically beginning at age 2 but before age 10

Clinical Presentation: This is the male equivalent of Rett. Childhood disintegrative disorder leads to the loss of language skills and social functioning with stereotyped interests and behaviors between the ages of 2 and 10.

Although it can be seen in females, 80% of those with childhood disintegrative disorder are males.

PPx: N/A

MoD: Can be precipitated by various conditions, including lipid storage diseases, subacute sclerosing panencephalitis, tuberous sclerosis, and leukodystrophy.

Dx: Same workup as ASD

Tx/Mgmt:
1. Behavioral therapy
2. Environmental therapy
3. Antipsychotics/antiepileptics

Genetic Disorders

Recognizing genetic disorders and understanding their mechanisms will be the extent to which you will be tested on the Pediatrics exam. Here, focus specifically on the Buzz Words above all else. Other important physician's tasks, if relevant, will be provided. Most of the diseases are discussed in other sections. This chapter focuses on these conditions only as they pertain to mental disorders.

Prader-Willi Syndrome

Buzz Words: Intellectual disability + obesity due to hyperphagia ("eats compulsively") + hypogonadism + almond-shaped eyes + skin picking + hypotonia + aggression, argumentative + narrow face

MoD: Chromosome 15 paternal deletion (can be boy or girl)

Angelman Syndrome

Buzz Words: Seizures + strabismus (heteropia; eyes are not properly aligned with one another) + sociable with episodic laughter

MoD: Deletion on maternal chromosome 15

Fragile X Syndrome

Buzz Words: Eleven years old + developmental delay, poor school and social performance, 50 IQ with macrocephaly + long face + macro-orchidism + autistic + delayed speech + "flapping hands"

Clinical Presentation: Patients with fragile X may suffer from complications such as seizures, mitral valve prolapse, dilation of the aorta, tremor, ataxia, and ADHD-like behavior. Fragile X is the **most common cause** of **inherited intellectual disability.**

MoD: X-linked dominant; CGG repeats with anticipation

MNEMONIC

(The 3 S's: seizures, strabismus, sociable)

QUICK TIPS

Associated with schizotypal personality disorder

Trisomy 21

Buzz Words: Simian crease + macroglossia + Brushfield spots + hypotonia + oblique palpebral fissures + epicanthal folds
MoD: Nondisjunction of chromosome 21

QUICK TIPS
Trisomy 21 is further covered in Chapter 12.

Neurofibromatosis 1

Buzz Words: Café-au-lait spots + seizures + large head
MoD: Autosomal dominant

Hurler Syndrome

Buzz Words:– Mucopolysaccharide defect + coarse facies + short stature + cloudy cornea
MoD: Autosomal recessive

Smith-Magenis Syndrome

Buzz Words: Broad, square face + short stature (like Hurler syndrome) + self-injurious (like Cornelia de Lange)
MoD: Deletion on chromosome 17

Williams Syndrome

Buzz Words: Elfin-appearance + friendly + increased empathy and verbal reasoning ability
MoD: Chromosome 7

Cornelia De Lange

Cornelia de Lange Syndrome

Buzz Words: Intrauterine growth restriction + hypertonia + distinctive facies + limb malformation + self-injurious behavior + hyperactive

CHARGE Syndrome

Buzz Words:
Coloboma of the eye (hole in one of the structures of the eye)
Heart defects
Atresia of the nasal choanae (back of nasal passage)
Retardation of growth and development
Genital and/or urinary abnormalities
Ear abnormalities and deafness
MoD: Abnormality on chromosome 8

Infectious Diseases in Pediatric Populations

Pediatric Autoimmune Neuropsychiatric Disorders Associated With Streptococcal Infections

Buzz Words: Patient who was recently "sick" with strep-related infection presents with **obsessive compulsive disorder (OCD)** symptoms and **tics**

Clinical Presentation: For PANDAS, recognize that strep infections can lead to OCD and tic symptoms in children. This is the extent to which you will be tested on this process.

PPx: N/A

MoD: N/A

Dx:

1. Antistrepolysin O (ASO) titer rises 3 to 6 weeks postinfection.
2. Antistreptococcal DNAaseB (AntiDNAse-B) titer rises 6 to 8 weeks postinfection.

Tx/Mgmt:

1. Intravenous immunoglobulin (IVIG)
2. Plasma exchange
3. Antibiotics
4. SSRIs + CBT for OCD
5. **Risperidone for tics**

GUNNER PRACTICE

1. A 15-year-old female is brought in for her annual well visit. According to Mom, she has not been eating in the last 4 weeks and has lost several pounds. This concerns her parents because she has appeared more tired than usual, had trouble concentrating in class and completing her homework, and has become very irritable over this same time frame. She used to enjoy hanging out with friends and playing soccer after class, but in the past few weeks has instead come home and gone straight to her room. Her vital signs are within normal limits, with a body mass index (BMI) of 19 kg/m^2. There were no abnormal findings on physical exam. Urinary drug screen was negative. What is the most likely diagnosis?
   A. Anorexia nervosa
   B. Bulimia
   C. Generalized anxiety disorder
   D. Major depressive disorder
   E. Normal behavior

2. A 3000-g female newborn born at 39 weeks' gestation to a 35-year-old G2P2 woman is found to have hypotonia. Apgar scores at 1 and 5 minutes after birth were 5 and 8, respectively. Examination shows a widened space between the first and second toes of both feet and single palmar creases. What is the next best step in managing this patient?
   A. Administration of ampicillin and cefotaxime
   B. Chromosomal analysis and echocardiogram

   C. Chromosomal analysis and blood glucose

   D. Magnetic resonance imaging (MRI) of the brain

   E. Administration of indomethacin

3. A 13-year-old male presents to the pediatrician with concerns of "weird behavior." Mom notices that the boy has been very repetitive with his tasks for the past 2 weeks. He used to hate making his bed and now is late to school because he wants to make sure his pillows are in the right place. Although he has a lot of friends, he has recently felt anxious hanging out with them because he has to wash his hands 30 to 40 times after high fives. He has no significant past medical history and is not currently taking any medication. Mom says he may have had a sore throat a few weeks earlier. His vitals are 98.7°F, 80 bpm, 115/85 mm Hg, 12 RR, 97% on RA. Examination shows no abnormalities. His urinary drug screen is negative. What is the most likely diagnosis?

   A. Obsessive compulsive disorder

   B. Obsessive compulsive personality disorder

   C. Avoidant personality disorder

   D. PANDAS

   E. Normal behavior

ANSWERS: What Would Gunner Jess/Jim Do?

1. WWGJD?

A 15-year-old girl is brought in for her annual well-visit. According to Mom, patient has not been eating in the last 4 weeks and has lost several pounds. This concerns her parents because she has appeared more tired than usual, had trouble concentrating in class and completing her homework, and has become very irritable over this same time frame. She used to enjoy hanging out with friends and playing soccer after class but in the past few weeks has instead come home and gone straight to her room. Her vital signs are within normal limits with a BMI of 19 kg/m². No abnormal findings were foundon physical exam. Urinary drug screen was negative. What is the most likely diagnosis?

Answer: D, Major depressive disorder

Explanation: This patient meets the clinical criteria for depression. In adolescents and children, being "irritable" is the code word for feeling sad and should raise concern about depressive symptomatology. This patient, for instance, has had 5/9 SIGECAPS criteria for more than 2 weeks: loss of interest, lack of appetite, fatigue, sad (aka irritable), and difficulty concentrating. Another key in the question stem is that the urinary drug screen was negative. Psychiatric disease cannot be newly diagnosed in patients who are under the influence of substances.

A. Anorexia nervosa → Incorrect. Although it may seem tempting because the parents' initial complaint was that patient was not eating, there are several clues that make anorexia less likely. Most importantly, the patient's BMI is within normal limits at 19 kg/m²; every patient on the exam who presents with anorexia will have a BMI <18 kg/m².

B. Bulimia → Incorrect. Patients with bulimia will usually present with some sort of physical exam abnormality on the exam, such as scars on knuckles or parotitis. This patient has a normal physical exam and has other findings that more likely point to MDD.

C. Generalized anxiety disorder → Incorrect. Patients with generalized anxiety disorder present as excessive worriers in question stems and will worry about work/school, home, and relationships. Although anxiety can make patients "irritable," anxious patients do not lose interest in hobbies or hanging out with friends, as the patient in this question stem does.

E. Normal behavior → Incorrect. Anything that disrupts one's ability to function at work and at school (e.g., "trouble concentrating in class") is likely pathologic on the exam and not normal behavior.

2. WWGJD?

A 3000-g female newborn born at 39 weeks' gestation to a 35-year-old G2P2 woman is found to have hypotonia. Apgar scores at 1 and 5 minutes after birth are found to be 5 and 8, respectively. Examination shows a widened space between the first and second toes of both feet and single palmar creases. What is the next best step in managing this patient?

Answer: B, Chromosomal analysis and echocardiography

Explanation: The Buzz Words in this question stem (e.g., "hypotonia," "widened space between first and second toes" and "single palmar creases") point to trisomy 21. Thus, the question becomes how to manage a patient with trisomy 21 as a neonate. The answer comes from an understanding of the potential medical complications that these patients can have. The most life-threatening are the cardiac complications, including endocardial cushion defects, such as a VSD. Thus, an echocardiogram would be a reasonable, noninvasive way of looking for any cardiac abnormalities. In addition, chromosomal analysis would allow the physician to make the definitive diagnosis of Down syndrome.

A. Administration of ampicillin and cefotaxime → Incorrect. This is the treatment for neonates suspected of having sepsis or meningitis.

C. Chromosomal analysis and blood glucose → Incorrect. Trisomy 21 patients do not have an increased risk of hypo- or hyperglycemia.

D. MRI of the brain → Incorrect. No brain abnormalities are expected in patients with trisomy 21.

E. Administration of indomethacin → Incorrect. This is the treatment for patients with coarctation of the aorta, which requires the ductus arteriosus to stay open for blood flow to continue.

3. WWGJD? A 13-year-old boy presents to the pediatrician with concerns of "weird behavior." Mom notices that they boy has been very repetitive with his tasks for the past week. He used to hate making his bed and now is late to school because he wants to make sure his pillows are in the right place. Although he has a lot of friends, he recently feels anxious hanging out with them because he has to wash his hands 30 to 40 times

after hi-fives. He has no past medical history and is not currently taking any medication. Mom said he may have had a sore throat a few weeks ago. His vitals are 98.7°F, 80 bpm, 115/85 mmHg, 12 RR, 97% on RA. Examination shows no abnormalities. His urine drug screen is negative. What is the most likely diagnosis?

Answer: D, Pediatric autoimmune neuropsychiatric disorder associated with streptococcal infections (PANDAS)

Explanation: The Buzz Words in the question stem that indicate PANDAS are (1) the age of the patient and (2) the recent history of strep-like illness ("sore throat") preceding OCD-like symptoms (e.g., disruptive, compulsive behavior adopted to reduce anxiety). This is a concept that is commonly tested on the Pediatrics and Psychiatry exams because it is so unique and affects only the pediatric population. Although there is an association with strep infections, the mechanism is unknown. PANDAS can be diagnosed with ASO and antistrep DNaseB titer. Treatment is with IVIG and SSRIs/CBT for the OCD symptoms.

A. Obsessive compulsive disorder → Incorrect. In kids with OCD-like symptoms, it is PANDAS until proven otherwise.

B. Obsessive compulsive personality disorder → Incorrect. OCPD is ego-syntonic, in that patients with this personality disorder will think that there is nothing wrong with their OCD-like tendencies. The patient in this question stem recognizes that his symptoms are not letting him hang out with his friends.

C. Avoidant personality disorder → Incorrect. Patients with avoidant personality disorder do not socialize with others owing to a pathologic fear of embarrassment. However, these patients deeply crave social interaction.

E. Normal behavior → Incorrect. On the exam, behavior that disrupts school/work (e.g., being "late to school") can never be considered normal.

Diseases of the Nervous System and Special Senses

Jacob Cox, Anne Fallon, Hao-Hua Wu, Leo Wang, and Rebecca Tenney-Soeiro

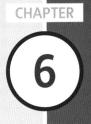

Introduction

Diseases of the nervous system and special senses often have a dramatic impact on patients' quality of life or even survival. Moreover, their assessment and management often involves complex anatomic and pathophysiologic concepts. As such, these diseases are often tested extensively on standardized exams.

The nervous system refers to the brain, spinal cord, sensory organs, and all the nerves that connect these organs with the rest of the body. Since it is so intimately intertwined with all the other organ systems, dysfunction in the nervous system can result in pain, disability, and death. Similarly, the special senses are the senses that are associated with a specialized organ or organ system (e.g., vision, hearing, balance, smell, and taste). These are essential to our ability to interact with the world around us. So while disorders of the special senses are rarely life-threatening, they are often debilitating and severely affect the individual's quality of life. Moreover, early detection and treatment of neurologic dysfunction in children can avert defects in neurodevelopment.

This chapter addresses a wide array of the most common and most severe diseases of the nervous system and special senses. They are categorized as infectious, immunologic and inflammatory, neoplastic, cerebrovascular, spinal, cranial, peripheral, pain-related, movement-related, paroxysmal, traumatic, mechanical, congenital, ocular, and disorders of the ear/nose/throat (ENT). All sections are high-yield, but infectious, congenital, ophthalmic, and ENT disorders are particularly high-yield. You should also become comfortable with the nervous system's unique vocabulary and basic concepts regarding the circulation and nerve pathways.

Only about 5%–10% of the National Board of Medical Examiners (NBME) Pediatrics exam will focus on diseases of the nervous system. These questions generally cover fundamental concepts and treatment plans rather than delving into nuanced specifics. As such, be sure to familiarize yourself with the presentation of various

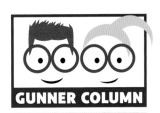

GUNNER COLUMN

diseases and the appropriate diagnostic and therapeutic steps, but don't stress about knowing every minor detail!

Infectious Diseases

Meningitis

Buzz Words: Nuchal rigidity + photophobia + headache + fever

Clinical Presentation:

- Infants and young children: Nonspecific symptoms (irritability or lethargy, high-pitched cry, poor feeding), fever, bulging fontanelle, opisthotonus position (severe hyperextension of the body).
- Older children and adolescents: nausea and vomiting, fever, nuchal rigidity, headache, purpura, photophobia. May lead to change in mental status, seizures, focal neurologic deficits, cranial nerve palsies. Long-term sequelae include sensorineural hearing loss, developmental delays, and hydrocephalus.

Prophylaxis (PPx): Immunizations

Mechanism of Disease (MoD): Inflammation of pia mater covering the brain. Usually due to hematogenous spread.

Diagnostic Steps (Dx):

1. Clinical: symptoms (see above), Brudzinski and Kernig signs.
2. Labs: leukocytosis, blood culture often positive.
3. Lumbar puncture (LP)—aim to obtain prior to intravenous (IV) abx but do not delay if ill. May consider computed tomography (CT) before LP if seizure or focal neurologic deficit, papilledema, immunocompromise, or hardware in place.

Treatment and Management Steps (Tx/Mgmt): Specific medications vary by pathogen, see Table 6.1.

Bacterial

Buzz Words: Elevated WBCs, decreased glucose, polymorphonucleocytes (PMNs) in cerebrospinal fluid (CSF)

Clinical Presentation: Same as above

PPx: Immunizations; airborne or contact precaution may be appropriate depending on bacterium.

MoD: Presence elsewhere in body or environment → bacteremia → translocation through blood-brain barrier (BBB) → bacteria in CSF attract neutrophils → acute meningitis

Dx: (Table 6.2)

1. Clinical exam

2. Lumbar puncture (LP) showing ↑ CSF protein and WBCs (neutrophils > lymphocytes); ↓ CSF glucose
3. Blood and CSF cultures

Tx/Mgmt:
1. Collect blood cultures prior to antibiotic initiation.
2. Empiric treatment if suspected but no culture yet (varies by age; refer to table). Narrow based on culture (varies by pathogen; refer below).

Listeria monocytogenes
Buzz Words: Soft cheese/deli meat consumption during pregnancy
Clinical Presentation: Neonatal meningitis
PPx: Dietary modifications during pregnancy
MoD: Same as above
Dx: Same as above with bacterial identification on culture
Tx/Mgmt:
1. Ampicillin ± gentamicin

Streptococcus agalactiae (Group B Streptococcus)
Buzz Words: Neonatal meningitis
Clinical Presentation: Same as above
PPx: Maternal screening during pregnancy and treatment during delivery
MoD: Same as above. Number one cause of neonatal meningitis (49%). Spreads from focus of infection in maternal vagina.
Dx: Same as above with bacterial identification on culture
Tx/Mgmt:
1. Penicillin G or ampicillin

Escherichia coli
Buzz Words: Neonatal meningitis
Clinical Presentation: Same as above
PPx: Maternal screening during pregnancy
MoD: Same as above. Number two cause of neonatal meningitis (18%). Spreads from focus of infection in maternal vagina.
Dx: Same as above with bacterial identification on culture
Tx/Mgmt:
1. Ampicillin (if susceptible) or third-generation cephalosporin (e.g., cefotaxime)

Streptococcus pneumoniae
Buzz Words: Symptoms of meningitis: nuchal rigidity + photophobia + headache + fever
Clinical Presentation: Same as above

PPx: Immunizations
MoD: Same as above
Dx: Same as above with bacterial identification on culture
Tx/Mgmt: Varies based on susceptibility
1. Penicillin G or ampicillin versus third-generation cephalosporins (cefotaxime or ceftriaxone).
2. Add vancomycin if patient is very ill or there is concern for resistance.

Haemophilus influenza
Buzz Words: Unvaccinated child
Clinical Presentation: Same as above
PPx: Immunization; Rifampin for intimate contacts with infected children
MoD: Same as above
Dx: Same as above with bacterial identification on culture
Tx/Mgmt:
1. Third-generation cephalosporin

Neisseria meningitides
Buzz Words: Outbreak in college dorm or military barracks, petechial rash
Clinical Presentation: Same as above. One of the most common cause of meningitis in those aged 1 month to 18 years.
PPx: Immunization; Rifampin/ciprofloxacin/ceftriaxone for close contacts of infected individuals
MoD: Same as above.
Dx: Same as above with bacterial identification on culture
Tx/Mgmt:
1. Third-generation cephalosporin

Mycobacterium tuberculosis
Buzz Words: International travel, immigrant, homeless, current or former prisoner
Clinical Presentation: Same as above. May occur in presence of TB pneumonia.
PPx: Negative-pressure isolation. Droplet precautions for health care providers with fitted N95 mask.
MoD: Same as above. Complication of primary tuberculosis. Involves base of brain. May lead to intracerebral vasculitis (infarction) and scarring (hydrocephalus).
Dx:
1. Clinical findings and risk factors.
2. CSF findings with ↑↑ protein and WBC (lymphocyte > neutrophils), ↓ glucose.
3. Growth on culture generally takes weeks, so begin treatment immediately if there is high clinical suspicion.

Signs of disseminated TB are diagnostically important but often absent.

Tx/Mgmt:
1. Isoniazid, rifampin, streptomycin, pyrazinamide all cross the BBB.
2. Ethambutol is less effective.
3. Dexamethasone (prevent scarring).
4. Assess for disease elsewhere in body.

Viral

Buzz Words: WBCs less than 100/mm^3, normal glucose, lymphocytes in CSF

Clinical Presentation: Similar to bacterial meningitis but may be more mild. May also cause encephalitis.
- Non-polio enteroviruses (coxsackie A and B, echoviruses)—most common cause
- Poliovirus—largely eradicated due to vaccination with inactivated poliovirus vaccine (IPV) or oral poliovirus vaccine (OPV). Still rarely seen in Africa and Asia. Associated with flaccid paralysis that may be irreversible and lead to death due to respiratory muscle paralysis.
- Arbovirus (West Nile, St. Louis, Western/Eastern Equine, La Crosse)—transmitted by mosquitoes
- Mumps—associated with parotitis
- Lymphocytic choriomeningitis virus (LCMV)—associated with exposure to rodent waste. Starts with influenza-like illness and then may develop meningitis. Other symptoms may include orchitis, parotitis, myopericarditis, or arthritis.

PPx: Airborne or contact precaution may be appropriate depending on virus. Vaccination for poliovirus, mumps, measles.

MoD: Presence of virus elsewhere in body or environment (more often fecal-oral than respiratory transmission) → viremia → crosses BBB → viral infection of host cells in subarachnoid space attracts neutrophils → acute meningitis

Dx:
1. Clinical exam.
2. LP showing ↑ CSF protein and WBCs, normal CSF glucose.
3. Negative bacterial culture.
4. Detection of virus on polymerase chain reaction (PCR) or antiviral antibodies, depending on virus. Cause is unidentified in 75% of aseptic meningitis cases.

Tx/Mgmt:
1. Usually supportive

Herpes Simplex Virus Encephalitis

Buzz Words: Newborn + elevated protein, normal glucose in CSF + mom had herpetic lesions prior to birth

Clinical Presentation: Herpes simplex virus (HSV) encephalitis is commonly seen in pediatrics in the setting of congenital localized HSV infection of the newborn. Only some patients with congenital HSV get encephalitis; others can have local involvement of skin, mouth, and eyes or disseminated involvement in visceral organs.

PPx:
1. Treat mom if lesions found prior to birth
2. C section

MoD: Transmission during vaginal delivery

Dx:
1. Clinical exam
2. LP showing ↑ CSF protein and normal CSF glucose
3. Negative bacterial culture
4. Detection of virus on PCR or antiviral antibodies, depending on virus

Tx/Mgmt:
1. Usually supportive

Spirochetal Diseases

There are two major spirochetes to consider: *Borrelia burgdorferi* and *Treponema pallidum.*

Borrelia burgdorferi

Buzz Words: Exposure to tick bites; travel history; Bell palsy; late summer, early fall

Clinical Presentation: Neurologic manifestations occur in second stage (1–4 months after bite). Include aseptic meningitis with symptoms similar to above, encephalitis, and facial nerve palsies (unilateral or bilateral).

PPx: N/A

MoD: *Ixodes* tick is the vector → spread to CSF or nerves leads to neurologic symptoms.

Dx:
1. Clinical exam. Other symptoms of Lyme disease are crucial in diagnosis, such as erythema migrans or Bell palsy.
2. Serologic testing for antibodies to *B. burgdorferi* (ELISA first as it is more sensitive).
3. Western blot for confirmation.

Tx/Mgmt:
1. Doxycycline is first-line (unless <8 years old, then amoxicillin).
2. IV ceftriaxone for meningitis.

Treponema pallidum

Buzz Words: Sexually active teenager + rash on palms and soles + meningitis → secondary syphilis
- Newborn + saddle nose + saber shins → congenital syphilis

Clinical Presentation:
- Meningitis—occurs during secondary syphilis with headache, malaise, and a disseminated rash (including palms/soles).
- Neurosyphilis—occurs during tertiary syphilis and is associated with rapidly progressive altered mental status and cranial nerve palsies along with other tertiary syphilis symptoms (tabes dorsalis, Argyll-Robertson pupils, gummas, aortitis). Very uncommon in the pediatric population.
- Congenital syphilis—neurologic symptoms include developmental delay, hearing loss, seizures; occurs in association with classic physical findings (rhinitis, rash, bone abnormalities leading to "saddle nose" and "saber shin" deformities).

PPx:
1. Avoidance of syphilis through safe sex practices
2. Treatment of maternal infection in utero

MoD: *T. pallidum* transmitted through sexual contact or through transplacentally if infection is congenital. Disseminates to central nervous system (CNS) during early infection but symptoms of neurologic involvement (meningitis, encephalitis, neurosyphilis) typically occur in setting of secondary or tertiary syphilis. Destruction of vasa vasorum (blood vessels that supply vessel wall) leads to necrosis.

Dx:
1. Clinical exam and risk factors
2. CSF demonstrates ↑ protein and WBC (lymphocytic), normal glucose
3. Serum or CSF VDRL

Tx/Mgmt:
1. Penicillin G, monitor for Jarisch-Herxheimer reaction (systemic response similar to shock occurring due to spirochete destruction)

Protozoal Diseases

Naegleria fowleri

Buzz Words: Swimming in freshwater lakes
Clinical Presentation: Rapidly progressive meningoencephalitis. Involves frontal lobes.

PPx: N/A

MoD: Protozoa are contracted while swimming in freshwater lakes. They travel through the cribriform plate to infect meninges and brain parenchyma, especially frontal lobes.

Dx:

1. Clinical exam
2. LP (amoebas visualized in CSF)

Tx/Mgmt:

1. Amphotericin B, although disease is rapidly progressive and almost universally fatal.

Congenital Toxoplasma gondii

Buzz Words: Mother consuming undercooked meat/handling kitty litter during pregnancy + chorioretinitis + hydrocephalus

Clinical Presentation: Most patients are asymptomatic or have symptoms similar to mono. Congenital infection associated with triad of hydrocephalus, seizures (due to intracranial calcification), and chorioretinitis but may cause miscarriage if it occurs early in pregnancy. Chorioretinitis also associated with CMV. Reactivation in immunosuppressed patients may cause encephalitis, focal seizures.

PPx: Avoidance of exposure (especially among seronegative women of childbearing age), maternal screening/treatment.

MoD: Primary maternal infection or reactivation in immunocompromised mother → transplacental transmission → enters fetal CNS, leading to abnormal neuronal development.

Dx:

1. Known risk factors/exposures and clinical findings.
2. Serologic testing (presence of immunoglobulin [Ig]M antibodies suggests active primary infection).

Tx/Mgmt:

1. Most infections do not require treatment.
2. Pregnant women with active primary infection, infants, or immunocompromised patients may be treated with antiparasitics (preferred regimen = pyrimethamine + sulfadiazine + leucovorin).

Immunologic and Inflammatory Disorders

Myasthenia Gravis, Including Thymoma

Buzz Words: Muscle weakness that gets WORSE with repeated muscle contractions + ptosis + eyes that fail to maintain prolonged upward gaze + large mass in the mediastinum on CXR

Clinical Presentation: Ocular symptoms (ptosis, diploplia) are the most common presenting symptoms but weakness in other muscle groups can be seen. Weakness WORSE later in day and with repeated or sustained muscle contractions.

There are three types of myasthenia gravis in the pediatric population: juvenile, congenital, and neonatal. In juvenile MG, symptoms begin during adolescence and there is a female predisposition. In contrast, patients with congenital MG, an autosomal recessive disease, show symptoms from birth. Last, neonatal MG is a transient MG of the newborn that occurs because autoantibodies to the acetylcholine (ACh) receptor (AChR) cross the placenta from mom to baby.

PPx: N/A

MoD: Autoimmune disease resulting from autoantibodies against AChR. Disease can range from generalized to focal, with ocular being the most common focal form. Thymic hyperplasia is common in pediatric MG but thymomas are rare.

Dx:
1. Clinical
2. CXR to look for evidence of thymoma
3. Tensilon test
4. Ice pack test
5. Serologic testing for autoantibodies (e.g., AChR)
6. Electrophysical testing (e.g., repetitive nerve stimulation testing, single-fiber electromyography [EMG])

Tx/Mgmt: Four categories of Tx:
1. Symptomatic → anticholinesterase (pyridostigmine). First-line therapy.
2. Chronic immunomodulators → glucocorticoids. Limited to severe disease when pyridostigmine fails due to significant side effects with chronic use (retardation of bone growth, osteoporosis, etc.). Other agents (azathioprine, mycophenolate, cyclosporine) have also been used but have more significant side effects (e.g., malignancy, impaired fertility).
3. Rapid immunomodulators → plasmapheresis/intravenous immunoglobulin (IVIG). Provide transient benefits.
4. Surgical → thymectomy → indicated in all patients with thymoma and beneficial even in nonthymoma cases.

Multiple Sclerosis

Buzz Words: Female predominance, associated with living at northern latitudes. Scanning speech, optic neuritis, internuclear ophthalmoplegia

Clinical Presentation: Episodic course featuring acute relapses and remissions (80%–90%). Wide variety of neuro sx's: Sensory (paresthesias, loss of sensation), motor (upper motor neuron [UMN] dysfxn → spasticity, ↑ deep tendon reflexes [DTRs], weakness), autonomic (bowel/bladder dysfunction), cerebellar (scanning speech, intention tremor, ataxia), ocular (optic neuritis → blurry vision, may be isolated symptom in pediatric MS; intranuclear ophthalmoplegia → inability to adduct ipsilateral eye + horizontal nystagmus in contralateral eye). More likely to present with encephalopathy in children.

PPx: N/A

MoD: Most common demyelinating disease. Predominance for white females of reproductive age, w/ greater prevalence at northern latitudes. Autoimmune disease targeting myelin sheath → focal inflammatory demyelinating lesions affecting the white matter of brain and spinal cord. Etiology related to environmental and genetic factors.

Dx: Magnetic resonance imaging (MRI) w/ gadolinium = best initial test + most accurate test → demyelinating lesions in brain and spine of various ages, often periventricular (e.g., "Dawson fingers"). LP → CSF with mild ↑ in protein and WBCs; oligoclonal bands in approximately 85% of patients (nonspecific).

Tx/Mgmt: High-dose IV steroids are best initial therapy for acute exacerbations of disease. Immunomodulatory agents prevent relapse/progression (glatiramer, interferon-beta initial therapies, natalizumab and other experimental agents considered for refractory disease).

Guillain Barré Syndrome (GBS)

Buzz Words: Ascending persistent paralysis + lower motor neuron [LMN] signs only + preceding infection + preceding bloody diarrhea (*Campylobacter jejuni*) + high protein, normal WBC/glucose on CSF analysis + autonomic dysfunction + <2 months

Clinical Presentation: GBS is less common in the pediatric than the adult population but is on the differential whenever paralysis is the chief complaint. On the shelf, it is associated with infectious organisms such as *C. jejuni*.

PPx: None

MoD: Viral or bacterial (*C. jejuni* or *Vibrio cholerae*) infx →
autoimmune attack of peripheral myelin due to molecular
mimicry → endoneural inflammation and demyelination of
peripheral nerves

Dx:

1. Physical exam
2. Electrodiagnostic testing
3. LP will show **albuminocytologic dissociation** (e.g.,
   normal WBC + normal glucose + high protein)
4. Measure **forced vital capacity** (FVC) to determine need
   for intubation
5. Head MRI to r/o stroke

Tx/Mgmt:

1. Fluids
2. IVIG
3. Plasmapheresis
4. Respiratory support/intubation if FVC less than 15 mL/kg

Seizure Disorders

Congenital Disorders Associated With Seizures

Tuberous Sclerosis (Tuberous Sclerosis Complex)

Buzz Words: Hypopigmented macules (ash-leaf spots) +
facial angiofibromas+ cardiac rhabdomyomas + renal
angioleiomyomas + MR + seizures + astrocytoma +
infantile spasms

Video of infantile spasms

Clinical Presentation: Tuberous sclerosis is a genetic disorder
characterized by tuberous sclerosis complex (TSC)1/2
mutations. It is most easily identified in a question stem
by ash-leaf spots and infantile spasms. Make sure to
differentiate from Sturge-Weber, which instead presents
with generalized seizures.

PPx: None

MoD: Do not memorize for the shelf; provided here for
background only. TSC1 and TSC2 gene mutations
(TSC1—chromosome 9—hamartin; TSC2—chromosome 16—tuberin) → impaired the mTOR (mammalian
target of rapamycin) pathway → tuberous sclerosis

Dx:

1. Look for ash-leaf spots and angiofibromas
2. Electroencephalogram (EEG)
3. MRI to r/o structural etiology
4. Pyruvate, lactate, amino acids, to r/o metabolic
   disorders
5. Consult ophtho to rule out TORCH infection

6. Genomewide sequencing to look for mutations like STXBP1, CASK and PNPO, v2
7. CXR to rule out TB (since that is a contraindication for adrenocorticotropic hormone [ACTH] therapy)

Tx/Mgmt:
1. Anticipatory guidance for parents
2. Treatment of infantile spasms (e.g., ACTH)

Sturge–Weber Syndrome

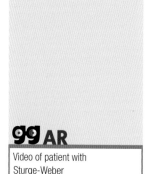

Video of patient with Sturge-Weber

Buzz Words: **Port wine stain** aka **nevus flammeus** + congenital unilateral cavernous hemangioma along trigeminal nerve distribution + intracranial calcifications that resemble a tram line + **generalized seizures** + mental retardation

Clinical Presentation: On the Pediatrics exam, Sturge-Weber syndrome is on the differential for children with generalized seizures and dermatologic findings. It is NOT THE SAME as tuberous sclerosis (infantile spasms = tuberous sclerosis = associated with adenoma sebaceum). Unlike tuberous sclerosis, patients with Sturge-Weber suffer from generalized seizures. The most common complications of this disorder are hemisensory disturbance, ipsilateral glaucoma, and hemianopia.

PPx: None
MoD: *GNAQ* gene mutation
Dx:
1. CT to r/o tumors
2. EEG to monitor seizures

Tx/Mgmt:
1. **Argon laser therapy** to remove skin lesions and reduce intraocular pressure
2. levetiracetam (Keppra) for generalized seizures

Partial Seizure

Simple Partial Seizure (Focal Seizure)

Buzz Words: Preserved consciousness + no postictal period + tonic or clonic movement involves only focal portion of body

Clinical Presentation: In simple partial seizures, consciousness is preserved and there is no postictal period. This entity is not commonly tested directly on the Pediatrics exam but will appear as a distractor answer.

PPx: None
MoD: Synchronized neuronal discharge

Dx:
1. EEG shows localized spike and sharp waves
Tx/Mgmt:
1. First-line: carbamazepine and valproic acid
2. Lamotrigine

Complex Partial Seizure (Focal Seizure With Consciousness Disturbance)

Buzz Words: Impaired consciousness + postictal period + tonic or clonic movement that involves focal part of body

Clinical Presentation: Complex partial seizures are characterized by tonic or clonic movements involving most of the face, neck, and extremities and lasting 10–20 seconds, accompanied by **impaired consciousness**.

PPx: None

MoD: Synchronized neuronal discharge

Dx:
1. EEG → anterior temporal lobe showing sharp waves or focal spikes

Tx/Mgmt:
1. First-line: valproic acid, carbamezepine
2. Lamotrigine

Generalized Seizures

By definition, generalized seizures impair consciousness. Most begin in childhood; thus these are high-yield for the Pediatrics shelf.

Absence Seizure (Petit Mal)

Buzz Words: Blank stare + pause in activities for a few seconds + induced by hyperventilation + no memory of event

Clinical Presentation: High-yield for the Pediatrics exam. Patients with absence seizures can present in the question stem as "a kid who does not pay attention" or "zones out easily in class." More common in girls, rare in children younger than 5 years, rarely last longer than 30 seconds. There is no aura or postictal state.

PPx: None

MoD: Dysfunction of T-type calcium channels

Dx:
1. EEG shows 3-per-second (3-Hz) typical spike-and-wave discharges.

Tx/Mgmt:
1. **Ethosuximide**
2. Valproic acid

Juvenile Myoclonic Epilepsy

Buzz Words: Quick, myoclonic jerks of arms + teenager + occurs in morning + followed by clonic-tonic generalized seizure

Clinical Presentation: Only type of seizure that occurs in the morning.

PPx: None

MoD: Synchronized neuronal discharge

Dx:
1. EEG

Tx/Mgmt:
1. Valproic acid

Idiopathic Generalized Epilepsy

Buzz Words: Loss of consciousness + skeletal muscles tense, alternating stiffening and movement + whole-body movement

Clinical Presentation: Idiopathic generalized epilepsy is characterized by frequent tonic-clonic seizures (aka grand mal) that involve the whole body. During the episode, patient's muscles will start to contract and relax rapidly, causing convulsions.

PPx: None

MoD: Synchronized neuronal discharge

Dx:
1. EEG

Tx/Mgmt:
1. Phenytoin
2. Valproic acid

Cranial and Peripheral Nerve Disorders

Cranial Nerve Injury/Disorders

Bell Palsy (CN VII)

Buzz Words: Unlike stroke, forehead is also paralyzed.

Clinical Presentation: Paralysis of entire side of face. (NOTE: stroke paralyzes only lower half of face.) Difficulty closing the eye, hyperacusis (sounds are extra loud because CN VII supplies stapedius muscle, which is a "shock absorber" on the ossicles), taste disturbances (b/c CN VII nerve provides taste to 2/3 of tongue).

PPx: N/A

MoD: Most cases = idiopathic. Some are due to Lyme disease, sarcoidosis, herpes zoster reactivation.

Dx:
1. Clinical exam: If patient CAN wrinkle forehead on affected side → worry about stroke. If patient CANNOT wrinkle forehead on affected side → Bell palsy.

Tx/Mgmt:
1. Some 60% recover fully without treatment.
2. Prednisone = best initial therapy.
3. Provide eye care (e.g., lubricant or suture lid closed temporarily).
4. Valacyclovir may be used for severe disease/if herpes is suspected as underlying cause.

Vestibular Neuritis, Labyrinthitis

Buzz Words: Viral infection + ataxia + nausea and vomiting (N/V)

Clinical Presentation: Vertigo often accompanied by acute N/V and gait impairment

PPx: N/A

MoD: Acute viral or postviral inflammation of vestibular branch of CN VIII (vestibular neuritis) or of both branches of CN VIII (labyrinthitis)

Dx: Clinical exam is diagnostic (ataxia, nystagmus, positive head-thrust test). MRI is necessary if headache present, focal neurologic signs, or stroke risk factors.

Tx/Mgmt: Steroids unless contraindications → aid short-term recovery, but long-term benefit is undetermined.

Peripheral Nerve/Plexus Injury/Disorders

Infant Botulism

Buzz Words: Infant + recent exposure to honey + constipation + descending paralysis (e.g., slowed feeding, weak muscle tone)

Clinical Presentation: Infant botulism occurs most commonly in patients who are younger than 12 months old and is associated with ingestion of foods such as honey that contain *Clostridium botulinum* spores. Constipation is usually the first sign.

PPx: Avoidance of honey

MoD: *C. botulinum* spores ingested → colonize large intestine → toxin produced

Dx:
1. Clinical
2. Stool tests to look for toxin

Tx/Mgmt:
1. Supportive care (to deter respiratory compromise)
2. Human botulism immune globulin

Peripheral Nerve Injury
Brachial Plexus Injury

Condition	Nerve Roots Injured	Causes	Muscles Affected	Functional Deficit
Erb palsy	C5–C6 (upper trunk)	Neonate → traction on neck during delivery	Deltoid, supraspinatus, infraspinatus, biceps brachii	Adducted + internally rotated upper arm with forearm extended
Klumpke palsy	C8–T1 (lower trunk)	Neonate → upward pull on arm during delivery	Intrinsic hand muscles	Total claw hand

Sleep Disorders
Narcolepsy

Buzz Words: Cataplexy + rapid eye movement (REM) during naps + hallucinations + sleep paralysis when waking up

Clinical Presentation: Excessive, irresistible sleepiness, cataplexy, hypnagogic/hypnopompic hallucinations, and sleep paralysis. Can present as young as 5 years old. Unique features of childhood-onset cases: cataplexy with prominent buccofacial involvement, daytime sleepiness manifested primarily as irritability, excessive napping, and hyperactivity. Depression is common, and children have greater risk of aggressive behavior, attention difficulties, poor school performance, and social/emotional stress. Obesity is common in affected patients, with onset often occurring around period where symptoms first appear.

PPx: N/A

MoD: Deficiency of hypocretin (peptide involved in alertness) in hypothalamus

Dx:
1. Sleep diary
2. Sleep EEG
3. LP to look for hypocretin levels in CSF

Tx/Mgmt: Tx options based on corresponding symptoms:
1. Daytime sleepiness → CNS stimulants (e.g., methylphenidate, amphetamines); wake-promoting agents (e.g., modafinil, armodafinil).
2. Cataplexy → if mild, no Tx necessary. If severe → sodium oxybate (first-line) or select antidepressants (e.g., clomipramine, protriptyline, fluoxetine, sertraline, venlafaxine).

Sleep Terror Disorder

Buzz Words: Child abruptly wakes from sleep with a scream + not responsive to comforting efforts + does NOT remember event.

Clinical Presentation: Child wakes abruptly with a scream, agitation, flushed face, perspiration, and tachycardia. May run from bed. Importantly, child is unresponsive to comforting efforts (and may seem "glassy-eyed") and does NOT remember this event.

PPx: N/A

MoD: Most common in ages 4–12 years. Occurs during first third of nocturnal sleep. There is a strong genetic predisposition.

Dx:
1. Clinical picture.
2. EEG may show high-amplitude rhythmic delta/theta activity.

Tx/Mgmt: Virtually always self-limiting. Ensure child is safe, w/ fall risks mitigated.

Sleepwalking

Buzz Words: Child wandering around home at night + confused when waking up

Clinical Presentation: Child is awake but unresponsive, wandering around home, and has no memory of event. More severe cases involve children becoming agitated, running, or demonstrating other inappropriate behaviors. Risk of injury, including hypothermia on cold nights.

PPx: N/A

MoD: Occurs during non-REM sleep. Seen in ~15% of children, with peak incidence at age 8–12 years.

Dx: Clinical picture is diagnostic.

Tx/Mgmt: Virtually always self-limiting. Ensure child is safe, with fall risks mitigated.

Traumatic and Mechanical Disorders and Disorders of Increased Intracranial Pressure

Epidural Hematoma (Cerebral and Spinal)

Buzz Words: "Lucid interval" + Biconvex (football-shaped) hematoma on CT

Clinical Presentation: Patient presents after trauma → lucid interval → lethargy, confusion, or obtundation. May demonstrate headache, vomiting, pupillary abnormalities, or focal neurologic deficits (e.g., seizures, hemiparesis).

PPx: N/A

MoD: Traumatic injury leading to rupture of middle meningeal artery

Dx:

1. Head CT without contrast → shows lentiform (biconvex) hematoma that does NOT cross suture lines (due to firm attachment of dura at these sites).

Tx/Mgmt:

1. Lower intracranial pressure (ICP) (temporary hyperventilation, mannitol, elevate head of bed) while awaiting emergent surgery to place burr holes, drain blood, and relieve ICP.

Subdural Hematoma (Cerebral and Spinal)

Buzz Words: Crescent-shaped hematoma on CT + history of abuse

Clinical Presentation: Gradual onset of symptoms over days to weeks. Infants present with seizures, lethargy, vomiting, apnea. Older children may have headache, vomiting, fluctuating levels of consciousness, somnolence. Herniation and death may occur. Chronic subdural hematoma can produce a reversible dementia-like state.

PPx: N/A

MoD: Traumatic event leads to shearing of bridging veins. Most commonly seen in children with shaken-baby syndrome.

Dx: Head CT without contrast → shows crescent-shaped hematoma (hyperdense if acute, hypodense if chronic) that CAN cross suture lines.

Tx/Mgmt:

1. If patient stable without neurologic deficits → supportive care

2. Monitoring. If patient deteriorating → craniectomy, drain blood, relieve ICP. File with protective services if consistent with nonaccidental trauma.

Subarachnoid Hemorrhage

Buzz Words: "Worst headache of my life" + "Crab of death" pattern on head CT

Clinical Presentation: Patient presents with sudden onset "worst headache of my life," often with no clear precipitating factor. Meningeal irritation present (stiff neck, photophobia) and fever common due to blood irritating meninges (can differentiate from meningitis based on sudden-onset of sx). Other complications include rebleeding + hydrocephalus (secondary to blockage of arachnoid granulations or foramina). Number-one cause is ruptured aneurysm, usually located in anterior circle of Willis. What provokes the rupture is not clear in the majority of cases, and the vast majority of aneurysms never rupture (present in 2% of routine autopsies). Increased risk of aneurysms in polycystic kidney disease, Ehlers–Danlos, and hypertension.

PPx: Detect and clip cerebral aneurysms in at-risk patients.

MoD: Idiopathic ruptured aneurysm

Dx:

1. Head CT showing "crab of death" pattern.
2. LP may still show xanthochromia (breakdown of blood in CSF into bilirubin pigment).
3. To determine which vessel ruptured → CT angiography, standard angiography with a catheter, or magnetic resonance angiography (MRA).

Tx/Mgmt: See above. Some 50% die shortly after onset. No treatment is able to reverse the hemorrhage.

1. Nimodipine (calcium channel blocker) → prevents subsequent ischemic stroke.
2. Catheter-directed embolization of site of bleeding → superior to surgical clipping in terms of survival and complications.
3. Ventriculoperitoneal shunt: needed only if hydrocephalus develops.
4. Antiepileptics.

Idiopathic Intracranial Hypertension (aka Pseudotumor Cerebri)

Buzz Words: Female + headaches + obesity + increased opening pressure with LP

Clinical Presentation: Headaches, often daily and pulsatile, worse during night or early morning. Possible retro-ocular pain worsened by eye movement, diplopia, blurry vision (due to papilledema), rhythmic tinnitus. Occasional cranial nerve deficits but no other focal neurologic signs or mental status changes. Worst complication is vision loss.

PPx: N/A

MoD: Unclear, may be due to ↓ CSF resorption in arachnoid granulations or cerebral venous outflow abnormalities → ↑ ICP. Most commonly seen in obese females of childbearing age. Other risk factors: hypothyroidism, Cushing disease, long-term tetracyclines (though rarely given to children), or isotretinoin (for acne).

Dx:

1. Exam—papilledema ± visual field loss, CN VI palsy.
2. MRI/magnetic resonance venography (MRV) preferred to CT → flattening of the posterior globe with normal ventricles + brain parenchyma; r/o central venous thrombosis or tumor or other CSF-obstructing lesion.
3. LP: elevated CSF pressure; normal CSF studies.

Tx/Mgmt:

1. Lifestyle changes: discontinue inciting agents (e.g., excess vit A); weight loss in obese patients.
2. Medical: carbonic anhydrase inhibitor (e.g., acetazolamide) = first-line. Loop diuretics as adjunct; systemic corticosteroids if visual loss only.
3. Procedural: serial LPs.
4. Surgical: lumboperitoneal shunt; optic nerve sheath fenestration.

Hydrocephalus

Buzz Words: Ventriculomegaly on MRI/CT

Clinical Presentation: Symptoms vary depending on etiology. Headache is common, usually worse at night or in early morning. Nausea, vomiting, behavioral, cognitive changes may be present. Infants demonstrate bulging fontanelles, enlarged head circumference.

PPx: N/A

MoD: Normal CSF life cycle: CSF production in choroid plexus of lateral ventricles → drainage through foramen of Monro into third ventricle → drainage through cerebral aqueduct to fourth ventricle → enters subarachnoid space → resorption by arachnoid granulations.

Hydrocephalus = error in process above leading to increased CSF volume and increased ICP. Two forms:
- Communicating (nonobstructive) hydrocephalus
  - No obstructions present in ventricular network
  - Causes: increased CSF production OR dysfunction in CSF reabsorption by arachnoid granulations
- Noncommunicating (obstructive) hydrocephalus
  - Any mass obstructing flow of CSF through ventricular network
  - Causes: tumor, Chiari type II malformation (downward displacement of cerebellum/medulla through foramen magnum), Dandy–Walker malformation (absent cerebellar vermis + cystic enlargement of fourth ventricle), scarring of base of brain (e.g., intrauterine infection). Congenital aqueductal stenosis. NOTE: Obstruction of aqueduct of Sylvius = #1 cause in newborns, leads to Parinaud phenomenon (upward gaze paralysis).

If untreated → edema and ischemia in periventricular brain tissue → white matter atrophy.

Dx: In adults/older children: MRI showing enlargement of ventricles; obstruction in noncommunicating hydrocephalus may be visible. In infants: head ultrasound.

Tx/Mgmt: Diuretics, external ventricular drain, + serial LPs are temporizing measures. Definitive: Communicating hydrocephalus → ventriculoperitoneal shunt or endoscopic third ventriculostomy. Noncommunicating hydrocephalus → remove obstructing lesions if possible; otherwise, use shunt.

Traumatic Brain Injury

Buzz Words: Headaches + lethargy + mental dullness + months after initial trauma → concussion and **postconcussive syndrome**

Clinical Presentation: Traumatic brain injury comprises the spectrum of injury caused to the brain by traumatic force. A mild traumatic brain injury is a "concussion." A moderate to severe traumatic brain injury is a "contusion."

PPx: N/A

MoD: Comes from stretching of the axons due to traumatic force

Dx:
1. CT/MRI to r/o hematoma
2. XR of cervical spine to r/o spinal injury

Tx/Mgmt:
1. Prevention of ICP increase.
2. Surgery if accompanying expanding hematoma that worsens ICP.
3. Supportive care; there is no direct treatment protocol right now that directly addresses traumatic brain injury (TBI).

Headache

Migraine

Buzz Words: Woman with unilateral pulsating pain + nausea + phonophobia + photophobia lasting 4–72 hours + usually with history of migraines in mother/grandmother
- Can be with or without aura (scotoma, teichopsia, numbness, tingling)

Clinical Presentation: On the Pediatrics exam, the typical patient with migraines is a teenage female who experiences sensory auras followed by intense headaches associated with photophobia.

PPx: N/A

MoD: Irritation of CN V, meninges, or blood vessels from vasodilation and due to release of substance P, CGRP, vasoactive peptides from cells in trigeminal nucleus:
- Familial migraine caused by deficits in ion channels

Dx:
1. Clinical diagnosis based on 2 or more repeated headaches for 4–72 hours.
2. CT/MRI only when sudden/severe, after age 40, to look for focal neurologic findings or rule out subarachnoid hemorrhage.

Tx/Mgmt:
1. Avoid triggers.
2. Abortive therapy for few attacks (less than 6 times per month): triptans (such as sumatriptan), ergotamine.
3. Prophylactic treatments for frequent attacks (if more than 6 times per month) beta blocker (propranolol), anticonvulsive medicines (i.e., topiramate).
4. Adjunct therapy: antidopaminergic drugs (antiemetics/neuroleptics—i.e., metoclopramide, promethazine, and prochlorperazine) for headache and nausea.

Tension Headache

Buzz Words: Stress-induced + bilateral, band-like pressure around the head

Clinical Presentation: Unlike the other types of headaches, tension headache is always stress-induced on the shelf and presents with a band-like pressure around the head. There are no accompanying features like nausea, vomiting, photophobia, or phonophobia.

PPx: N/A

MoD: Unknown, thought to relate to pain filter in brain secondary to stress

Dx: Clinical history

Tx/Mgmt:
1. Nonsteroidal anti-inflammatory drugs (NSAIDs)
2. Tricyclic antidepressants (TCAs)
3. Behavioral approaches for stress

Cluster Headache

Buzz Words: 1–8 per day + **teenage males** + extreme irritability and pain + alcohol trigger + autonomic symptoms (**lacrimation,** pupillary constriction in periorbital and sinus region, **unilateral**)

Clinical Presentation: The classic cluster headache patient on the Pediatrics exam is a male teenager who complains of unilateral headaches that cause his eyes to water. Treatment modalities for cluster headaches are frequently tested.

PPx: N/A

MoD: Dilation of blood vessels → pressure on trigeminal nerve

Dx: Clinical history and features

Tx/Mgmt:
1. Acute treatments (abortive treatments) — 100% oxygen and subcutaneous (SC) sumatriptan
2. Transitional treatment — steroids
3. Prophylactic treatment — verapamil, topiramate, gabapentin

QUICK TIPS

Headache + Aura = Migraine
Headache + unilateral + tears in one eye = Cluster
Headache + bilateral + vise-like grip = Tension

Congenital Disorders

Friedreich Ataxia

Buzz Words: Hammer toes + ataxia + pes cavus + hypertrophic cardiomyopathy

Clinical Presentation: Progressive neurologic deficits: ataxia (universal symptom), loss of deep tendon reflexes (DTRs), leg weakness, dysarthria, loss of sensations from dorsal columns (vibration and proprioception). Skeletal: hammer toes, high pedal arches, + kyphoscoliosis. Other complications: hypertrophic cardiomyopathy (#1 cause of death) + type 1 diabetes mellitus (DM) (in 10%).

PPx: Genetic counseling for parents

MoD: Autosomal recessive trinucleotide repeat disorder (GAA) affecting Frataxin gene on chromosome 9 → impaired iron homeostasis in mitochondria → cells more prone to apoptosis due to oxidative damage. Neuronal cells cannot regenerate, therefore leads to degeneration of:

- Dorsal columns → UMN; disrupts fine touch, vibrioception, proprioception, pressure sense
- Spinocerebellar tract → upper motor neurons (UMNs); disrupts fine movements, leads to ataxia
- Lateral corticospinal tracts → UMNs; disrupts fine movements
- Dorsal root ganglia
- Large sensory peripheral neurons

Dx:
1. Genetic testing confirms mutation in Frataxin gene.
2. MRI shows spinal atrophy.

Tx/Mgmt:
1. Supportive

Neural Tube Defects

Buzz Words: Maternal folate deficiency + dimple ± tuft of hair at base of spine

Clinical Presentation: Typically affects lumbosacral spine leading to neurologic deficits, learning disabilities, attention issues, reading comprehension difficulties, and orthopedic issues.

PPx:
1. Maternal folate supplementation
2. Discontinue teratogenic medications
3. Prenatal care and screening

MoD: Results from (1) failure of fusion of lateral folds of neural plate in gestational weeks 3–4 or (2) rupture of a previously closed neural tube. Due to environmental and genetic risk factors (e.g., maternal folate deficiency, tricyclic antidepressants, valproate). Three forms (in order of least to most severe):

- Spina bifida occulta → small gap between 2+ vertebrae, but meninges and spinal cord do not protrude through vertebral defect. No neurologic deficits.
- Meningocele → spina bifida with cystic mass containing meninges and CSF; spinal cord does not protrude through defect. Sx are varied, may be asymptomatic.
- Myelomeningocele → spina bifida with cystic mass containing meninges, CSF, spinal cord, and nerve roots protruding through defect. Neuro sx nearly universal. Also ↑ risk of infection.

Dx:
1. Prenatal exam shows ↑ alpha-fetoprotein (AFP) in maternal serum or amniotic fluid; defect may be visible on maternal ultrasound if severe.
2. Physical exam of neonate shows either small dimple ± tuft of hair (spina bifida) or lumbar sac (meningocele, myelomeningocele) at base of spine.

Tx/Mgmt:
1. Provide prenatal counseling.
2. Cover defect, provide prophylactic antibiotics, assess for additional congenital anomalies.
3. Initiate clean, intermittent catheter for likely bladder dysfunction (reduces risk of UTI and progressive renal disease).
4. Surgical repair of defect w/in 72 hours if possible.
5. Monitor for hydrocephalus → if present place ventriculoperitoneal shunt.
6. Serial, lifelong neurologic evaluations, including signs of spinal cord/brain stem compression due to risk of Chiari II malformation.
7. Orthopedic consult to correct deformities, maintain posture, and promote ambulation.

Holoprosencephaly

Buzz Words: Intellectual disability and developmental delay + midline facial abnormalities

Clinical Presentation: Holoprosencephaly occurs when the brain fails to develop into two hemispheres. Facial defects are common. Relatively mild facial defects include microcephaly, microphthalmia, midfacial hypoplasia, cleft lip, and cleft palate. More severe facial defects include cyclopia (single midline eye), midfacial clefting, and proboscis (an underdeveloped nasal structure). Severe disease is incompatible with life.

PPx: Genetic counseling for parents with family Hx of this disease

MoD: Developmental defect in differentiation of embryonic forebrain. Exact etiology remains unknown.

Dx:
1. Prenatal ultrasound within first trimester.
2. Fetal MRI can detect and characterize milder features.

Tx/Mgmt:
1. Children with milder disease are treated with supportive measures.

Anencephaly

Buzz Words: Absence of major portion of brain and skull

Clinical Presentation: Some 75% of patients are stillborn. Live-born infants are permanently unconscious but usually maintain brain stem function w/ spontaneous breathing and primitive reflexes (e.g., root, suck). Rarely, the infant may live up to a few days following delivery.

PPx:

1. Maternal screening

MoD: Results from neural tube defect in which developing forebrain and portions of brain stem are exposed to amniotic fluid during embryogenesis, leading to developmental failure or destruction. Characterized by open defect in calvaria and skin, leaving cranial neural tube exposed, usually with complete absence of brain tissue.

Dx:

1. Elevated maternal AFP.
2. Findings on ultrasound are diagnostic. Mother often has polyhydramnios.

Tx/Mgmt:

1. Provide prenatal counseling.
2. Referral to clinical geneticists, pediatric neurologist is generally warranted.

Duchenne Muscular Dystrophy

Buzz Words: Child 2–3 years old + Gower sign + toe walk + male

Clinical Presentation: Duchenne muscular dystrophy (DMD) is an X-linked recessive myopathy that occurs due to a defect in dystrophin, a protein crucial in muscle function. Characterized by proximal muscle weakness and is eventually fatal.

PPx: N/A

MoD: Defect in dystrophin gene

Dx:

1. Clinical
2. Muscle biopsy staining for dystrophin

Tx/Mgmt:

1. Bracing
2. Physical therapy
3. Prednisone
4. Deflazacort
5. Ventilator support (nasal mask, elective tracheotomy if severe)

Becker Muscular Dystrophy

Buzz Words: Teenager + Gower sign + toe walk + male

Clinical Presentation: Becker muscular dystrophy (BMD) is also an X-linked recessive myopathy that can be thought of as the late-presenting version of DMD.

PPx: N/A

MoD: Defect in dystrophin gene

Dx:
1. Clinical
2. Muscle biopsy staining for dystrophin

Tx/Mgmt:
1. Bracing
2. Physical therapy
3. Ventilator support (nasal mask, elective tracheotomy if severe)

Neoplasms of the Nervous System

Benign Neoplasms

Meningioma

Buzz Words: Occipital headache + slurred speech + atrophy/fasciculation of tongue + weakness in b/l body + Babinski sign b/l + "**streak**"/"**tail**" (dural attachment) seen on MRI → meningioma of the foramen magnum

Clinical Presentation: Meningioma is one of the most common brain tumors in the pediatric population. For the shelf, you do not need to know the histology. It is often asymptomatic in real life but will likely present on the shelf with symptoms.

PPx: Reduce ionizing radiation

MoD: Arises from arachnoid cells of the meninges:
- Extra-axial

Dx:
1. MRI
2. Biopsy

Tx/Mgmt:
1. Resection
2. Radiation

Von Hippel-Lindau Disease

Buzz Words: Hemangiomas of brain/spinal cord/eye + cysts in kidney/liver/pancreas

Clinical Presentation: Characterized by multiple hemangioblastomas (benign vascular tumor) in medulla, retina, and cerebellum → headaches, ataxia, weakness, and vision problems. Multiple cysts in kidney, liver, and pancreas. Risk of bilateral renal cell carcinoma, pheochromocytomas.

PPx: Genetic counseling for parents

MoD: Autosomal dominant mutation of Von Hippel–Lindau (VHL) tumor-suppressor gene on chromosome 3

Dx:

1. Multiple hemangioblastomas in CNS or eye
2. Single hemangioblastoma in CNS or eye + one of following: renal cancer, pheochromocytoma, multiple renal/pancreatic/hepatic cysts
3. Positive family history plus any one of the above clinical manifestations
4. Deleterious mutation of VHL gene on genetic testing

Tx/Mgmt:

1. Referral to clinical genetics, pediatric neurology, and oncology is generally warranted.

Neurofibromatosis I (aka Von Recklinghausen Disease)

Buzz Words: Optic nerve glioma + café-au-lait spots + iris hamartomas (Lisch nodules) + pheochromocytoma + dermal neurofibromas

Clinical Presentation: Neurofibromatosis I (NF I) is among the most high-yield diseases in this chapter. It is easily recognizable with its combination of café-au-lait spots and Lisch nodules. It is likely to be tested on the pediatrics, neurology, Medicine shelf and Surgery shelf.

PPx: N/A

MoD: Tumor arises from neural crest cells (don't have to memorize for shelf, learn for own interest only):

- Due to mutation of neurofibromin on chromosome 17, a tumor suppressor gene and downregulator of RAS

Dx:

1. Head CT
2. Urine metanephrites to dx pheochromocytoma

Tx/Mgmt:

1. Surgery

Neurofibromatosis II (aka Vestibular Schwannomas)

Buzz Words:

- Hearing loss + tinnitus + dizziness + Schwannoma + enlarged internal auditory canal extending into cerebellopontine angle → vestibular schwannomas
- Bilateral vestibular schwanomma → NF II

Clinical Presentation: Bilateral vestibular schwannomas are NF II until proven otherwise.

PPx: N/A

MoD: Arises from Schwann cells, most typically in CN8

Dx: CT

Tx/Mgmt:
1. Surgery
2. Radiation

Craniopharyngioma

Buzz Words: Bilateral **temporal hemianopsia** (aka no peripheral vision OR traffic accident because patient didn't see oncoming car) + calcifications in Rathke pouch + headaches + urinary frequency

Clinical Presentation: This diagnosis should be considered whenever a patient presents with temporal hemianopsia. Calcifications in Rathke pouch are also pathognomonic.

PPx: N/A

MoD: Tumor cells from remnants of Rathke pouch:
- Tumor compresses medial side of optic tract at chiasm, leading to b/l hemianopsia.
- Urinary frequency due to posterior pituitary compression (no ADH).

Dx: Head CT, MRI

Tx/Mgmt:
1. Surgery
2. Radiation

Pituitary Adenoma

Buzz Words: Bilateral **temporal hemianopsia** (aka no peripheral vision OR traffic accident because patient didn't see oncoming car) + prolactinoma + other overactive/underactive pituitary conditions

Clinical Presentation: Pituitary adenoma is similar to craniopharyngioma but has pituitary side effects and no calcifications in Rathke pouch.

PPx: N/A

MoD: Tumor cells from pituitary cells (can be any of them). Tumor compresses medial side of optic tract at chiasm, leading to bilateral hemianopsia.

Dx:
1. Head CT, MRI

Tx/Mgmt:
1. Surgery
2. Radiation

QUICK TIPS

Prolactinoma is the most common finding from pituitary adenoma; look for galactorrhea.

Pilocytic Astrocytoma

Buzz Words: Seizures + cystic appearance on imaging and gross exam + posterior fossa (e.g., cerebellum) + GFAP-positive + children

Clinical Presentation: Pilocytic astrocytoma is the most common posterior fossa tumor in children. It may appear on answer choice as simply "astrocytoma."

PPx: Reduce ionizing radiation.

MoD: Arises from astrocytes; a subtype of astrocytoma (grade I)

Dx:
1. Head CT/MRI
2. Biopsy

Tx/Mgmt:
1. Surgery

Malignant Neoplasms

Medulloblastoma

Buzz Words: Cerebellar location + ataxia + children + hydrocephalus + drop metastases to spinal cord

Clinical Presentation: Medulloblastoma is seen in children and puts the patient at risk for drop metastases in the spinal cord. The most common chief complaint is ataxia.

PPx: N/A

MoD: Arises from primitive neuroectodermal cells, making it a type of primitive neuroectodermal tumor (PNET).

Dx:
1. Head CT/MRI
2. Biopsy

Tx/Mgmt:
1. Radiotherapy
2. Surgery
3. Chemotherapy

Ependymoma

Buzz Words: Fourth ventricle tumor + hydrocephalus + children

Clinical Presentation: Rarely tested but is frequently used as a distractor answer.

PPx: N/A

MoD: Arises from ependymal cells of the fourth ventricle

Dx:
1. Head CT/MRI
2. Biopsy

Tx/Mgmt: Surgery

Disorders of the Eyes, Ears, Nose, Throat

Ophthalmologic Disorders

Retinoblastoma

Buzz Words: White reflex (white instead of red seen when light in eye)

Clinical Presentation: Child age less than 2 with leukocoria (white reflex rather than red reflex) and/or strabismus

PPx: Genetic screening in families with history of disease

MoD: #1 intraocular neoplasm of children (10%–15% of cancers seen before age 1 year). Fatal if untreated, but survival greater than 95% if treated promptly. Heritable and nonheritable forms exist, both due to mutations in *RB1* gene (tumor suppressor gene on chromosome 13). Inherited disease usually presents with bilateral disease, whereas sporadic, nongermline cases are often unilateral.

Dx: Clinical picture of leukocoria and/or strabismus is common. Intraocular calcified mass can be seen on ultrasound/CT in most cases.

Tx/Mgmt: Radiotherapy, chemotherapy, and/or enucleation. Also assess for masses elsewhere in body, as retinoblastoma is also associated with neoplasms of bone.

Strabismus

Buzz Words: "Wandering/crossed eyes"

Clinical Presentation: Irregular alignment of one or both eyes. Esotropia = nasal deviation, exotropia = temporal deviation. May lead to amblyopia if untreated. Pseudostrabismus refers to false appearance of strabismus due to prominent epicanthal folds.

PPx: Childhood eye exams

MoD: Cause usually unknown. Prevalence of ~3% in children.

Dx: Clinical exam = sufficient. Hirschberg test → light reflex test in which light is shone in both eyes and light reflects off both eyes symmetrically in nonstrabismus + pseudostrabismus patients. Light reflects from nasal aspect of cornea in exotropia and temporal aspect of cornea in esotropia. "Cover–uncover test" demonstrates movement of eyes in patients with strabismus → this test involves point-fixing gaze on an object and examiner alternating between covering one eye and the other repeatedly and in rapid succession. The misaligned eye will appear to deviate inward or outward.

Tx/Mgmt: Ocular patching is first-line. Surgery may be needed. Corrective lenses if concurrent amblyopia.

Amblyopia

Buzz Words: Child having trouble seeing the board in school + poor vision in one eye

Clinical Presentation: Amblyopia is colloquially known as "lazy eye." Leads to poor visual acuity of one eye, generally not due to a structural defect alone.

PPx: Childhood eye exams

MoD: Decreased visual acuity in one eye relative to the other due to abnormal visual experience in childhood that causes the mind to favor one eye during neurodevelopment. Some 50% of cases are due to strabismus. Other causes: uncorrected refractive errors in vision, structural defects of one eye.

Dx:

1. Clinical exam maneuvers: Test visual acuity of each eye separately; in early childhood, this may be done using specific pediatric visual acuity tests that involve shapes/games rather than letters.

Tx/Mgmt: Varies depending on cause. Treatments options include:

1. Patching of good eye.
2. Corrective lens.
3. Surgery. Good restoration of visual acuity in 90% of children treated before age 10. Prognosis decreases w/ aging, but treatment should always be attempted regardless of age.

Cellulitis (Preseptal and Orbital)

Buzz Words: Erythema and tenderness of eyelid + eye movements intact + no proptosis → preseptal (aka preorbital) cellulitis

Erythema and tenderness of eyelid + impaired ocular movement (painful) + proptosis + decreased visual acuity

Clinical Presentation: Cellulitis of the eye in the pediatric population is most commonly either preseptal or orbital. Preseptal (aka periorbital) cellulitis is infection of the eye anterior to the orbital septum, whereas orbital cellulitis is infection posterior to the septum. Most common mechanism is spread from an adjacent infection (e.g., sinusitis).

PPx: N/A

MoD: Spread from adjacent infection (e.g., sinusitis) or infection from local trauma

Dx:

1. Clinical
2. CT/MRI to rule out orbital cellulitis

Tx/Mgmt: Antibiotics targeted at nasal pathogens (e.g., *S. pneumoniae, S. aureus, Moraxella*)

Disorders of the Ear

Otitis

Otitis Media Versus Otitis Externa

Condition	Common Causes	Treatment
Otitis media = inflammation of middle ear (erythema and bulging of tympanic membrane [TM], loss of landmarks), usually due to infection. Viral causes are usually self-limiting. Bacterial causes should be treated as outlined in this table. —Serous otitis = serous fluid behind TM, often described as "straw-colored." —Suppurative otitis = purulent fluid behind TM.	*Streptococcus pneumoniae, H. influenzae, Moraxella catarrhalis,* viral URI > group A strep	Age: <6 months → Tx (10-day course); 6–24 months → watchful waiting for 72 h w/ f/u; >24 months → Tx if worsens after 72 h (5-day course). Tx: first-line → amoxicillin; second (or w/ concurrent conjunctivitis) → amoxicillin + clavulanic acid; third → cefuroxime/clarithromycin.
Otitis externa = inflammation of external auditory canal (EAC) (swelling/redness and discharge of EAC), usually due to infection. Often bacterial. Progression of *Pseudomonal* disease can lead to **malignant otitis externa** → necrotic disease of auditory canal/skull base → emergent ENT consult!	*Pseudomonas aeruginosa, S. aureus;* acute otitis media (AOM) organisms if due to eardrum perforation	Tx: (1) Thoroughly clean ear canal. (2) Rx: mild disease → acetic acid + corticosteroid; moderate/severe disease → topical fluoroquinolones ± corticosteroid (cortisporin = cheaper alternative).

TABLE 6.1 Most Common Organism for Meningitis by Age

Age of Patient	Most Common Organism	Treatment
<1 month	(1) Group B streptococci, (2) *Escherichia coli*, (3) *Listeria*	Ampicillin + gentamicin or cefotaxime
1–3 months	(1) Group B streptococci, (2) gram-negative bacilli, (3) *Streptococcus pneumoniae*, (4) *Neisseria meningitidis*	Third-generation cephalosporin (cefotaxime or ceftriaxone) + vancomycin
3 months–6 years	(1) Viral (primarily entero), (2) *N. meningitidis*, (3) *S. pneumoniae* (4) *Haemophilus influenzae*	Third-generation cephalosporin (cefotaxime or ceftriaxone) + vancomycin
6–18 years	(1) Viral (entero > HSV), (2) *N. meningitidis* (#1 in teens), (3) *S. pneumoniae*	Third-generation cephalosporin (cefotaxime or ceftriaxone) + vancomycin

TABLE 6.2 Cerebrospinal Fluid Findings in Mengingitis

Test	Bacterial	Viral	Fungal
White blood cell (WBC) count	High (e.g., >1000/mm^3)	<100/mm^3	Variable
Protein	Elevated	Normal to elevated	Elevated
Opening pressure	High	Normal	Variable
Cell differential	Polymorphonucleocytes (PMNs)	Lymphocytes	Lymphocytes
Glucose (compared with blood serum)	Decreased	Normal	Decreased

GUNNER PRACTICE

1. A 25-day-old boy who was born at 38 weeks' gestation is brought to the emergency department because of fever. He had an uncomplicated birth, although mom missed several prenatal visits. He has a fever of 101.5°F. On exam, he is fussy and difficult to console, particularly when you move his neck, and his anterior fontanelle seems somewhat full. Urine culture is negative and CXR does not show signs of infection. Results of a lumbar puncture are pending. What is the most appropriate treatment for this patient?
   A. Cephalexin
   B. Ceftriaxone
   C. Vancomycin and ceftriaxone
   D. Ampicillin and gentamicin
   E. Metronidazole

Notes

ANSWER: What Would Gunner Jess/Jim Do?

1. WWGJD? A 25-day-old boy who was born at 38 weeks' gestation is brought into the emergency department because of fever. He had an uncomplicated birth, although mom missed several prenatal visits. He has a fever of 101.5°F. On exam, he is fussy and difficult to console, particularly when you move his neck, and his anterior fontanelle seems somewhat full. Urine culture is negative and CXR does not show signs of infection. Results of a lumbar puncture are pending. What is the most appropriate treatment for this patient?

Answer: D, Ampicillin and gentamicin

Explanation: Given the patient's fever, irritability, and full fontanelle, it is likely that he has meningitis, which is a life-threatening cause of fever in a neonate. Bacterial meningitis is most common, and in a newborn, the organisms to watch out for are those that populate mom's reproductive tract (e.g., *E. coli*, group B strep, and *Listeria*). The key word here is that **ampicillin** is needed for treatment of patients under 1 month of age who are suspected of meningitis in order to treat *Listeria* and GBS. This concept is frequently tested on the exam.

A. Cephalexin → Incorrect. Cephalexin (aka Keflex) is a first-generation cephalosporin that is often given to patients preoperatively to decrease rates of surgical site infection.

B. Ceftriaxone → Incorrect. Ceftriaxone is a third-generation cephalosporin that can be used in the treatment of bacterial meningitis but is usually given in conjunction with another drug (e.g., vancomycin). It is also not used in neonates because it can displace bilirubin from albumin and increase the risk of kernicterus.

C. Vancomycin and ceftriaxone → Incorrect. Vancomycin provides coverage for methicillin-resistant *S. aureus* (MRSA) and is more commonly used in older patients, though it may be considered in very ill-appearing infants. Ceftriaxone is not used in neonates because it can displace bilirubin.

E. Metronidazole → Incorrect. Metronidazole is typically used for anaerobic bacteria and is commonly used for to treat bowel infections.

Cardiovascular Disorders

Anup Bhattacharya, Sila Bal, Daniel Gromer, Hao-Hua Wu,
Erika Mejia, Leo Wang, and Rebecca Tenney-Soeiro

Introduction

The heart is essential for pumping oxygenated blood to the vital organs of the body. The embryonic development of the heart follows a specific sequential course; when there are errors in this progression, the newborn faces significant difficulties. For the Pediatrics shelf, questions about the congenital disorders are particularly high-yield because they require significant understanding of the associated clinical findings, especially heart sounds and age at presentation. Additionally, you will be expected to understand the physiology of these disorders. For example, a patient with a patent ductus arteriosus (PDA) will have a widened pulse pressure; however, questions will often bury this finding in a lengthy physical exam. Associations are often made with genetic syndromes and cardiac anomalies as well. You will be required to distill important laboratory and exam data.

There are several organizing principles to this chapter. First, use a consistent framework to understand the cyanotic heart lesions as opposed to the noncyanotic heart lesions, which have the potential to become cyanotic if there is reversal of the direction of the shunt. This reversal is known as Eisenmenger syndrome. If you use this framework, deciphering the answers to shelf questions will be much easier and you will be able to begin to narrow down your choices.

This chapter is divided into two main sections: (1) a brief background review of embryonic development, fetal maturation, and perinatal transitional changes, and (2) congenital heart disorders, which is the most high-yield portion of this chapter.

Development

Embryonic Development

The heart spontaneously beats at week 4 of development and is the first functional organ in human development. In week 4 of gestation, the left-right polarity of the heart is established.

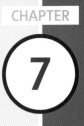

GUNNER COLUMN

QUICK TIPS

The congenital abnormalities that begin with a "T" will cause cyanosis. Remembering them is as easy as 1, 2, 3, 4, 5: (1) One trunk, Truncus arteriosus (persistent). (2) Transposition of the TWO vessels. (3) Tricuspid atresia. (4) Tetralogy of Fallot. (5) Five words for Total anomalous pulmonary venous return.

QUICK TIPS

The rest of the shunts are left-to-right; use "VAP" to remember them: (1) VSD, (2) ASD, and (3) PDA.

QUICK TIPS

There are four chambers in the heart, which beats spontaneously at week 4 of development.

QUICK TIPS

Dextrocardia can be caused by a deficiency in dynein. This is seen in primary ciliary dyskinesia (Kartegener syndrome).

Atria

The septum primum and septum secundum help separate the left and right atria. When they fail to fuse, the condition is known as a patent foramen ovale, which is discussed later in this chapter.

Ventricles

The ventricular septum is formed by three components: (1) the muscular interventricular septum, (2) the aorticopulmonary septum, and (3) the endocardial cushions. Problems with this process can lead to a ventricular septal defect (VSD), which is discussed later in this chapter.

Fetal Maturation

The heart undergoes a large transformation in the fetal period. Physiologically, there is a tremendous increase in the number of membrane-bound tubules in the sarcoplasmic reticulum, in the number of myofibrils, and in the contractile ability of the heart itself.

Perinatal Transitional Changes

During the first 2 days after birth, the patent ductus arteriosus (PDA), which in the womb shunts oxygen-rich blood from the right side of the heart to the organs of the lower extremity via the descending aorta, closes.

The ductus venosus, which allows blood to bypass the fetal liver, becomes the remnant known as the ligamentum venosum. The foramen ovale becomes the fossa ovalis. The umbilical vein, which provides oxygenated blood to the fetus, becomes the ligamentum teres hepatis, contained in the falciform ligament. Finally, the umbilical arteries, which carry deoxygenated blood back to the placenta, become the medial umbilical ligaments (Fig. 7.1).

Congenital Disorders

Anomalous Left Coronary Artery From the Pulmonary Artery

Buzz Words: Anomalous coronary vessel, coronary steal, heart attack

Clinical Presentation: Myocardial infarction in baby, crying or sweating during feeding, rapid breathing, pale skin, and poor feeding in first 2 months of life.

Prophylaxis (PPx): N/A

Mechanism of Disease (MoD): Left coronary artery starts at the pulmonary artery instead of at the aorta and therefore carries deoxygenated blood to the heart.

Fetal circulation

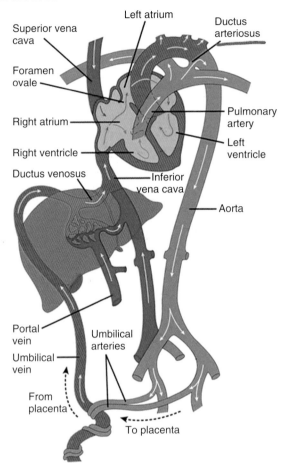

FIG. 7.1 Fetal circulation.

Diagnostic Steps (Dx):
1. Electrocardiogram (ECG)
2. Coronary arteriography
3. Cardiac catheterization.
4. Echocardiography

Treatment and Management Steps (Tx/Mgmt): Surgical intervention necessary to correct origin of anomalous left coronary artery. Can manage with:
1. Diuretics
2. Inotropes
3. Beta blockers
4. Angiotensin-converting enzyme inhibitors (ACEIs) for symptomatic relief

Atrial Septal Defect

Buzz Words: Fixed, split S2 and left-to-right shunt, diastolic murmur

Clinical Presentation: Often asymptomatic; older children may experience shortness of breath or a murmur may be detected on exam.

PPx: N/A

MoD: There are several types, including primum defect (seen in trisomy 21) as well as secundum defect due to failure of the interatrial septum to appropriately fuse.

Dx: Echocardiography is the gold standard. Will show defect in interatrial septum.

Tx/Mgmt:

1. If asymptomatic, consider watchful waiting.
2. If symptomatic, surgical intervention to repair defect in interatrial wall.

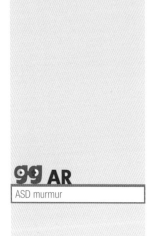

ASD murmur

Coarctation of the Aorta

Buzz Words: Rib notching on CXR, reduced perfusion in lower extremities (radiofemoral delay), turbulence bruit on the back, systolic blood pressure (BP) in upper extremity (UE) is greater than 10 mm Hg higher than lower extremity (LE).

Clinical Presentation: Turner syndrome patient with elevated upper extremity blood pressures → think coarctation of aorta. Early on patients will have widened pulse pressure due to a PDA.

PPx: N/A

MoD: Congenital condition due to mechanism not fully understood

Dx:

1. Upper and lower extremity blood pressures
2. CXR to identify possible rib notching
3. Echocardiogram

Tx/Mgmt: Balloon angioplasty/surgical intervention often necessary

Endocardial Cushion Defect

Buzz Words: AV canal defect, aorticopulmonary septum malformation, neural crest migration defect

Clinical Presentation: Often seen in trisomy 21; associated with cyanosis, tachypnea, failure to grow.

PPx: N/A

MoD: Failure of migration of neural crest cells from aortic arches

Dx: Echocardiography

Tx/Mgmt: Surgical repair if symptomatic

Patent Foramen Ovale

Buzz Words: Stroke from emboli to the heart

Clinical Presentation: Patent foremen ovale (PFO) is not classically considered a congenital defect because the foramen ovale normally takes a little time to close after birth. However, there are some whose foramen ovale does not close. These patients are asymptomatic and largely incidentally discovered on echocardiography. The most important clinical correlate is that emboli that would otherwise end up in the lung can travel through the PFO to the left circulation and end up in the brain.

PPx: N/A

MoD: At birth, the influx of oxygen into the lungs results in a decrease in pulmonary vascular resistance and right heart pressure. Conversely, the influx of oxygenated blood into the left heart causes an increase in left heart pressure. Although the exact mechanism behind failed complete fusion remains unknown, genetic and environmental factors have been shown to play a role. Most individuals with Ebstein abnormality (maternal lithium use) have a PFO.

Dx: Echocardiography

Tx/Mgmt: Treated only when symptomatic; patch placed via catheter/surgical repair

Patent Ductus Arteriosus

Buzz Words: Continuous machine-like murmur, brisk pulses, widened pulse pressure

Clinical Presentation: Premature Infant who is found to have continuous murmur.

PPx: N/A

MoD: The ductus arteriosus connects the pulmonary artery to the descending aorta in the womb. Normally, it closes shortly after birth. Failure to close results in a PDA.

Dx:
1. Echocardiogram to confirm diagnosis
2. Auscultation of continuous machine-like murmur

Tx/Mgmt: Indomethacin (nonsteroidal anti-inflammatory drug [NSAID]) helps to close the ductus arteriosus; may require surgical clip.

Tetralogy of Fallot

Buzz Words: Most common cyanotic heart lesion and most common cause of a blue baby

Clinical Presentation: Cyanotic infant with holosystolic murmur. Any decrease in systemic vascular resistance such as exercise or dehydration or any process that increases right-sided pressure in the heart, such as crying or tachy-cardia, will result in right-to-left shunting and subsequent cyanosis. Toddlers will then try to fix this with Valsalva maneuvers such as squatting.

PPx: N/A

MoD: Possibly due to maternal malnutrition or in-utero viral illness; exact etiology unknown.

Dx:
1. Echocardiogram
2. ECG
3. CXR
4. Pulse oximetry
5. Cardiac catheterization

Tx/Mgmt: Surgical repair

Transposition of the Great Arteries

Buzz Words: Poor feeding, lethargy, and cyanosis during perinatal period. No murmur.

Clinical Presentation: Transposition of the great arteries (TGA) is associated with maternal diabetes during gestation. Neonates will be cyanotic at birth.

PPx: N/A

MoD: Switching of positions of pulmonary artery and aorta; in TGA, the pulmonary artery comes off the left ventricle while the aorta comes off the right ventricle.

Dx: Echocardiography is the gold standard.

Tx/Mgmt:
1. Prostaglandins to maintain patent ductus arteriosus to enable mixing of oxygen rich and oxygen-poor blood.
2. More definitive treatment is surgical repair.

Ventricular Septal Defect

Buzz Words: Holosystolic murmur exacerbated by inspiration

Clinical Presentation: Continuous murmur that may present at any time, often incidentally discovered, is the most common congenital heart defect.

PPx: N/A

MoD: Defect in interventricular septum allowing blood to travel freely between right and left ventricles, creating an initial left-to-right shunt. If left unattended, can reverse (Eisenmenger syndrome), causing a right-to-left shunt reversal and cyanosis.

Dx: Echocardiography

Tx/Mgmt: Surgical repair if large. Note that smaller VSDs have louder murmurs.

GUNNER PRACTICE

1. A newborn male is noted to have a cardiac murmur in the well baby nursery. He was born 11 hours earlier, after a 39-week pregnancy, to a healthy 36-year-old woman. She recently immigrated to this country and does not have medical records or prenatal screening test information available. The delivery proceeded without complication, and Apgar scores were 7 at 1 minute and 9 at 5 minutes after birth. The infant's vital signs are T 98.2°F, HR 142, BP 65/32, RR 39 SpO$_2$ 95% on room air. On exam, he is interactive with a lusty cry, but his palpebral fissures are upslanting and there is an increased distance between his great and second toes. His ears appear low-set and slightly rotated as well. Cardiac auscultation yields multiple murmurs of distinct quality, duration, and timing. What is the most likely diagnosis?
   A. Atrial septal defect
   B. Transposition of the great arteries
   C. Infective endocarditis
   D. Tetralogy of Fallot
   E. Endocardial cushion defect

2. A 7-year-old female is brought to the ED by her mother. Her past medical history is significant for mild reactive airway disease and eczema. She was kept home from school for 2 days last week with low-grade fevers, abdominal pain, and loose stools, but had made a brief recovery before developing shortness of breath and abdominal pain yesterday. Her symptoms progressed quickly, and her mother was alarmed to find that this morning she was struggling to breathe. The child's vital signs are T 99.4°F, HR 131, BP 70/49, RR 26, SpO$_2$ 85% on room air. On examination, she appears to be in severe respiratory distress. Her extremities are cool and clammy, pulmonary auscultation yields crackles bilaterally in the lower lung lobes, cardiac auscultation yields an S3, and the liver edge is palpable 3 cm below the costal margin. Echocardiography reveals global hypokinesis. What is the most likely diagnosis?
   A. Infective endocarditis
   B. Viral myocarditis
   C. Tetralogy of Fallot
   D. Anaphylaxis
   E. *Mycoplasma pneumoniae* pneumonia

3. A 14-year-old female is brought to the pediatrician's office by her mother for a delayed vaccination and checkup. She has had sporadic clinical follow-up throughout her lifetime, and does not have medical records available. She has no complaints. Her mother mentions that she has previously been found to have "a single big kidney across her belly" and "bad hearing," but has otherwise been healthy. Her weight and height are both below the 3rd percentile, and she has not yet had her menses. Her vital signs are T 98.3°F, HR 85, BP 139/88, RR 16, SpO$_2$ 98% on room air. Blood pressure in the lower extremities is 83/51. Physical exam reveals small ears and a delay between her upper extremity and femoral pulses. What is the most likely diagnosis and the most appropriate next step in management?

A. Fibromuscular dysplasia; MRI of the renal arteries

B. Coarctation of the aorta in Turner syndrome; echocardiography and karyotype analysis

C. Patent ductus arteriosus in trisomy 21; echocardiography and karyotype analysis

D. Lupus nephritis; antinuclear antibody and anti-dsDNA antibody titer measurement

E. Abdominal aortic aneurysm; ultrasound of the abdomen

Notes

ANSWERS: What Would Gunner Jess/Jim Do?

1. WWGJD? A newborn male is noted to have a cardiac murmur in the well baby nursery. He was born 11 hours ago, after a 39-week pregnancy, to a 36-year-old healthy woman. She recently immigrated to this country and does not have medical records or prenatal screening test information available. The delivery proceeded without complication, and Apgar scores were 7 at 1 minute and 9 at 5 minutes after birth. The infant's vital signs are T 98.2°F, HR 142, BP 65/32, RR 39, SpO_2 95% on room air. On exam, he is interactive with a lusty cry, but his palpebral fissures are upslanting and there is an increased distance between his great and second toes. His ears appear low-set and slightly rotated as well. Cardiac auscultation yields multiple murmurs of distinct quality, duration, and timing. Echocardiography reveals a common AV valve annulus. What is the most likely diagnosis?

Answer: E, Endocardial cushion defect

Explanation: This is a newborn male in no acute distress who appears to have trisomy 21 and a cardiac murmur. The details about the palpebral fissures, toes, and ears are classic features of patients with trisomy 21 (there are many others, and questions will often mention only a few). Additionally, his mother's age is greater than 35, at which point the risk of trisomy 21 increases. The most common associated cardiac malformation is an endocardial cushion defect, also known as an atrioventricular canal defect, which is a catch-all term for defects involving the atrioventricular (AV) septum and valves. The multitude of murmurs described in the question are concordant with the pulmonary outflow obstructions, diastolic rumbles, and mitral and tricuspid regurgitation (among others) that can occur with these defects. Finally, the echocardiogram reveals a joint AV defect, which suggests an endocardial cushion defect.

A. Atrial septal defect → Incorrect. Atrial septal defects (ASDs) are associated with trisomy 21, but less commonly than endocardial cushion defects. Additionally, and more helpful for answering the question, is the fact that an ASD less commonly causes multiple murmurs. Finally, the echocardiogram is inconsistent with an ASD.

B. Transposition of the great arteries → Incorrect. Transposition of the great arteries (TGA) is one of the five cardiac malformations most commonly associated with cyanosis (mnemonic below). This infant, who is not hypoxemic, cyanotic, or in any acute distress, is less likely to have TGA, especially given the echocardiographic findings consistent with another malformation and the presence of multiple murmurs. The five most common cardiac malformations are:

  i. Truncus arteriosus (single outflow tract)
  ii. Transposition of the great arteries (two switched arteries)
  iii. *Tri*cuspid atresia
  iv. *Tetra*logy of Fallot
  v. Total anomalous pulmonary venous return (five words)

C. Infective endocarditis → Incorrect. Infective endo-carditis can be diagnosed using the Duke criteria. Here—in an infant with no fever, no tachycardia, no signs of distress, no embolic signs of endocar-ditis, and no further history or imaging information indicating a cardiac vegetation—suspicion is low.

D. Tetralogy of Fallot → Incorrect. This is one of the cardiac malformations listed above. It is unique in that the cyanosis associated with tetralogy of Fallot can be intermittent. This condition can be accom-panied by a pulmonic stenosis–like murmur or pat-ent ductus arteriosus murmur if the pulmonary valve is atretic. It is, however, not the most likely diagno-sis in a patient with trisomy 21, and the echocardio-gram is again suggestive of another malformation.

2. WWGJD? A 7-year-old female is brought to the ED by her mother. Her past medical history is significant for mild reactive airway disease and eczema. She was kept home from school for 2 days last week with low-grade fevers, abdominal pain, and loose stools, but had made a brief recovery before developing short-ness of breath and abdominal pain yesterday. Her symptoms progressed quickly, and her mother was alarmed to find that this morning she was struggling to breathe. The child's vital signs are T 99.4°F, HR 131, BP 70/49, RR 26, SpO_2 85% on room air. On examination, she appears to be in severe respiratory distress. Her extremities are cool and clammy, pulmo-nary auscultation yields crackles bilaterally in the lower lung lobes, cardiac auscultation yields an S3, and the liver edge is palpable 3 cm below the costal margin. Echocardiography reveals global hypokinesis. What is the most likely diagnosis?

Answer: B, Viral myocarditis

Explanation: This is a child with a recent "viral prodrome" who presents with shortness of breath. Her tachycardia, hypotension with low pulse pressure, hypoxemia, and cool extremities indicate that she is in shock. The physical exam findings of bilateral pulmonary crackles, a cardiac S3, and hepatomegaly are suggestive of cardiogenic shock due to heart failure. Echocardiography shows decreased wall motion throughout the heart muscle. This presentation is classic for viral myocarditis, which involves inflammation of the heart muscle and often occurs shortly after a respiratory or gastrointestinal illness.

A. Infective endocarditis → Incorrect. Although it is important to consider bacterial infection in this patient, the echocardiographic findings in a patient presenting with a recent viral syndrome and current heart failure are more suggestive of myocarditis.

C. Tetralogy of Fallot → Incorrect. We are given no history that would indicate tetralogy of Fallot, and the echocardiography is not suggestive of this diagnosis.

D. Anaphylaxis → Incorrect. This is a common cause of distributive shock in children. Although dyspnea and hypoxemia may be present, the patient will classically have warm extremities and should not have the history presented by the mother in this case.

E. *Mycoplasma pneumoniae* pneumonia → Incorrect. Although this might cause dyspnea and pulmonary crackles, it does not otherwise fit with the clinical picture.

3. WWGJD? A 14-year-old female is brought to the pediatrician's office by her mother for a delayed vaccination and checkup. She has had sporadic clinical follow-up throughout her lifetime, and does not have medical records available. She has no complaints. Her mother mentions that she has previously been shown to have "a single, big kidney across her belly" and "bad hearing," but has otherwise been healthy. Her weight and height are both below the 3rd percentile, and she has not yet had her menses. Her vital signs are T 98.3°F, HR 85, BP 139/88, RR 16, SpO$_2$ 98% on room air. Blood pressure in the lower extremities is 83/51. Physical exam reveals small ears and a delay between her upper extremity and femoral pulses. What are the most likely diagnosis and most appropriate next step in management?

Answer: B, Coarctation of the aorta in Turner syndrome; echocardiography and karyotype analysis

Explanation: This is an adolescent female with growth failure, primary amenorrhea, bad hearing, and what sounds suspiciously like a horseshoe kidney. These are classic features of Turner syndrome, which this patient has. Additionally, the patient has upper extremity hypertension and lower extremity hypotension with brachial-femoral pulse delay, indicating that she may have coarctation of the aorta. Coarctation of the aorta (as well as other cardiac anomalies, including bicuspid aortic valve) are common in Turner syndrome as well and should be investigated with an echocardiogram. The karyotype analysis is warranted in this patient due to suspicion of Turner syndrome.

A. Fibromuscular dysplasia; MRI of the renal arteries → Incorrect. Although fibromuscular dysplasia can classically involve the renal arteries of young women and lead to hypertension, it should not cause lower extremity hypotension or brachial–femoral pulse delay.

C. Patent ductus arteriosus in trisomy 21; echocardiography and karyotype analysis → Incorrect. This patient has historic and phenotypic features of Turner syndrome, not trisomy 21.

D. Lupus nephritis; antinuclear antibody and anti-dsDNA antibody titer measurement → Incorrect. The patient does not have any complaints, nor does she have a clinical syndrome resembling nephritic syndrome or nephrotic syndrome. She simply has asymmetric blood pressure measurements.

E. Abdominal aortic aneurysm; ultrasound of the abdomen → Incorrect. This would not explain most of the patient's phenotype, nor would it truly explain the cardiovascular findings. Additionally, these are most commonly seen in elderly smokers.

Diseases of the Respiratory System

Lauren Briskie, Daniel Gromer, Hao-Hua Wu, Garrett P. Keim, Leo Wang, and Rebecca Tenney-Soeiro

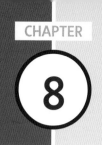

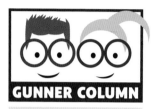

GUNNER COLUMN

Introduction

This chapter covers a wide variety of both pulmonary conditions and ear/nose/throat (ENT) pathologies. About 10%–15% of the National Board of Medical Examiners (NBME) Pediatrics exam questions come from this chapter. This chapter is divided into infectious, immunologic, and inflammatory disorders of both the upper and lower airways. It also covers benign neoplasms, asthma, traumatic and mechanical disorders, and congenital conditions.

The infectious diseases covered in this chapter are critically important, as you can be asked questions about them in multiple ways. For example, a child presenting with stridor and fever requires you to work through multiple different infectious pathologies that can cause these symptoms.

The examiners may then ask for simply the diagnosis, or second-order questions regarding pathophysiology or treatment. Therefore it is important to thoroughly learn this information and the common associations of these conditions.

You may have noticed in the overview that asthma has an entire section to itself. It is really important to be able to determine the classification of asthma from a clinical vignette as well as to decide on appropriate treatment in the outpatient setting. Additionally, the examiners will often test your ability to recognize and manage an acute exacerbation. This is a bread-and-butter topic and is commonly tested.

If you are crunched for time, there are some areas that are lower-yield but still fair game for the exam; these include benign neoplasms and congenital cysts. Congenital diaphragmatic hernia and primary ciliary dyskinesia (PCD) are more frequently tested and of greater value. For those who have completed the surgery rotation, the trauma section may cover material that you have already studied. Good luck!

Need-to-Know Embryology

Respiratory tract and lung embryology will not be directly tested on the exam but reviewing it may help you to understand some of the congenital disorders. Feel free to skip this subsection if you already have a solid foundation from step 1 studying.

The first appearance of the fetal lung occurs at approximately 26 days' gestation. The initial branching of the lung occurs at 33 days, forming the prospective main bronchi. Further branching forms the segmental bronchi. From weeks 5 to 16 of gestation, additional generations of airway branching occur, starting from the main segmental bronchi and progressing toward the terminal bronchioles. From the 16th to 25th weeks of gestation, the transition to viable lung occurs, as the respiratory bronchioles and alveolar ducts begin to form. At 20 weeks' gestation, the cuboidal epithelial cells begin to differentiate into alveolar type II cells with formation of lamellar bodies. The presence of lamellar bodies indicates the production of surfactant. A count of lamellar bodies can be performed to help gauge fetal lung maturity.

At approximately 24 weeks' gestation, gas exchange becomes possible due to the presence of large and primitive forms of future alveoli. At this stage, the alveoli begin to form by the outgrowth of the septa that subdivide terminal saccules into anatomic alveoli, where gas exchange occurs. A lecithin/sphingomyelin ratio is used to assess fetal lung maturity. These are in equal concentration until about week 32–33. When their ratio is greater than 2, the risk of respiratory distress syndrome due to surfactant deficiency is very low.

Because sinusitis is covered in this chapter, we include a quick review of the development of the sinuses. Maxillary and ethmoid sinuses are present at birth. The maxillary sinuses become pneumatized at 4 years of age. Frontal sinuses begin developing at age 7 and are not completely developed until adolescence. The sphenoid sinuses are present by 5 years of age. By age 12, the paranasal sinuses have reached nearly adult proportions. Sinusitis most commonly affects the paranasal sinuses.

Infectious, Immunologic, and Inflammatory Disorders of the Upper Airways

Acute Upper Respiratory Infection

Buzz Words: Rhinorrhea + sore throat + nontoxic appearance

Clinical Presentation: Peak incidence from early fall through late spring. The annual number of colds decreases with age. Children in day care and with siblings are at increased risk. Prominent symptoms of rhinorrhea, nasal obstruction, sore throat, absent or mild fever. On exam, nasal turbinates are edematous and erythematous. Usually persists for about 1 week.

Prophylaxis (PPx): N/A

Mechanism of Disease (MoD): Most commonly caused by rhinoviruses

Diagnostic Steps (Dx): Clinical

Treatment and Management Steps (Tx/Mgmt): Symptomatic. Antihistamines and decongestants are not recommended for children <6 years of age as risk outweighs benefit.

Influenza ("Flu")

Buzz Words: Lack of vaccinations + sniffling + runny nose/congestion + sneezing + sore throat + winter + **muscle ache** + fatigue **+** high fever + chest tightness

Clinical Presentation: Flu is caused by the influenza virus. Differentiate a cold from influenza by the presence of a high fever and **myalgias.** In children, flu can also cause vomiting and diarrhea. Some prominent complications include viral pneumonia, bacterial pneumonia, or superinfections leading to bacterial sinusitis (Fig. 8.1).

PPx: Frequent handwashing + annual influenza vaccine + surgical mask

MoD: Respiratory droplet transmission of influenza A, B, or C. Influenza A is most common and includes the H1N1 to H7N9 viruses. Viruses bind to **hemagglutinin** on epithelial cells → replication. **Neuraminidase** leads to release of viral particles from host cells.

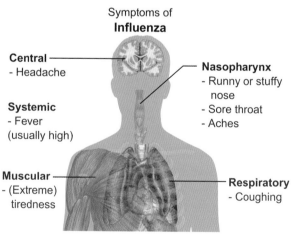

Symptoms of
Influenza

Central
- Headache

Nasopharynx
- Runny or stuffy nose
- Sore throat
- Aches

Systemic
- Fever
(usually high)

Muscular
- (Extreme) tiredness

Respiratory
- Coughing

FIG. 8.1 Symptoms of influenza (Wiki).

Dx:
1. Clinical
2. Rapid influenza test only in severe cases:
   - Variable sensitivity (10%–70%)
3. Other tests exist (polymerase chain reaction [PCR], antigen detection, viral culture) but are used only when absolutely critical to make influenza Dx (as in health care worker, etc.).

Tx/Mgmt:
1. Tylenol/nonsteroidal anti-inflammatory drugs (NSAIDs) (avoid NSAIDs in children <6 months) for symptoms
2. Neuraminidase inhibitors (oseltamivir, zanamivir):
   - Should be given to patients presenting with fever AND lower respiratory tract infections within 48 hours of symptom onset while awaiting testing
3. M2 inhibitors (amantadine, rimantadine):
   - Influenza resistance to these is high; they are rarely used in clinical practice.

Hand, Foot, and Mouth Disease

Buzz Words: Vesicular rash of palms and soles + children + decreased intake by mouth (PO)

Clinical Presentation: Presents with vesicular lesions on the palms and soles. Patient will complain of mouth or throat pain due to vesicular lesions in back of mouth.

PPx: N/A

MoD: Coxsackie virus

Dx: Clinical

Tx/Mgmt: Supportive. Important to ensure that child is not dehydrated due to pain with oral intake.

Bacterial Sinusitis

Buzz Words: Rhinorrhea for 10–14 days + cough + headache

Clinical Presentation: Viral upper respiratory infection (URI) is the most important risk factor for development of acute bacterial sinusitis. The persistence and severity of symptoms distinguishes bacterial sinusitis from viral URI. Commonly presents as an unresolving URI with persistent mucopurulent rhinorrhea, nasal stuffiness, and cough. May develop headache, fever, sore throat, and halitosis. Another common presentation is biphasic illness, where the child appears to be recovering from URI but then becomes acutely worse on day 6 or 7.

PPx: N/A

MoD: Often a complication of URI or allergic rhinitis. Suppurative infection of the paranasal sinuses. Common causes are *Streptococcus pneumoniae,* nontypeable

Haemophilus influenzae, Moraxella, and *Staphylococcus aureus.*

Dx: Clinical. Definitive Dx can be made with sinus aspirate, but this is not routinely performed. Computed tomography (CT) is unable to differentiate acute from chronic or allergic pathologies.

Tx/Mgmt: Amoxicillin/clavulanate 10–14 days

Epiglottitis

Buzz Words: Child + no *Haemophilus influenzae* B (HiB) vaccination (or foreign immigrant) + difficulty swallowing, hoarse voice + stridor

Clinical Presentation: Typically occurs in children with fever + difficulty swallowing. Is caused by HiB or other bacterial infections of the epiglottis. Stridor is upper airway obstruction and is a **surgical emergency.** Since advent of HiB vaccination, now mostly occurs in older children and adults.

PPx: Vaccinate against HiB; can also use rifampin for people who may have been exposed.

MoD: Traditionally caused by HiB, but if immunized, suspect *S. pneumoniae, Streptococcus pyogenes, S. aureus.* Also linked to cocaine use.

Dx:

1. Laryngoscopy to rule out croup, peritonsillar abscess, retropharyngeal abscess.
2. X-ray shows "thumbprint sign."
3. CT shows "Halloween sign" (Fig. 8.2).

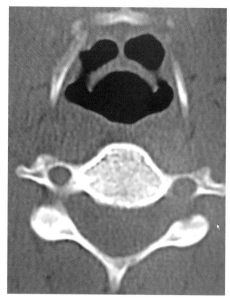

FIG. 8.2 "Halloween sign" on CT (Wikipedia).

Tx/Mgmt:
1. Endotracheal intubation
2. Ceftriaxone + vancomycin
3. Corticosteroids

Croup (Laryngotracheobronchitis)

Buzz Words: Barking cough + stridor + "steeple sign" on anteroposterior (AP) neck x-ray (XR)

Clinical Presentation: Most common in children 6 months to 3 years old. Peaks in fall and early winter. Onset is gradual and often begins with rhinorrhea, congestion, and coryza. Proceeds to fever, barking cough, and inspiratory stridor within next 12–48 hours. Patient will have increased difficulty breathing when lying down.

PPx: N/A

MoD: Most commonly caused by parainfluenza virus types 1, 2, and 3. Respiratory syncytial virus (RSV) second most common cause.

Dx:
1. Clinical, may be assisted by finding of narrowed airway on AP neck radiograph.

Tx/Mgmt: Dexamethasone to decrease inflammation; racemic epinephrine to help with respiratory distress (short-term)

Acute Laryngitis

Buzz Words: Hoarseness with upper respiratory infection (URI) symptoms

Clinical Presentation: Commonly seen in children from 5 years through adolescence. Presents with hoarseness, sore throat, rhinorrhea, cough.

PPx: N/A

MoD: Acute infection causing inflammation of the mucosa of the larynx. Most commonly due to viral respiratory tract infections.

Dx: Clinical

Tx/Mgmt: Usually self-limited process; supportive care only

Bacterial Tracheitis

Buzz Words: Stridor + respiratory distress after viral URI/croup

Clinical Presentation: Most commonly occurs following a viral URI or in a child with croup. Most often seen in children younger than 6 years old. Presents with stridor, cough, respiratory distress, high fever, and rapid deterioration. Radiographic features include ragged, irregular tracheal border.

PPx: N/A

MoD: Rare but serious superinfection of the trachea. Most commonly caused by *S. aureus.*

Dx:

1. Endoscopy needed for definitive Dx

Tx/Mgmt:

1. In cases of severe obstruction or pending respiratory failure, airway management precedes diagnostic testing.
2. Treatment with antimicrobials.

Streptococcal Pharyngitis

Buzz Words: Pharyngeal exudates + fever + dysphagia

Clinical Presentation: Presents with pain on swallowing, pharyngeal exudates, cervical adenopathy, tonsillar petechiae, fever. Uncommon to have cough or hoarseness. Uncommon in children younger than 3 years of age.

PPx: N/A

MoD: Inflammation of the pharynx and adjacent structures. Most commonly caused by group A beta hemolytic strep.

Dx:

1. Rapid strep test.
2. Throat culture is the gold standard for diagnosis.

Tx/Mgmt:

1. Oral/IM penicillin or amoxicillin. Treatment is necessary to prevent acute rheumatic fever.

Viral Pharyngitis

Clinical Presentation: More gradual in onset than bacterial pharyngitis. Symptoms more often include rhinorrhea, cough, and diarrhea.

Peritonsillar Abscess

Buzz Words: Muffled voice + severe sore throat + drooling + trismus + deviation of the uvula

Clinical: Most frequent in adolescents and young adults. Presents with severe sore throat, drooling, trismus, "hot potato"/muffled voice. Commonly presents with high fever.

PPx: Prompt treatment of strep pharyngeal infections

MoD: Collection of pus located between the palatine tonsil and the pharyngeal muscles. Often polymicrobial, predominantly caused by group A streptococcal infection, *Staphylococcus*, and respiratory anaerobes.

Dx:

1. Clinical. May see deviation of the uvula to the opposite side of abscess.

Tx/Mgmt:

1. Drainage of abscess and antimicrobial therapy

QUICK TIPS

The term *tonsillitis* may be used in cases when involvement of the tonsils is prominent.

Allergic Rhinitis

Buzz Words: Nasal itching watery eyes + sneezing

Clinical Presentation: More common in children with personal or family history of eczema or asthma. Presents with nasal itching, itchy/watery eyes, watery rhinorrhea, nasal congestion, and sneezing. On exam nasal turbinates are pale and edematous. May see allergic shiners—blue/gray discoloration under the eyes and a transverse nasal crease ("allergic salute"). Symptoms are usually intermittent in response to specific exposures such as cats, pollen, or dust.

PPx: Avoidance of allergens

MoD: Histamine release by mast cell degranulation in response to allergens

Dx:
1. Immunoglobulin (Ig)E testing

Tx/Mgmt: Symptomatic treatment with:
1. Antihistamines
2. Intranasal steroids
3. Immunotherapy

Infectious, Immunologic, and Inflammatory Disorders of the Lower Airways

Pneumonia

Clinical Presentation: Has a wide variety of causes including bacterial, viral, and fungal. It can be classified into different categories based on patient status in regard to recent hospital stays or interactions with the healthcare system. Importantly in children, the most common pathogens vary by age group.

Presents as fever, cough, tachypnea and exam with focal decreased breath sounds or crackles. Patient may have dyspnea and hypoxemia. In neonates and infants, may present with difficulty feeding or emesis.

PPx: Influenza vaccine recommended for all children over 6 months. Vaccination against *H. influenzae* and *S. pneumoniae* also recommended.

Dx:
1. Clinical diagnosis!
2. Chest x-ray (CXR) can be used to provide supportive information.

Tx/Mgmt:
1. Community-acquired pneumonia treated with amoxicillin.
2. More severe cases treated with other combinations of antibiotics.

Hospital-Acquired Pneumonia
Pneumonia developing more than 48 hours after admission or after hospitalization in the last 90 days. These patients have a higher incidence of gram negative organisms such as *Pseudomonas* and *Escherichia coli*. Cannot treat these patients with macrolides. Require anti-pseudomonal coverage.

Ventilator-Associated Pneumonia
Pneumonia developing in a patient on a ventilator. Can be difficult to diagnose as these patients often have many concurrent illnesses. Consider in patients with fever, new infiltrate, purulent secretions from ET tube. Respiratory culture and gram stain from an endotracheal tube (ETT) to help diagnose though may be difficult to differentiate colonization from causative agent.

Tx/Mgmt: Coverage with antipseudomonal agent + agent for methicillin-resistant *Staphylococcus aureus* (MRSA)

Community-Acquired Pneumonia (CAP)
Occurring before hospitalization or within 48 hours of hospitalization. *Streptococcous pneumoniae* is the most common cause of CAP.

Within CAP fall two large classifications: typical and atypical.

Typical Community-Acquired Pneumonia
Clinical Presentation: Acute onset of fever and chills. Productive cough. Patient will often complain of pleuritic chest pain, tiredness, and dyspnea. Tachycardia, tachypnea, decreased breath sounds are common. May have increased tactile fremitus and dullness to percussion.

MoD: Most common agents include *Streptococcus pneumoniae*, followed by *H. influenzae*, aerobic gram-negative rods (*Klebsiella*) and *S. aureus*. *S. pneumoniae* is the most common cause of bacterial pneumonia in children of all ages.

Dx:
1. Clinical.
2. CXR with typical pneumonias will have lobar consolidation.

Tx/Mgmt:
1. Antimicrobial therapy—amoxicillin/ampicillin first-line for uncomplicated CAP

Atypical Community-Acquired Pneumonia
Atypical refers to organisms not visible on Gram stain and not culturable on standard blood agar.

Clinical Presentation: Insidious onset of headache, sore throat, fatigue, myalgias, dry cough, and fever. Patient will have normal vital signs but may have a fever.

MoD: In children older than 5 years, *Mycoplasma pneumoniae* is the most common cause of atypical pneumonia, followed by *Chlamydia pneumoniae*. Others less commonly seen but frequently tested are *Coxiella burnetti and Legionella*.

Dx:

1. CXR will show diffuse reticulonodular infiltrates with absent or minimal consolidation.

Tx/Mgmt:

1. Azithromycin or doxycycline. Can usually be treated on an outpatient basis.

Fungal Infections

Allergic Bronchopulmonary Aspergillosis

Buzz Words: Asthma or CF + new or worsening cough + brown mucous plugs

Clinical Presentation: Found most commonly in patients with asthma or CF. Characterized by recurrent pulmonary infiltrates and bronchiectasis. Presents with cough, dyspnea, increased sputum production, expectoration of brown-black mucous plug, wheezing.

PPx: N/A

MoD: Hypersensitivity of the lungs to fungal antigens that colonize the bronchial tree

Dx:

1. Peripheral blood eosinophilia
2. Skin test reactivity to *Aspergillus* antigen
3. Elevated IgE
4. Antibodies against *Aspergillus*

Tx/Mgmt:

1. Oral steroids
2. Itraconazole for recurrent episodes

Pneumocystis jirovecii Pneumonia (PJP)

Buzz Words: HIV + low CD4 count + dry cough

Clinical Presentation: Occurs almost exclusively in AIDS patient with a CD4 count less than 200. Presents with dyspnea on exertion, dry cough, and fever. In Pediatrics, can also be seen in patients with cancers (especially liquid cancers), post–stem cell transplant, and in patients with inherited immunodeficiencies.

PPx: Trimethoprim-sulfamethoxazole (TMP-SMX) in any patient with CD4 count under 200, active treatment for cancers

MoD: Caused by *Pneumocystis jirovecii*
Dx:
1. CXR showing bilateral interstitial infiltrate.
2. Elevated LDH levels.
3. Most accurate test is bronchoalveolar lavage.
Tx/Mgmt:
1. TMP-SMX.
2. Add steroids if P_{O_2} is less than 70 or A-a gradient is greater than 35.

Acute Bronchiolitis

Buzz Words: Wheezing in infant younger than 2 years old with fever + respiratory distress

Clinical Presentation: Most commonly seen in infants and young children. Leading cause of hospitalization among infants, occurring almost exclusively during the first 2 years of life. Presents as progressive respiratory illness beginning with cough and rhinorrhea. Progresses over 3–7 days to noisy, raspy breathing and audible wheezing with low-grade fever. Prolonged expiratory phase, nasal flaring, intercostal retractions, and air trapping are common. In more severe cases, grunting and cyanosis can be present.

PPx: Monthly injection of palivizumab, a monoclonal antibody specific to respiratory syncytial virus (RSV), can be used for high-risk infants such as those with chronic lung disease, very low birth weight, and those with hemodynamically significant congenital heart disease.

MoD: Increased mucous production and occasional bronchospasm. Most commonly caused by a viral lower respiratory tract infection. The primary cause is RSV.

Dx:
1. Clinical.
2. Can use antigen tests of nasopharyngeal secretions or PCR to identify specific virus.

Tx/Mgmt:
1. Treatment is supportive.

Bordetella pertussis: "Whooping Cough"

Buzz Words: Inspiratory whoop + post-tussive emesis

Clinical Presentation: Classically seen in children 1–10 years old.

Catarrhal stage: Severe congestion and rhinorrhea for 1–2 weeks

Paroxysmal stage: Severe coughing episodes with extreme gasp for air = inspiratory whoop. Can have posttussive emesis. Lasts 2–4 weeks

Convalescent stage: Decrease of frequency of coughing—
  1–2 weeks
PPx: DTap vaccine
MoD: Caused by infection with *B. pertussis*
Dx:
1. PCR of nasal secretions.
2. Lymphocytosis is commonly present but not diagnostic.
Tx/Mgmt:
1. Azithromycin or erythromycin in the catarrhal stage
   may decrease severity and length of illness.
2. Azithromycin in paroxysmal stage to lessen duration of
   shedding.
3. Give macrolides to all close contacts.

Pulmonary Tuberculosis

Buzz Words: Chronic cough, prolonged fever, weight loss,
  night sweats, immigrant, incarceration
Clinical Presentation: Patient with risk factors presenting with
  fever, chronic cough, sputum, weight loss, hemoptysis,
  and night sweats. More commonly seen in foreign-born
  children, having a foreign-born parent, or having lived
  outside the US for more than 2 months. Commonly seen
  in patients with H1.
PPx: N/A
MoD: Infection with *Mycobacterium tuberculosis*
Dx:
1. Often clinical.
2. PPD or IGRA used for screening test in groups at risk.
3. If suspicious for acute TB, sputum stain + culture for
   acid-fast bacilli must be done 3 times to fully exclude TB.
Tx/Mgmt:
1. Rifampin, isoniazid, pyrazinamide, and ethambutol.
   For positive PPD without signs of active disease, treat
   with isoniazid for 9 months.

MNEMONIC
Mnemonic for the TB drugs: RIPE

Benign Neoplasms

FOR THE WARDS
Remember to supplement isoniazid with pyridoxine, as isoniazid
can cause vitamin B6 deficiency.

Vocal Cord Nodules/Polyps

Buzz Words: Chronic hoarseness
Clinical Presentation: Vocal nodules are the most common
  cause of chronic hoarseness in school-aged children.
  More common in boys. Nodules tend to appear bilaterally. Polyps tend to appear unilaterally, usually at junction of anterior third and posterior two-thirds of the vocal
  folds. Trauma, chronic irritation, reflux, and smoking may
  contribute to their formation.
PPx: N/A

MoD: Repeated trauma and abuse of the vocal cords from screaming and shouting or prolonged intubation cause an inflammatory reaction with fibrotic healing.

Dx: Stroboscopy

Tx/Mgmt:

1. Surgical treatment depending on the severity of voice complaint.
2. Voice therapy can be attempted.

Nasal Polyps

Buzz Words: Grape-like mass, rhinorrhea, swelling of nasal mucosa

Clinical Presentation: Rarely occur in children (prevalence 0.1%). More common in patients with aspirin and NSAID intolerance, asthma, cystic fibrosis (CF), allergic rhinitis. Presents with rhinorrhea, sneezing, postnasal drip. On exam, bilateral edematous swelling of nasal mucosa is seen.

PPx: N/A

MoD: Unknown

Dx:

1. Grape-like structure found on physical exam, usually with rhinoscopy

Tx/Mgmt:

1. Intranasal steroids for at least 3 months
2. If no improvement, obtain CT scan
3. Consider endoscopic sinus surgery

Juvenile Papillomatosis

Buzz Words: Hoarseness + biphasic stridor + infancy

Clinical Presentation: Rare condition of benign tumors caused by HPV 6 and 11 acquired at birth from maternal genital warts. Manifestations begin in infancy with biphasic stridor and hoarse cry/voice. Lesions most commonly in larynx.

PPx: Maternal treatment or C section to avoid exposure

MoD: HPV 6 and 11

Dx: Clinical

Definitive Dx with endoscopy

Tx/Mgmt:

1. Limited, rarely curative, include laser therapy and interferon

Obstructive Airway Disease

Asthma

Buzz Words: Reversible + cough + wheezing + prolonged expiratory phase + chest pain/tightness + tachypnea + dyspnea

Clinical Presentation: Most common chronic disease of childhood. Exacerbated by viral infections, exposure to allergens and irritants, exercise, changes in weather. Nighttime symptoms are common. Symptoms reversible with bronchodilator therapy differentiates from chronic obstructive pulmonary disease (COPD). Acute exacerbation presents with wheezing, prolonged expiratory phase, chest tightness, tachypnea, and dyspnea. Associated with eczema and seasonal allergies (allergic triad).

Classifications of Asthma

Intermittent
Symptoms ≤2 days/week
Nighttime awakenings ≤2× per month
Short-acting beta agonist (SABA) use ≤2 days/week
No interference with normal activity
Normal FEV_1 between exacerbations, FEV_1 >80% predicted, FEV_1/FVC normal
Step 1 treatment: albuterol (SABA) as needed

Mild Persistent
Symptoms ≥2 days/week but not daily
Nighttime awakenings 3–4× per month
SABA use more than 2 days/week, but not daily. Not more than once per day
Minor limitation with activity
Step 2 treatment: SABA + low-dose inhaled glucocorticoid

Moderate Persistent
Symptoms daily
Nighttime awakenings >1× per week but not nightly
SABA use daily
Some limitation with activity
Step 3: SABA + medium-dose inhaled corticosteroid

Severe
Symptoms throughout the day
Nighttime awakenings: nightly
SABA use several times per day
Extreme limitation of activity
Step 4: SABA + medium-dose inhaled glucocorticoid + LABA
Step 5: SABA + high-dose inhaled glucocorticoid + LABA or montelukast (leukotriene antagonist)
In severe cases, can move up to step 6 and add oral systemic glucocorticoids

PPx: Avoid exposure to triggers, careful adherence to medications

MoD: Inflammatory cells, chemical mediators, and chemotactic factors mediate underlying inflammatory response. Inflammation contributes to airway hyperresponsiveness. Results in edema, increased production of mucus, and influx of inflammatory cells. Chronic inflammation leads to airway remodeling.

Dx:

1. Clinical diagnosis based on symptoms!!
2. Pulmonary function tests (PFTs) can assist with diagnosis but may be normal between exacerbations and are difficult to obtain in young children.

    PFTs: Decreased FEV_1/FVC, increase in FEV_1 >12% with use of albuterol, decrease in FEV_1 >20% with methacholine challenge, increased diffusion capacity for the lung for carbon monoxide (DLCO).

    Acute exacerbation: Peak expiratory flow can be used; it is an approximation of FVC.
3. CXR can be obtained to exclude pneumonia, congestive heart failure (CHF).

    Management of Asthma: To determine treatment, must first determine classification of asthma. Use stepwise method of treatment as described under "Clinical Presentation." Patient can be moved up or down based on severity and control of symptoms.

    Treatment of Acute Exacerbation:

    Best initial therapy = albuterol via inhaler or nebulizer, systemic steroids, oxygen if there is hypoxemia:

    1. Ipratropium can be given and is often given in combination with albuterol; it has been shown to decrease hospitalization rate for pediatric patients presenting to emergency department (ED) with asthma exacerbation. Ipratropium does not work as quickly as albuterol.
    2. Magnesium can be used to help relieve bronchospasm and may be useful in refractory status asthmaticus.
    3. If patient is not responding to treatment and has an increasing P_{CO_2} on ABG, need to consider noninvasive ventilation or intubation.

Traumatic and Mechanical Disorders

Upper Airways
Epistaxis
Buzz Words: Nosebleed + fall/winter season

Clinical Presentation: A fancy word for a nosebleed. Most common in children from 2 to 10 years old. Usually benign and self-limited. Commonly caused by digital trauma (nose picking) or dry nasal mucosa. Can be seen in the setting of a rhinitis, foreign-body insertion, vascular malformation (Osler–Weber–Rendu), and tumors. Typically the bleeding is from the anterior vessels.

PPx: Humidified air, ointment such as Vaseline to nares, keep fingernails trimmed to decrease trauma.

MoD: Usually not associated with underlying disorder. Most commonly due to trauma or dry mucosa. About 90% originates from the anterior nasal vessels, specifically Kiesselbach plexus. Posterior bleeding occurs in about 10% of cases.

Dx:
1. Clinical

Tx/Mgmt:
1. Assess airway. Advise patient to lean forward. Direct pressure by pinching nostrils for 10–15 minutes.
2. Can conservatively manage with topical vasoconstrictors or cautery. If not resolving, nasal packing can be used. Finally, surgical intervention is an option if unable to control bleeding.

> **QUICK TIPS**
> Prolonged epistaxis can be a sign of underlying hematologic disorder in children.

Laryngeal/Pharyngeal Obstruction

Airway can become narrowed or blocked for many reasons including anaphylaxis, chemical burns, epiglottis, smoke inhalation, foreign bodies, infections, peritonsillar abscess, retropharyngeal abscess, cancer, tracheomalacia, vocal cord prolapse. These can all present in similar fashion with cough, wheezing/stridor. These are explored in further detail below and their unique features are discussed.

Tracheoesophageal Fistula

Buzz Words: Excessive salivation + inability to feed/vomiting with first feeding + unable to pass nasogastric (NG) tube, CXR—coiling of the NG tube, gastric bubble and esophageal bubble

Clinical Presentation: Connection between the trachea and esophagus, most commonly in the setting of esophageal atresia. Presents with polyhydramnios in utero, increased oral secretions, inability to feed, gagging, chronic cough, recurrent aspiration pneumonia, respiratory distress. Recurrent aspiration pneumonia is due to food and secretions traveling into the lungs via the tracheoesophageal fistula (TEF).

PPx: N/A

MoD: Esophagus and trachea develop in close proximity; defects in mesenchyme separating the structures result in TEF. Most common type is blind proximal esophagus with distal TEF. Associated with other anomalies of VACTERL syndrome; single-artery umbilical cord is often present.

Dx:

1. CXR showing an NG tube coiled in the esophagus.
2. Suggested by air in the GI tract, and can be confirmed by bronchoscopy. May also see a gastric bubble and esophageal bubble on CXR.

Tx/Mgmt:

1. Surgical repair

Tracheal Stenosis

Buzz Words: Biphasic stridor following acute injury + abnormal tracheal rings on imaging

Clinical Presentation: Narrowing of the trachea that can be acquired or congenital. More commonly found as subglottic stenosis, which specifically refers to narrowing immediately below the vocal cords. Symptoms include biphasic stridor, recurrent pneumonia, wheezing, cyanosis, and chest congestion. May occur shortly after birth or develop after acute injury or prolonged intubation.

PPx: N/A

MoD: Acquired stenosis occurs due to repeated irritation or injury, as in repeated or long-term intubation. Causes include ongoing irritation from an ETT and injury from external factors such as smoke inhalation. Congenital form is a rare condition, in which cartilaginous structures are abnormal causing a narrowing.

Dx: X-ray/CT/MRI all can provide information about the extent of airway narrowing. Bronchoscopy can differentiate tracheal stenosis from other lesions causing stridor and respiratory distress.

Tx/Mgmt:

1. Milder forms—observation, balloon dilation
2. More severe—surgical treatment

Tracheomalacia

Buzz Words: Floppy trachea + wheezing/stridor + normal voice + cough

Clinical Presentation: Floppy trachea presents with expiratory monophonic wheezing and a prolonged expiratory phase. Exacerbated by respiratory infections. Infants with severe tracheomalacia can have complete collapse during agitation, resulting in cyanotic episodes.

PPx: N/A

MoD: Abnormal cartilaginous rings that do not extend as far around the trachea, are absent, or are damaged and cause excessive collapse of the trachea. Most pronounced during expiration.

Dx:

1. Bronchoscopy

Tx/Mgmt:

1. Mild to moderate can be observed, as it usually improves with airway growth.
2. For older children, management is aimed at preventing exacerbation by infection.
3. Ipratropium bromide inhaler can help increase smooth muscle tone and may be used in a scheduled fashion or as needed when child is sick.
4. Infants with severe disease may require tracheostomy tubes.

Foreign-Body Aspiration

Buzz Words: Acute-onset stridor + playing with small objects or unsupervised

Clinical Presentation: Commonly given is a scenario where a toddler was playing with small objects and develops acute respiratory distress and stridor or wheezing. More common in children younger than 4 years of age. Objects can lodge in upper or lower respiratory tract. In some cases small object can be present for a long time and cause persistent cough, recurrent wheezing unresponsive to bronchodilator therapy, or unilateral pneumonia.

PPx: Careful supervision, educating parents on not giving children items such as nuts before molars have erupted

MoD: Due to the anatomy of the right mainstem bronchus, objects tend to lodge on that side. Possible for smaller objects to lodge more proximally in larynx, completely occluding the airway.

Dx:

1. Expiratory and lateral decubitus films to examine for air trapping. May see object on imaging if radiopaque, such as a coin. Button battery in airway or esophagus requires emergent removal (seen on x-ray to be radiopaque with a radiolucent ring near edge).

Tx/Mgmt:

1. Rigid bronchoscopy. In cases of acute airway occlusion and choking, Heimlich maneuver or back slaps for infant should be performed.

Airway should be inspected for visible foreign body, but do not perform finger sweep so as to not lodge object further back.

Lower Airways and Pleura

Atelectasis

Buzz Words: Postoperative day 1 + fever + patchy areas on CXR

Clinical Presentation: Common cause of day 1 postoperative fever. Can present with mild cough, low oxygen saturation, and fast, shallow breathing. Expect to see in clinical context of prior abdominal surgery or foreign-body aspiration.

MoD: Collapse or closure of an area of the lung due to reduced or absent gas exchange. It is usually seen in a person taking restricted breaths due to pain, such as following abdominal surgery. However, this can also be seen in cases of foreign-body aspiration.

Dx:
1. CXR—seen as volume loss caused by opacification (ribs pulled together)

Tx/Mgmt:
1. Directed at underlying cause, airway recruitment with incentive spirometry or positive end-expiratory pressure (PEEP) devices

Diaphragmatic Rupture

Buzz Words: Blunt trauma + bowel sounds in chest + NG tube in the chest cavity

Clinical Presentation: Diaphragmatic rupture is an uncommon injury occurring after significant blunt trauma, usually a motor vehicle collision (MVC). Presents with chest pain radiating to the shoulder, shortness of breath, and abdominal pain. Auscultation of bowel sounds in the chest and diminished breath sounds are common physical exam findings.

MoD: Blunt trauma causing rupture of the diaphragm. More common on the left side because of the protective effect of the liver on the right.

Dx:
1. CT most commonly. May be shown via CXR with NG tube coiled in the chest cavity.

Tx/Mgmt:
1. Stabilization of the patient.
2. NG tube placement may be useful to decompress the stomach, allowing for better lung expansion.
3. Surgical management is the definitive treatment.

Drowning and Near Drowning

Buzz Words: Drowning—death by suffocation from submersion in liquid

Near drowning—survival after a submersion event

Clinical Presentation: Incidence of drowning is highest in two groups, teenagers and toddlers. Among teenagers, male victims are more common and alcohol is frequently involved. Toddlers are at increased risk due to their inquisitive nature and inability to get themselves out of water. Following near-drowning, the presentation can range from asymptomatic to cardiac arrest, depending on the time of submersion and the temperature of the water.

PPx: Adequate supervision, efforts to safeguard access to water, use of flotation devices, public awareness

MoD: Hypoxemia as a result of laryngospasm and aspiration. Respiratory distress may also develop secondary to pulmonary endothelial injury, increased capillary permeability, and destruction of surfactant.

Dx:
1. Often witnessed or victim found submerged

Tx/Mgmt:
1. ABCs!
2. Aim is to correct hypoxia, acidosis, and hypotension.

Penetrating Chest Wounds/Chest Trauma

Tension Pneumothorax

Buzz Words: Tracheal deviation away from side of lesion, mediastinal shift, unilateral absence of breath sounds, increased percussion

Clinical Presentation: Patient presenting with shortness of breath and hemodynamic instability after a penetrating injury to the chest. On exam, tracheal deviation and unilateral absence of breath sounds are classic findings.

PPx: N/A

MoD: Progressive buildup of air in the pleural space. The positive pressure pushes the mediastinum to the opposite side and obstructs venous return to the heart.

Dx:
1. Clinical. Can be seen on CXR, but patient needs emergent treatment and cannot afford time for x-ray.

Tx/Mgmt:
1. Needle decompression/chest tube

Pericardial Tamponade

Buzz Words: Beck triad—distended neck veins + muffled heart sounds + hypotension

QUICK TIPS

Consider tracheobronchial injury if chest tube fails to reexpand the lung.

QUICK TIPS

Chest wall is more elastic and pliable in children, making rib fractures rare. Be suspicious for abuse, especially with posterior rib fractures.

Clinical Presentation: Patient presents with signs of shock and hemodynamic instability. Will have distended neck veins and muffled heart sounds. Breath sounds will be intact and no tracheal deviation will be present, differentiating this from tension pneumothorax.

PPx: N/A

MoD: Pericardial sac fills with blood. The pressure prevents the heart from contracting normally and essentially causes an obstructive shock.

Dx:

1. Clinical

Tx/Mgmt:

1. Pericardiocentesis

Obstructive Sleep Apnea

Buzz Words: Habitual snoring + daytime sleepiness + poor school performance + behavior problems

Clinical Presentation: Affects 2%–3% of children, most commonly 2–8 years old. Presents as episodes of respiratory pauses, gasping, and restless sleep. Commonly children may have difficulty awakening, daytime sleepiness, poor school performance, behavioral problems, and poor growth. Nighttime hypoxia and hypercarbia can lead to morning headaches and, in chronic cases, pulmonary hypertension.

MoD: Airway obstruction due to excessive tissue, loss of pharyngeal tone, or abnormal anatomy. Most commonly due to adenotonsillar hypertrophy. Other risk factors include obesity, craniofacial malformations (Pierre Robin, trisomy 21), and neuromuscular diseases.

Dx:

1. Polysomnography

Tx/Mgmt:

1. Tonsillectomy and adenoidectomy (T&A)
2. Continuous positive airway pressure (CPAP)

Congenital Disorders

Cystic Fibrosis

Buzz Words: Bronchiectasis + pneumonia with staph/pseudo + hypoxia = barrel chest + clubbing + **chronic rhinosinusitis +b/l nasal polyps** leading to nasal obstruction/chronic rhinosinusitus + foul-smelling stool (failure to absorb vitamins A, D, E, K [ADEK]) + failure to thrive (due to low fat absorption) → CF:

- Clubbing = bulbous enlargement of the tips of the digits
- Nasal polyps in 40% of CF

Cystic fibrosis + **Infertility!!** (95% of males, 20% females) + osteopenia/kyphoscoliosis/digital clubbing + meconium ileus/distal obstruction syndrome + **exocrine pancreatic insufficiency** + **diabetes** + recurrent pulm pathology → complications of CF

Clinical Presentation: Cystic fibrosis is a congenital multiorgan disorder that primarily affects the lung and pancreas. The chloride channels in CF are defective, meaning that fluid is not sent toward the respiratory or gastrointestinal lumen, and secretions that were meant to be cleared are stuck, leading to infection and digestive abnormality. CF is one of the most high-yield diseases on the shelf because it can present in so many different ways in many different age groups (mostly peds, but now patients are living into adulthood). Most notably, patients with CF frequently get pneumonia infected by organisms associated with immunocompromised patients, such as *Pneumocystis jirovecii*. Also, CF patients may have difficulty with digestion owing to a lack of exocrine secretions from the pancreas. Importantly, the treatment of patients with CF is multifaceted and requires a lot of work on the part of the patient. Chest PT, for instance, requires the patient's care provider to tap methodically on the patient's chest to loosen up secretions every single day. Last, for the purposes of the shelf, remember that CF is associated with infertility due to no semen production (male) or obstruction of semen entrance (female).

PPx: N/A (although avoid sick contacts if you have disease)

MoD: Mutation of the CFTR protein → defective chloride ion channels → increased loss of sodium in sweat

For mechanism of infertility → **congenital bilateral absence of vas deferens** in males, inspissated mucus in the fetal genital tract obstructs developing vas deferens:

- Even if the testes are descended and spermatogenesis is normal → **sperm cannot be ejaculated,** resulting in no semen production (obstructive azoospermia); in females, viscous cervical mucus can obstruct sperm entry.

Dx:

1. CXR.
2. Spirometry.
3. **Quantitative pilocarpine iontophoresis** for measurement of sweat chloride concentration (pilocarpine = cholinergic drug that induces sweating).

4. A chloride level >60 mmol/L on 2 occasions confirms diagnosis, DNA test to identify two CF mutations.
5. F/u with DNA analysis.
6. Nasal potential difference (defective nasal epithelial ion transport) → perform if sweat testing and DNA analysis equivocal.
7. Sputum culture if pneumonia.

Tx/Mgmt:
1. Supportive (steroids for rhinosinusitis or surgery for nasal polyps)
2. Antibiotics for infections (i.e., gentamicin)
3. Lung physiotherapy

Bronchogenic Cysts

Buzz Words: Wheezing + neck mass + chronic pneumonia

Clinical Presentation: May be asymptomatic. Can have cough, fever, sputum production, hemoptysis, chest pain, dyspnea. More common in males. Palpable neck mass often found in infants.

MoD: Congenital anomaly of the embryonic foregut resulting in cyst formation, typically in the middle mediastinum or lung—leads to tracheobronchial compression and infection.

Dx:
1. Round smooth bordered density on imaging, palpable neck mass.
2. Confirm with histopathology from fine needle aspiration (FNA) or biopsy.

Tx/Mgmt:
1. Surgical excision

Congenital Cysts

Thyroglossal duct cysts, branchial cleft cysts

There are many different types of congenital cysts that can be found in the neck and lead to trouble with the respiratory system. We will cover only the most likely to appear on your exam.

Thyroglossal Duct Cyst

Buzz Words: Mass moves upward with swallowing or protrusion of tongue

Clinical Presentation: Most common **midline** congenital neck anomaly. Painless, soft, mobile midline mass near hyoid bone. If symptomatic, may present with pain, dyspnea, dysphagia, or discharge. Most commonly diagnosed in children younger than 5 years old.

MoD: Failure of thyroglossal duct to involute completely during development

Dx:
1. Imaging
2. FNA

Tx/Mgmt:
1. If infected, requires antibiotics followed by incision and drainage (I&D).
2. Definitive treatment is surgical resection.

Branchial Cleft Cyst

Buzz Words: Neck mass along anterior border of sternocleidomastoid muscle (SCM)

Clinical Presentation: (1) Commonly found at **mandibular angle**, can present along anterior border of SCM. (2) Usually found in older children and young adults. (3) Symptoms are nonspecific and include swelling, inflammation, recurrent infection.

MoD: Aberrant development, incomplete obliteration, or incomplete fusion of the branchial cleft or pouch during fetal development

Dx:
1. Imaging
2. FNA

Tx/Mgmt:
1. Resection

Congenital Diaphragmatic Hernia

Buzz Words: Scaphoid abdomen, bowel sounds in chest, may see heart shifted to right, respiratory distress

Clinical Presentation: (1) Identified prenatally. (2) Neonates present with severe respiratory distress. (3) If allowed to persist, symptoms include recurrent infection, recurrent vomiting, cough, wheezing/stridor, irritability, feeding difficulty, failure to thrive, apneic spells. (4) On exam, signs of increasing work of breathing, barrel-shaped chest, heart sounds shifted to the right. (5) Associated with CHARGE syndrome, Beckwith–Wiedemann syndrome, Cornelia de Lange and trisomy 13, 18, 21.

MoD: Incomplete formation of the diaphragm. Allows herniation of abdominal contents into the thoracic cavity. Does not allow lungs to grow normally, causing pulmonary hypoplasia.

Dx:
1. Prenatal ultrasound. Classically, NG tube in the thoracic cavity on CXR.

Tx/Mgmt:
1. Respiratory support, surgical repair

Pulmonary Sequestration

Clinical Presentation: Rare. Respiratory distress, pneumonia, feeding difficulties, hemorrhage, and heart failure. Extralobar more likely to be diagnosed prenatally or in infancy. Intralobar typically present later in childhood or adulthood.

MoD: Cystic mass of nonfunctioning pulmonary tissue not communicating with the tracheobronchial tree:
1. Intralobar sequestration: incorporated into normal surrounding lung tissue
2. Extralobar sequestration: completely discrete from normal lung and enveloped by separate parenchyma

Dx:
1. Doppler US for prenatal. CXR, may require additional imaging to confirm.

Tx/Mgmt:
1. Ventilatory support. More severe cases may require surgery.

Immotile Cilia Syndrome = Primary Ciliary Dyskinesia = Kartagener Syndrome

Buzz Words: Recurrent otitis media, chronic sinusitis, and bronchiectasis

Clinical Presentation: Presents with recurrent otitis media, chronic sinusitis, and bronchiectasis, infertility in males. Due to cilia not beating upward → recurrent infection → bronchiectasis.

MoD: Inherited disorder in which abnormal ciliary structure results in absent or disordered movement of cilia. Most common defect is in the dynein arms.

Dx:
1. Electron microscopy of respiratory cilia
2. Can screen with nasal nitric oxide, low levels consistent with PCD

Tx/Mgmt:
1. Preventing infections and improving clearance of respiratory secretions
2. CT to monitor progression of bronchiectasis

TABLE 8.1 Common Respiratory Viruses

Organism	Syndrome/Associations
Adenovirus	Pharyngitis, conjunctivitis, URI, pneumonia
Coronavirus	URI, more common in winter and in adults
Coxsackie virus	Hand, foot, mouth disease, herpangina
Influenza virus	"Flu," pneumonia
Parainfluenza virus	Croup
Rhinovirus	"The common cold" (URI)
Respiratory syncytial virus	Bronchiolitis

URI, Upper respiratory infection.

TABLE 8.2

Organism	Associated Syndrome	Dx/Treatment
HSV-1	Herpetic gingivostomatitis—common between 6 months and 5 years of age. Prodromal symptoms followed by oral vesicles with generalized edematous and bleeding gingiva.	Clinical Dx Acyclovir
Coxsackievirus	Herpangina—abrupt onset of high fever with hyperemia and yellow/gray vesicular lesions on the anterior pillars, soft palate, tonsils, and uvula.	Clinical Dx Supportive treatment
Epstein–Barr virus	Mononucleosis—severe fatigue, malaise, headache, low-grade fever, tonsillitis and/or pharyngitis, cervical node enlargement	Dx with heterophile test (good in patients ≤12 years old; not as sensitive in patients <12 years). Supportive treatment with avoidance of contact sports (due to risk of splenic rupture).

TABLE 8.3 Highly Tested Associations

Organism	Association
Burkholderia cepacia complex	CF
Chlamydophila pneumoniae	Hoarseness, staccato cough pattern, insidious onset of rhinorrhea
Coxiella burnetti	Animals at time of birth, farmers
Klebsiella	DM, alcoholism, currant-jelly sputum, hemoptysis
Legionella	Standing water/AC systems, hyponatremia, diarrhea, headache, confusion; diagnose with urinary antigen test
MSSA/MRSA	Recent viral infection, commonly with influenza
Mycoplasma	Young, healthy patients, "walking pneumonia" Diagnose with PCR, cold agglutinins
Pseudomonas	Acquired by hospital/chronic-care facility patients, CF, DM

CF, Cystic fibrosis; *DM,* diabetes mellitus; *MSSA,* methicillin-sensitive *S. aureus.*

TABLE 8.4 Common Etiologies of Pneumonia by Age Group

Age Group	Common Pathogens	Treatment
Neonates to 1 month	*Group B streptococcus, Escherichia coli*, other GNRs	Ampicillin + cefotaxime
Febrile pneumonia 1–3 months	RSV, other respiratory viruses, *Streptococcus pneumoniae, Haemophilus influenza*	Amoxicillin or ampicillin if fully immunized Cefotaxime if not immunized
Afebrile pneumonia 1–3 months	*Chlamydia trachomatis, Mycoplasma, Bordetella*	Azithromycin or erythromycin
3 months to 5 years	RSV, other respiratory viruses, *S. pneumoniae, H. influenzae,* influenza viruses	Ampicillin (plus macrolide if atypical pneumonia suspected)
5–18 years	*Mycoplasma, S. pneumoniae, Chlamydia pneumoniae,* influenza viruses	Ampicillin (plus macrolide if atypical pneumonia suspected or oseltamivir if influenza virus suspected)

GNR, Gram-negative rod; *RSV*, respiratory syncytial virus.

TABLE 8.5

	Blastomycosis	Coccidioidomycosis (aka San Joaquin Fever or Valley Fever)	Histoplasmosis
Buzz Words	• Pneumonia • Granulomas in skin and bone • Central America/Great Lakes/East Coast	• Mild respiratory sx → pneumonia • Granulomas in skin (erythema nodosum) and musculoskeletal pain (arthralgia) • s/p earthquakes • SW US or Central/South America	• Pneumonia • Mississippi/Ohio River Valleys • Cave (e.g., contact with bats) • Hiking (e.g., contact with birds)
Clinical presentation (all three can form **granulomas**)	Blastomycosis is an inflammatory lung disease that can disseminate to skin and bone. Geographically, patients are either from the Great Lakes, the East Coast of the US, or Central America.	Coccidioidomycosis is usually asymptomatic, but patients can present with mild respiratory symptoms and concomitant skin and bone involvement. Infection can occur after earthquakes that shake up fungal spores. Geographically, patients are from SW US, San Joaquin Valley, South America.	Histoplasmosis is usually asymptomatic but can present with mild respiratory symptoms or pneumonia. Disease is associated with contact with bats (e.g., caves) and birds (e.g., hiking). Geographically, patients are from Mississippi and Ohio.
PPx (No human-to-human transmission)	Avoid endemic areas	Avoid endemic areas	Avoid endemic areas
MoD	*Blastomyces dermatitidis*	*Coccidioides immitis/ posadasii*	*Histoplasma capsulatum*

TABLE 8.5—cont'd

	Blastomycosis	Coccidioidomycosis (aka San Joaquin Fever or Valley Fever)	Histoplasmosis
Dx **Do not need to know in detail for the clinical subject exam** (however, important for step 1)	• Biopsy shows single broad-based bud, thick-walled budding yeast at 37°C + hyphae w/ small conidia at 25°C. • Dimorphic systemic fungi (e.g., mold outside body but yeast within body).	Biopsy shows huge **spherule** w/ endospores. • Fungal endospores w/ spherules at 37°C + branched hyphae at 25°C. • Only fungus that is not dimorphic because it exists as a spherule.	Biopsy shows spores seen **within the macrophage.** • Dimorphic systemic fungi.
Tx/Mgmt	(1) Itraconazole (or another azole such as ketoconazole). (2) Amphotericin B.	(1) Itraconazole. (2) Amphotericin B.	(1) Itraconazole. (2) Amphotericin B.

GUNNER PRACTICE

1. A 30-month-old male is brought to the pediatrician's office by his mother. She says that he became cranky and began to have nasal congestion 2 days earlier, and now she is worried because of his "noisy breathing and coughing." He was born at 38 weeks 2, days with no apparent complications; since then he has had diaper dermatitis with a candidal superinfection and a single right-arm cellulitis. His family history is notable for asthma in his father and breast cancer in his mother and maternal grandmother. His vital signs are T 99.6°F, HR 125, BP 80/47, RR 30, SpO_2 98% on room air. Examination yields an uncomfortable child with a hoarse voice, harsh barking cough, rhinorrhea, and inspiratory stridor when agitated. What is the most likely diagnosis and best next step in management?
A. Bronchiolitis; nasal suctioning and reassurance
B. Community-acquired pneumonia; amoxicillin treatment
C. Cystic fibrosis; chloride sweat test
D. Croup; dexamethasone and reassurance
E. Asthma exacerbation; albuterol

2. A 3-year-old male is brought to the ED by his father, who says that his son became cranky and complained of a sore throat early that morning. By midafternoon, the boy was refusing food and drink and seemed to be having difficulty breathing. Both parents have a history of asthma. The child's vital signs are T 103.2°F, HR 155, BP 75/43, RR 44, SpO$_2$ 94% on room air. He is ill-appearing, drooling, and leaning forward with head extended, with audible inspiratory stridor. What is the best next step in management?

A. Intravenous fluid administration
B. Operating room intubation
C. Vancomycin and ceftriaxone administration
D. Albuterol administration
E. Rapid strep test

3. A female neonate experiences respiratory distress minutes after delivery. She was born after 38 weeks and 1 day of gestation and had an uncomplicated spontaneous vaginal delivery. There is no family history of cardiac or respiratory problems and this is the mother's first child. The infant's vital signs are T 98.8, HR 190, RR 81, SpO$_2$ 82% on room air. The child is intubated immediately. Examination yields an infant with normal facies, a scaphoid-shaped abdomen, and decreased breath sounds, especially on the right side. Her CXR is shown below. What is the likely diagnosis?

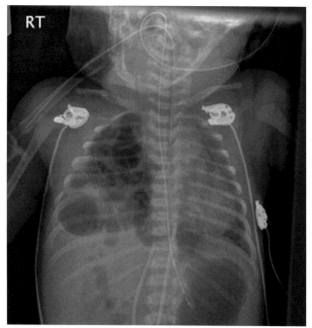

(Chiu PPL, Langer JC: Surgical conditions of the diaphragm: posterior diaphragmatic hernias in infants. *Thorac Surg Clin* 19(4):451–461, 2009, Copyright © 2009 Elsevier Inc.)

A. Meconium aspiration syndrome
B. Group B streptococcal pneumonia
C. Congenital diaphragmatic hernia
D. Tracheoesophageal fistula
E. Renal hypoplasia

ANSWERS: What Would Gunner Jess/Jim Do?

1. WWGJD? A 30-month-old male is brought to the pediatrician's office by his mother. She says that he became cranky and began to have nasal congestion 2 days earlier, and now she is worried because of his "noisy breathing and coughing." He was born at 38 weeks, 2 days with no apparent complications; since then he has had diaper dermatitis with a candidal superinfection and a single right-arm cellulitis. His family history is notable for asthma in his father and breast cancer in his mother and maternal grandmother. His vital signs are T 99.6°F, HR 125, BP 80/47, RR 30, SpO_2 98% on room air. Examination yields an uncomfortable child with a hoarse voice, harsh barking cough, rhinorrhea, and inspiratory stridor when agitated. What is the most likely diagnosis and best next step in management?

Answer: D, Croup; dexamethasone and reassurance

Explanation: This question tests your ability to differentiate between common clinical syndromes of respiratory disease in young children. This is a 2.5-year-old male with hoarseness, rhinorrhea, a barking cough, and inspiratory stridor, which is the presentation of croup (or laryngotracheitis). Croup is a common syndrome in children, usually between 6 months and 6 years of age, characterized by the symptoms listed above and caused by a viral upper respiratory infection (especially parainfluenza). Although this is a *clinical* Dx and does not require imaging, occasionally a neck x-ray showing a "steeple sign" will be given to match a question about a croup patient. Although several home remedies may improve symptoms as the infection clears, dexamethasone is commonly given to alleviate symptoms in those with croup who are brought to medical attention. Note that this patient has inspiratory stridor only when agitated and has no signs of respiratory distress.

A. Bronchiolitis; nasal suctioning and reassurance → Incorrect. Bronchiolitis is another common viral syndrome in children that can be differentiated from croup in several ways. First, this patient is older than most patients with bronchiolitis, which is usually seen in children under age 2. Second, bronchiolitis often presents with wheezing, and physical examination usually yields adventitious sounds on pulmonary auscultation. Bronchiolitis is classically caused by respiratory syncytial virus (RSV), or RS5.

B. Community-acquired pneumonia; amoxicillin treatment → Incorrect. This patient has croup, which is caused by a viral infection. The rhinorrhea, along with the clinical syndrome of croup, identify this as a viral process as opposed to a bacterial process. Additionally, we are given no information about adventitious lung sounds and the patient is not tachypneic or in respiratory distress.

C. Cystic fibrosis; chloride sweat test → Incorrect. This patient does not have the historic symptoms and signs of cystic fibrosis (CF), which include failure to thrive (FTT), frequent sinus and respiratory infections, and delayed meconium passage as an infant. We are also given no relevant family history.

E. Asthma exacerbation; albuterol → Incorrect. This patient does not exhibit asthma flare symptoms, which include a prolonged expiratory phase, wheezing, and respiratory distress.

2. WWGJD? A 3-year-old male is brought to the ED by his father. He says that his son became cranky and complained of a sore throat early in the morning. However, by the midafternoon, the boy was refusing food and drinks and seemed to be having difficulty breathing normally. Both parents have a history of asthma. The child's vital signs are T 103.2°F, HR 155, BP 75/43, RR 44, SpO_2 94% on room air. He is ill-appearing, drooling, and leaning forward with head extended, with audible inspiratory stridor. What is the best next step in management?

Answer: B, Operating room intubation

Explanation: This question tests your ability to recognize an emergent medical condition by clinical observation. This 3-year-old male with high fever, ill appearance, drooling, odynophagia, stridor, and respiratory distress, in the "tripod" position, displays the clinical features of epiglottitis. Epiglottitis can lead to life-threatening airway compromise, so the initial management of a patient with suspected epiglottitis should be securing the airway. Attempts to treat the patient otherwise can increase anxiety and worsen the respiratory distress. Thus, even noninvasive examination maneuvers and treatment modalities should be avoided, if possible. Of note, the incidence of epiglottitis has drastically decreased in children due to the *Haemophilus influenzae* type

B vaccine. This patient's vaccination (and immuno-competence) status is unknown.

A. Intravenous fluid administration → Incorrect. This is not the first priority in stabilizing the patient with epiglottitis.

C. Vancomycin and ceftriaxone administration → Incorrect. This is not the first priority in stabilizing the patient with epiglottitis.

D. Albuterol administration → Incorrect. The clinical concern for epiglottitis is higher than the concern for asthma exacerbation.

E. Rapid strep test → Incorrect. See above.

3. WWGJD? A female neonate experiences respiratory distress minutes after delivery. She was born after 38 weeks and 1 day of gestation and had an uncomplicated spontaneous vaginal delivery. There is no family history of cardiac or respiratory problems and this is the mother's first child. The infant's vital signs are T 98.8°F, HR 190, RR 81, SpO$_2$ 82% on room air. The child is intubated immediately. Examination yields an infant with normal facies, a scaphoid-shaped abdomen, and decreased breath sounds, especially on the right side. Her CXR is shown below. What is the likely diagnosis?

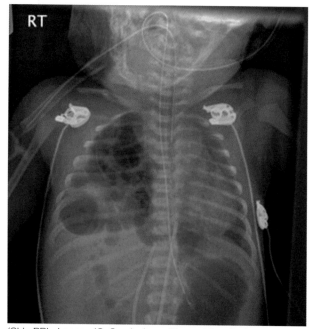

(Chiu PPL, Langer JC: Surgical conditions of the diaphragm: posterior diaphragmatic hernias in infants. *Thorac Surg Clin* 19(4):451–461, 2009, Copyright © 2009 Elsevier Inc.)

Answer: C, Congenital diaphragmatic hernia
  Explanation: This question tests your knowledge of
    common causes of neonatal respiratory distress
    and your ability to differentiate between them. This
    is a newborn with respiratory distress, a scaphoid-
    shaped abdomen, and decreased breath sounds,
    especially on one side. The provided image depicts
    an infant with abdominal contents in the right
    hemithorax and the mediastinum shifted into the left
    hemithorax. This is an example of congenital dia-
    phragmatic hernia. A defect in the diaphragm allows
    abdominal contents to leave the abdomen (so that
    it appears more empty) and puts pressure on the
    budding respiratory tree, which becomes hypo-
    plastic. The hypoplasia can be largely contained
    to the side of the defect or can be bilateral due to
    decreased space in the contralateral hemithorax as
    the mediastinum shifts. The identification of bowel
    in the thorax is key to solving this problem.
  A. Meconium aspiration syndrome → Incorrect. This
    is certainly a cause of neonatal respiratory distress
    but would not result in the described physical exam
    findings or imaging.
  B. Group B streptococcal pneumonia → Incorrect. This
    would not explain the physical findings or imaging.
  D. Tracheoesophageal fistula → Incorrect. This would
    also not explain the physical exam findings or
    imaging. Additionally, note that the endotracheal
    and nasogastric tubes in the CXR appear to be
    located appropriately, which decreases the likeli-
    hood of a tracheoesophageal fistula.
  E. Renal hypoplasia → Incorrect. This would not explain
    the physical findings or imaging. Additionally, note
    that renal hypoplasia causing oligohydramnios
    can lead to respiratory distress due to pulmonary
    hypoplasia, but in this case it can also yield charac-
    teristic physical exam findings known as the Potter
    sequence. We are given no indication that the mother
    of the child had oligohydramnios prior to delivery.

Nutrition and Digestive Disorders

Diana Kim, Daniel Gromer, Alejandro Suarez Pierre, Hao-Hua Wu, Elana B. Mitchell, Leo Wang, and Rebecca Tenney-Soeiro

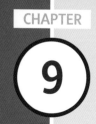
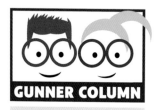

GUNNER COLUMN

Introduction

Nutritional and digestive disorders will make up 10%–15% of your Pediatrics shelf and will correspond to 10–15 questions. As such, it is one of the most important sections in this book. Luckily, if this is not your first rotation, you will have seen many of these diseases in your medicine, surgery, or even family medicine rotations. Food poisoning is ubiquitous among all shelves and will thus be one of the most high-yield topics in this chapter. In children, food poisoning can be particularly debilitating, so the ability to differentiate between various etiologies and their treatments will go a long way (e.g., even though hemolytic uremic syndrome [HUS] is caused by bacteria, you almost never give antibiotics!). Unlike other shelves, the Pediatrics shelf will place high emphasis on diseases such as Meckel diverticulum that occur as a result of failure of obliteration of an embryonic structure, the omphalomesenteric duct. Always, always try to tie anatomical abnormalities back to embryogenesis as this will aid in your understanding of why and how they develop.

This chapter is organized into several sections: (1) Embryonic Development, Fetal Maturation, Perinatal Changes; (2) Infectious Disorders; (3) Immunologic and Inflammatory Disorders; (4) Disorders of Oral Cavity; (5) Disorders of Stomach, Small Intestine, and Colon; (6) Disorders of the Liver; (7) Congenital Disorders; and (8) Disorders of Jaundice. The diseases in each section are already the most important and relevant to the clinical subject exam. As always, remember the four physician tasks: Prophylaxis (PPx), Mechanism of Disease (MoD), Diagnostic Steps (Dx), and Treatment and Management Steps (Tx/Mgmt). The most important tasks on this shelf will be Dx and Tx/Mgmt, although MoD will also be important for diseases that develop from defective embryogenesis such as Meckel's.

Embryonic Development, Fetal Maturation, Perinatal Changes

The most high-yield portion of gastrointestinal (GI) embryonic development is the formation of the intestine. An umbilical loop is formed in the fourth week of gestation, allowing the midgut to extend into the umbilical coelom. From the apex of extension, a connection to the umbilical vesicle will form, leading to the omphalomesenteric duct. This is obliterated soon, but if it is not, this can lead to **Meckel diverticulum**. The umbilical loop will then experience a rotation of 90 degrees clockwise and the cranial pedicles will form. As the loop further extends, the cecum will develop (~between 5 and 6 weeks). Between weeks 6 and 7, the loop turns around on its own axis and a physiologic naval hernia remains here until the ninth week of pregnancy. Beyond this, it is considered an **omphalocele**. Next, loops of the small intestine formed from all the aforementioned processes return into the abdomen to be surrounded by parts of the colon. When the intestinal loop returns to the abdominal cavity, a 270-degree rotation must occur. When no rotation or incomplete rotation occurs, this can lead to **volvulus** or **strangulation** (Fig. 9.1).

Very good video of intestinal rotation

Infectious Disorders

Bacterial

Pseudomembranous Colitis

Buzz Words: Antibiotic use + clindamycin + *Clostridium difficile*

Clinical Presentation: Pseudomembranous colitis is inflammation of the colon due to an overgrowth of *C. difficile* secondary to antibiotic use or in the setting of immunosuppression. This is an extremely high-yield disease on any clinical subject exam. Presents as profuse watery diarrhea ± blood, abdominal cramps, fever. Toxic megacolon, acute toxic colitis with dilatation of the colon, is a major complication with risk of perforation.

PPx: Hand hygiene, minimizing antibiotic use in patients with history of pseudomembranous colitis

MoD: Antibiotic use kills normal bacteria flora that normally live in the intestine and inhibit overgrowth of *C. difficile*. This leads to overgrowth of *C. difficile* and toxin production, causing inflammation and disruption of the intestinal mucosa.

Dx:

1. Clinical presentation and history + leukocytosis are sufficient.
2. Immunoassay for *C. difficile* toxin in stool is diagnostic (95% sensitivity) but takes at least 24 hours. Colonoscopy for visualization.

Tx/Mgmt:

1. Stop the inciting antibiotic.
2. Oral metronidazole is first-line.
3. Oral vancomycin is second-line for 2-week course.

Enteritis/Enteric Infections

Staphylococcus aureus

Buzz Words: Nausea/vomiting without diarrhea + recent ingestion of dairy product → *S. aureus*

Clinical Presentation: Fast onset (1–6 hours); nausea, vomiting, abdominal cramps. Self-limited disease.

PPx: Adequate refrigeration of food products, hand hygiene

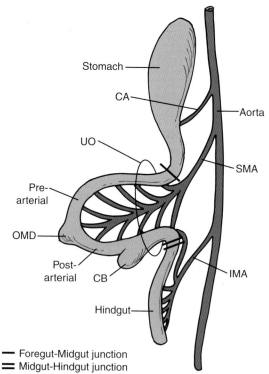

— Foregut-Midgut junction
= Midgut-Hindgut junction

FIG. 9.1 Intestinal tract development at 6 weeks. (Javors et al: *Applied Embryology of GI Tract, Textbook of GI Radiology*, 2015, Elsevier.)

MoD: Heat-stable enterotoxin B acts as a superantigen. *S. aureus* is likely to grow in dairy products, meats, and mayonnaise-based salads that are kept at room temperature. β-Hemolytic, catalase (+), coagulase (+), Gram-positive coccus.

Dx:

1. Clinical diagnosis

Tx/Mgmt:

1. Supportive therapy

Escherichia coli

Buzz Words: HUS + schistocytes + bloody diarrhea + recently ate undercooked meat (e.g., hamburgers)

Clinical Presentation: There are four types of *E. coli* that can be tested by the NBME (see below). Enterohemorrhagic *E. coli* (EHEC), enteropathogenic *E. coli* (EPEC), and enterotoxigenic *E. coli* (ETEC) are all high-yield on the peds shelf. Skip enteroinvasive *E. coli* (EIEC) if pressed for time.

1. EHEC—Shiga-like toxin from undercooked meat that may lead to HUS (see below)
2. EPEC—Predominates in children, non-bloody diarrhea
3. ETEC—Traveler's diarrhea, non-bloody diarrhea
4. EIEC—Inflammatory bowel, bloody diarrhea

PPx: Hand washing, adequate sanitization of water, and avoiding food contamination

> **QUICK TIPS**
> Triad of HUS: anemia + thrombocytopenia + acute kidney injury

TABLE 9.1 Most Common Diarrheal Illnesses Caused by *Escherichia coli*

	ETEC (i.e., Traveler's Diarrhea)	EHEC (*O157:H7 Serotype*)	EIEC
Presentation	Watery diarrhea	Hemorrhagic colitis and HUS in 8% of cases	Dysentery 12–72 h after ingestion
MoD	Heat-labile (LT) and heat-stable (ST) toxins activate adenylate and guanylate cyclase respectively → secretory diarrhea	Shiga toxin (verotoxin) → endothelial damage (gut, kidney, lung) → hemorrhage	Mucosal cell invasion causing membrane disruption
Clinical cues	Traveler's and children <5 years old	Children and elderly; transmitted through undercooked ground beef	Developing countries; invasion rarely goes beyond submucosa
Management	Fluid replacement Ciprofloxacin	Fluid replacement Avoid antibiotics! These may precipitate HUS	Fluid replacement

EHEC, Enterohemorrhagic *E. coli*; *EIEC*, enteroinvasive *E. coli*; *ETEC*, enterotoxigenic *E. coli*; *HUS*, hemolytic uremic syndrome.

MoD:

For **EHEC**: Shiga-like toxin (verotoxin) causes endothelial damage leading to hemorrhage **EHEC**, and
EIEC: Invade and inflame gut mucosa → bloody diarrhea

ETEC and EPEC: Do not invade and inflame gut mucosa → non-bloody diarrhea

Dx:

1. Stool culture and Gram stain (Motile, encapsulated gram-negative rod, catalase (+), and oxidase (–)
2. MacConkey's agar (pink; lactose fermenter)

Tx/Mgmt:

1. Supportive therapy.
2. Avoid antiperistaltic agents (loperamide) as these might prolong duration of infection.
3. For EHEC, **avoid antibiotics**, which may precipitate HUS by releasing more Shiga-like toxins.

Hemolytic Uremic Syndrome

Buzz Words: Hemolytic anemia + thrombocytopenia + renal dysfunction

Clinical Presentation: Triad of hemolytic anemia, thrombocytopenia, and renal dysfunction due to *E. coli*. Do not usually see purpura despite the thrombocytopenia. Recent infection with abdominal pain, diarrhea (usually bloody), and low urine output or pallor.

PPx: None

MoD: Shiga toxin binds to glomerular vascular endothelium, most commonly due to *E. coli* (**EHEC 0157:H7**) but also seen following Shigella infection.

Dx:

1. Clinical picture
2. Urinalysis
3. Complete blood count (CBC)
4. May culture for blood infection though not always present at the time of presentation

Tx/Mgmt: DO NOT give antibiotics as they may increase the release of shiga toxin and cause worsening renal dysfunction. Supportive care only.

Listeria Monocytogenes

Buzz Words: Unpasteurized dairy + dark/cloudy amniotic fluid + newborn meningitis

Clinical Presentation: Can be maternally acquired from unpasteurized dairy or raw foods. May see brown murky amniotic fluid. May result in abortion, stillbirth, or neonatal sepsis and meningitis.

Listeria is the third most common cause of meningitis in newborns and is the reason why ampicillin is added to the treatment regimen for ≤3-month-olds with sepsis.

PPx: N/A

MoD: Transmitted through contaminated dairy products and raw foods.

Dx:
1. Stool culture and Gram stain (shows tumbling motility, catalase [+], gram-positive, facultative anaerobe).
2. Infants younger than 3 months old may also require blood and cerebrospinal fluid (CSF) cultures.

Tx/Mgmt:
1. Ampicillin

Yersinia enterocolitica

Buzz Words: Gram-negative coccobacillus with bipolar staining ("safety-pin" appearance)

Clinical Presentation: A child with mesenteric lymphadenitis that simulates acute appendicitis. May also see enterocolitis, resulting in bloody diarrhea and fever.

PPx: Avoid contact with canine feces and use hand washing after touching pets.

MoD: Organism courses through the stomach, attaches and invades the gut wall to end up localizing in regional lymphoid tissue.

Dx:
1. Culture isolation from stool, pharynx, or mesenteric nodes

Tx/Mgmt:
1. Supportive therapy.
2. Severe cases may use fluoroquinolones or TMP-SMX.

Campylobacter spp.

Buzz Words: Bloody diarrhea + fever + cramping periumbilical abdominal pain

Clinical Presentation: Bloody diarrhea, fever, and cramping periumbilical abdominal pain. Children may manifest abdominal pain that mimics appendicitis or colitis. Much more commonly affects children and adolescents than adults.

PPx: Avoid eating raw/undercooked meat

MoD: Poultry. Puppies are the most common source of infection for children. Disease is self-limited with a mean duration of 7 days.

Dx:
1. Stool culture

Tx/Mgmt:
1. Supportive therapy
2. Azithromycin, or erythromycin in setting of severe symptoms

Vibrio cholera

Buzz Words: Rice-water stools + comma-shaped, gram-negative rod

Clinical Presentation: High-volume secretory diarrhea ± vomit, significant hypovolemia, electrolyte abnormalities that may occur hours after onset of disease.

PPx: Adequate hygiene and keeping a clean water supply

MoD: Fecal-oral transmission

Dx:
1. Clinical suspicion, confirmation may come from stool cultures

Tx/Mgmt:
1. Supportive, including aggressive oral or intravenous (IV) rehydration therapy

Salmonella Species

Buzz Words: Poultry/milk ingestion + exposure to lizards or turtles + "pea-soup" diarrhea

Clinical Presentation: Diarrhea with abdominal cramps, nausea, vomiting, and fever. Diarrhea can be bloody or non-bloody ("pea-soup" appearance is common).

MoD: Transmission through ingestion of poultry, eggs, and milk products or handling of lizards or turtles. Chronic carriage state (>1 year) is typically not seen in children.

Dx:
1. Stool culture (H_2S [+], motile, gram-negative bacilli, black colonies on Hektoen agar)

Tx/Mgmt:
1. Supportive therapy
2. Third-generation cephalosporin for severe disease only

Shigella spp.

Buzz Words: Bloody diarrhea + HUS+ seizures

Clinical Presentation: Patient with frequent, bloody stools with fever and abdominal cramps. Thrombocytopenia and HUS are common in young children (similar to EHEC). Neurological complications, mainly **seizures**, may also occur.

PPx: Adequate hygiene

MoD: Fecal-oral, hand-hand transmission

Dx: Stool culture to isolate bacteria (immotile, gram-negative bacilli; green colonies on Hektoen agar)

Tx/Mgmt:
1. Supportive therapy.
2. Severe cases may use fluoroquinolones, Ceftriaxone or azithromycin depending on local resistance patterns.

Viral

Hepatitis A

Buzz Words: Travel to rural area or developing country + jaundice + elevated LFTs + no history of HAV vaccine + ingestion of uncooked shellfish + daycare

Clinical Presentation: Hepatitis A is the most common viral cause of hepatitis worldwide.

It is commonly asymptomatic in children, especially if younger than 6 years of age. When symptomatic, it typically presents as an acute, self-limited illness with nonspecific symptoms such as fever, anorexia, GI discomfort, and diarrhea. May or may not present with jaundice. Symptoms last longer and are more severe in older children.

PPx: (1) Inactivated vaccine. (2) Hygienic practices such as handwashing and heating food.

MoD: Fecal-oral transmission (contaminated water supplies or food). Uncooked shellfish is a common source of infection in developed countries.

Dx:
1. Serum immunoglobulin (Ig)M anti-HAV antibodies

Tx/Mgmt:
1. Supportive treatment

Hepatitis B

Buzz Words: Exposure to endemic areas + jaundice + IV drug use

Clinical Presentation: The majority of children with hepatitis B virus (HBV) infection are immigrants from endemic areas or are exposed via perinatal transmission (Table 9.2). Adolescents who engage in high-risk behaviors such as IV drug use or multiple sexual partners are also at high risk.

Acute HBV infection: Variable ranging from asymptomatic infection to fulminant hepatitis. Incubation period of 1–4 months is followed by constitutional symptoms, jaundice, and right upper quadrant discomfort. These will disappear in 1–3 months.

Chronic HBV infection: Mostly asymptomatic. However, right upper quadrant discomfort and fatigue occur in some children.

TABLE 9.2 Hepatitis B Virus Serologic Studies

Interpretation	HBsAg	HBV DNA	Anti-HBc IgM	Anti-HBc IgG	Anti-HBs	HBeAg	Anti-HBeAg
Early infection	+	–	–	–	–	+	–
Acute infection	+	+	+	–	–	+	–
Window phase	–	–	+	–	–	–	+
Recovery	–	–	–	+	+	–	+
Immunized	–	–	–	–	+	–	–
Healthy carrier	+	–	–	+	–	–	+
Infective carrier	+	+	–	+	–	+	–

HBV surface antigen (HBVsAg) indicates active disease. HBV core IgM (anti-HBc-IgM) is IgM against core HBV antigen and indicates acute/early infection. HBV core IgG (anti-HBc-IgG) occurs with infection but not with immunization. Hepatitis B envelope antigen (HBeAg) rises very early then decreases as the immune system produces immunoglobulins (anti-HBeAg) against it. HBeAg indicates HBV infectivity while anti-HBe indicates low transmissibility.
HBV, Hepatitis B virus.

PPx: HBV vaccination. In infants born to hepatitis B positive mother, should receive HBIG and hepatitis B vaccine within first 12 hours of life.

MoD: Vertical transmission, parenteral or sexual transmission

Dx:

1. Acute HBV infection: presence of hepatitis B surface antigen (HBsAg) and IgM antibody to hepatitis B core antigen (IgM anti-HBc) (Table 9.1).
2. Chronic HBV infection: persistence of HBsAg for more than 6 months; presence of IgG anti-HBc; absence of IgM anti-HBc.

Tx/Mgmt:

1. Interferon is first-line for short-term treatment.
2. For long-term treatment, entecavir or lamivudine.

Hepatitis C

Buzz Words: Mother with hx of IV drug use/hepatitis C virus (HCV) infection + liver failure

Clinical Presentation: Hepatitis C is caused by the HCV. Maternal-fetal transmission is the most common source of infection in children (vs. parenteral transmission in adults). Suspect hepatitis C in children of mothers with known HCV infection or with a history of IV drug use. Acute infection is rarely symptomatic. Chronic infection, which occurs in 80% of infected patients, becomes more symptomatic over time. However, disease progression is slow. Advanced fibrosis, cirrhosis, and jaundice are only occasionally seen in children with chronic hepatitis C.

PPx: No vaccine or immunoglobulin is available to reduce perinatal or parenteral transmission. Avoid needle sharing to address parenteral transmission concerns.

MoD: Perinatal (more common) or parenteral transmission. The virus lacks proofreading enzymes, which allows for significant antigenic variability and causes it to be a challenging vaccination and immunologic target. The virus has six different genotypes.

Dx:
1. Anti-HCV antibodies or HCV RNA in serum.
2. ALT rises during symptomatic infection (ALT > AST).
3. Chronic HCV infection is diagnosed by detectable HCV viral level greater than 6 months. Also, LFTs are decreased with chronic HCV 2/2 cirrhosis.

Tx/Mgmt:
1. Defer treatment for most children/adolescents until availability of new drugs, namely direct-acting antiviral agents (DAA).
2. For patients who choose to proceed with treatment, use pegylated interferon with ribavirin.

Hepatitis D

Buzz Words: Concomitant HBV infection

Clinical Presentation: Hepatitis D is caused by hepatitis D virus (HDV), which is a virus that requires HBsAg for infection. Superinfection upon preexisting HBV is more severe than co-infection, which is simultaneous infection with HBV and HDV. Severity of infection is dependent on viral genotype. Infection may be asymptomatic, may cause progression of hepatitis B infection, or may lead to fulminant liver failure.

PPx: Because HDV cannot be transmitted without HBV, hepatitis B vaccine in newborn infants is protective.

MoD: Parenteral, sexual, and vertical transmission. Although HDV can replicate autonomously, it requires HBsAg for virion assembly and secretion.

Dx:
1. Serum HDAg, HDV RNA or anti-HDV antibodies (both IgM and IgG).

Tx/Mgmt: Treat hepatitis B infection as above.

Hepatitis E

Buzz Words: Similar presentation as hepatitis A + hepatitis E virus (HEV) in serum/stool + contaminated water

Clinical Presentation: Hepatitis E is caused by HEV. It is responsible for 50% of acute hepatitis in adolescents in endemic countries. It is typically a mild, self-limiting disease with a very similar presentation to that of hepatitis A. Self-limited acute viral hepatitis. However, fulminant hepatitis and mortality can occur in pregnant patients or those with pre-existing liver disease.

PPx: Hand-washing and avoiding consumption of untreated water and insufficiently cooked food.

MoD: Fecal-oral transmission (contaminated water supplies or food).

Dx:

1. Detection of HEV in serum or stool by PCR
2. Anti-HEV IgM antibodies in serum

Tx/Mgmt:

1. Supportive therapy

> Hepatitis E: Expectant mothers, Endemic areas

> HEV and HAV: via EAting (fecal-oral transmission)

Non-Polio Enterovirus Enteritis/Colitis (Echovirus, Coxsackievirus)

Buzz Words: Sick contacts + mild watery diarrhea + absence of other symptoms

Clinical Presentation: Frequently asymptomatic or presents as an undifferentiated febrile illness. If GI symptoms are present, may produce a mild watery diarrhea.

PPx: N/A

MoD: Fecal-oral transmission. Virus replicates in the pharynx and intestines. Secreted in stool.

Dx:

1. Clinical diagnosis

Tx/Mgmt:

1. Supportive treatment.
2. Be watchful for non-GI involvement such as aseptic meningitis, encephalitis, myocarditis, petechiae/purpura, and others.

Rotavirus Enteritis

Buzz Words: Daycare + watery, non-bloody diarrhea + winter

Clinical Presentation: Rotavirus is the most common cause of viral gastroenteritis in children worldwide. A child, usually between 6 months to 2 years of age, who attends daycare and presents with watery, nonbloody diarrhea, abdominal cramps, vomiting, and fever. In severe cases, dehydration, seizures, and death can occur. Occurs usually in winter months. After recovery, some may develop transient lactose intolerance.

PPx: Live-attenuated vaccine is given at 2 and 4 months (and 6 months if three-dose series).

MoD: Rotavirus leads to loss of brush border enzymes, which leads to malabsorption of carbohydrates. Rotavirus enterotoxin stimulates Ca^{2+}-dependent cell permeability and disrupts epithelial cell integrity, leading to increased water and electrolyte loss $\rightarrow$ osmotic diarrhea.

Dx:
1. Enzyme-linked immunosorbent assay (ELISA) and latex agglutination of the stool are most commonly used.

Tx/Mgmt:
1. Supportive treatment. Rehydration is particularly important due to extreme fluid loss.
2. Breastfeeding can continue through diarrhea.
3. Hospital admission with refusal of oral fluids, clinical deterioration, and/or neurologic abnormalities.

Mumps

Buzz Words: limited vaccination history + parotid swelling (chipmunk facies) + testicular pain

Clinical Presentation: Mumps is an acute, self-limited viral syndrome most commonly associated with parotitis and orchitis. Presents with nonspecific prodromal symptoms (fever + constitutional symptoms) of 2–3 days followed by parotid tenderness and swelling. Ninety-percent of symptomatic cases of mumps involve parotid swelling (bilateral > unilateral). Complications include orchitis, aseptic meningitis, encephalitis, and pancreatitis.

PPx: Measles-mumps-rubella (MMR) vaccine is given (two-dose series; 12–15 months and 4–6 years).

MoD: Transmitted via respiratory droplets or direct contact. Highly infectious. Neuraminidase and hemagglutinin are the main virulence factors.

Dx: Clinical features + CBC (leukopenia with a relative lymphocytosis) + increased serum amylase

Tx/Mgmt:
1. For isolated parotitis and/or orchitis, symptomatic treatment with analgesics and antipyretics.
2. If meningitis or pancreatitis, hospitalization with IV fluids (Fig. 9.2).

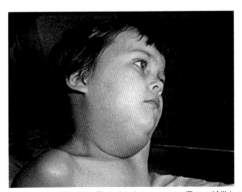

FIG. 9.2 Parotitis in mumps. (From Wikipedia.)

Herpetic Gingivostomatitis

Buzz Words: "Dew drops on a rose petal" appearance, Cowdry bodies, multinucleated giant cells in Tzanck smear, dsDNA virus

Clinical Presentation: Herpetic gingivostomatitis is an inflammation of the gingiva and oral mucosa that most commonly occurs as the initial presentation of primary herpes simplex virus (HSV) infection during childhood (particularly 6 months to 5 years of age). Presents with a viral prodrome (fever + constitutional symptoms) followed by gingivae that bleed easily and vesicular clusters on erythematous base. Vesicles will coalesce to form large, painful ulcers on the gingiva and oral mucosa. They bleed easily and can become covered with a black/grayish crust. Patient will refuse to drink and eat. Regional lymphadenitis will be present.

PPx: Contact precautions with affected children

MoD: HSV-1. After the resolution of symptoms, the virus migrates to the trigeminal ganglion, where it will remain latent. Reactivation can occur with stressors such as sunlight, trauma, cold, emotional stress, and immunosuppression.

Dx:

1. Clinical diagnosis

Tx/Mgmt:

1. Supportive treatment.
2. Use oral acyclovir in immunocompetent children, use IV acyclovir in infants and immunocompromised patients (Fig. 9.3).

Fungal

Thrush (Oropharyngeal Candidiasis)

Buzz Words: White plaques on oral mucosa that are easily scrapable

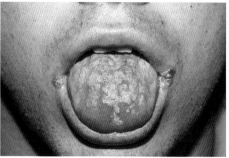

FIG. 9.3 Herpetic gingivostomatitis. (From Buttaravoli et al., *Oral Herpes Simplex, Minor Emergencies,* 2012, Elsevier.)

Clinical Presentation: Irregular white plaques on oral mucous membranes that are easily scraped off with a tongue depressor, revealing inflamed and friable mucosa. Occurs in neonates, due to immaturity of their host defenses, and immunocompromised children and adults.

PPx: N/A

MoD: Oropharyngeal overgrowth of *Candida albicans*. Infection may be transmitted by the passage through the birth canal, breastfeeding, or the environment.

Dx:

1. Physical exam is adequate.

Tx/Mgmt:

1. Nystatin (topical) as it is not absorbed from the GI tract.
2. If the mother's breasts are also infected, treat at the same time.

Parasitic

Entamoeba histolytica

Buzz Words: Flask-shaped ulcers in colon + travel history to a developing country + bloody diarrhea + spherical cysts

Clinical Presentation: While most patients are asymptomatic, symptoms range from mild diarrhea to dysentery with severe abdominal pain and bloody stools. May see amebic liver abscesses.

PPx: Avoiding consumption of untreated water and undercooked food when traveling to developing countries

MoD: Transmission occurs via ingestion of cysts in contaminated food/water; cysts become trophozoites in the cecum and secrete agents that produce flask-shaped ulcers. Trophozoites can invade into hepatic veins and produce a liver abscess or systemic disease.

Dx:

1. Stool antigen test

Tx/Mgmt:

1. Metronidazole is the mainstay of therapy.

Enterobius vermicularis (Pinworm)

Buzz Words: Perianal itching + positive Scotch Tape test

Clinical Presentation: Presents with perianal itching, especially at night. In prepubertal females, it can present as vulvovaginitis.

PPx: Hand hygiene and regular cleaning of objects/surfaces

QUICK TIPS

Be able to differentiate *Giardia* cysts, which are oval-shaped and cause **non-bloody** diarrhea.

MoD: Eggs of the gravid female worm are deposited in the perianal folds. Autoinfection occurs with scratching the perianal area and inadvertently ingesting with contaminated hands. Person-to-person transmission can occur by handling contaminated objects/surfaces.

Dx:

1. Scotch Tape test, in which enterobius eggs can be detected on tape after pressing to the perianal skin

Tx/Mgmt:

1. Albendazole, mebendazole, or pyrantel pamoate

Immunologic and Inflammatory Disorders

Celiac Disease (Gluten-Sensitivity Enteropathy)

Buzz Words: Atrophic intestinal villi + steatorrhea

Clinical Presentation: This is an autoimmune disease of the small intestine caused by sensitivity to gluten and similar proteins, resulting in malabsorption and steatorrhea. Often seen with other autoimmune diseases such as type 1 diabetes mellitus, IgA deficiency, and autoimmune thyroid disease, and may be associated with trisomy 21. Due to a genetic predisposition.

May present at any age with irritability, steatorrhea, failure-to-thrive, and sometimes signs of nutrient/vitamin deficiency (e.g., microcytic anemia from Fe^{2+} deficiency).

PPx: N/A

MoD: Inappropriate T-cell and IgA-mediated response to gluten and related proteins. Duodenum is the most commonly damaged site.

Dx:

1. Anti-tissue transglutaminase and anti-endomysial antibodies
2. Mucosal biopsy demonstrating villous atrophy

Tx/Mgmt:

1. Gluten-free diet will induce resolution within a few weeks to months.

Inflammatory Bowel Disease

Inflammatory bowel disease (IBD) is the collective term for Crohn disease (CD) and ulcerative colitis (UC). IBD typically presents between 15 and 30 years of age and occurs most frequently in people of Caucasian and Ashkenazi Jewish origin. This disease should be considered in a child or adolescent with bloody diarrhea, abdominal pain, growth failure, or perianal disease. Extraintestinal manifestations include erythema nodosum, pyoderma gangrenosum, migratory polyarthritis, aphthous ulcers, uveitis, and ankylosing spondylitis. IBDs are extremely high yield for all subject exams.

Crohn Disease

Buzz Words: Skip lesions + non-caseating granulomas + "string-sign" from narrowing of the ileum + young adult female

Clinical Presentation: CD is characterized by a chronic transmural inflammation of any part of the GI tract, from the mouth to anus. Most commonly involves the terminal ileum.

Can present with postprandial diarrhea, abdominal pain, weight loss, low-grade fever in a young adult (female > male). Perianal disease, fistulas (e.g., enterocutaneous or colovesical), fissures, abscesses, kidney stones, and gallstones are characteristic and help differentiate from UC.

PPx: Avoid smoking

MoD: Segmental, transmural inflammation of the GI tract resulting from combination of the individual's genetic susceptibility, external environment, intestinal microbial flora, and immune responses.

Dx:
1. FOBT
2. Colonoscopy
3. Biopsy
4. Fecal calprotectin

Tx/Mgmt:
1. Initial treatment: For mild disease, use aminosalicyates. For moderate to severe disease, use glucocorticoids or exclusive enteral nutrition.
2. Maintenance therapy: Aminosalicylates, methotrexate, azathioprine, infliximab, adalimumab.

Ulcerative Colitis

Buzz Words: "Lead-pipe" radiographical appearance + sclerosing cholangitis + young adult male

Clinical Presentation: UC is characterized by chronic inflammation of the rectal mucosa with or without colon involvement (Table 9.3). Associated with sclerosing cholangitis. Can present with rectal bleeding, abdominal cramping, diarrhea, tenesmus in a young adult (male > female). A major complication is toxic megacolon, which is caused by disruption of the mucosal barrier that allows bacterial invasion. This

QUICK TIPS

Both types of **stones** (kidney stones and gallstones) are seen in **Crohn's.**

TABLE 9.3 Comparison of Crohn Disease (CD) Versus Ulcerative Colitis (UC)

	CD	UC
Origin	Terminal ileum	Rectum
Age of onset	10–40 years	10–30 years
Progression	"Skip lesions"	Uniform spread proximally
Thickness of inflammation	Transmural	Mucosal/submucosal
Symptoms	Crampy pain	Bloody diarrhea
Complications	Fistulas, abscesses, obstruction, anemia, arthritis, skin changes, not many extraintestinal manifestations	Toxic megacolon, hemorrhage, weight loss, ulceration, primary sclerosing cholangitis, erythema nodosum, pyoderma gangrenosum
Serological markers	ASCA+	p-ANCA+
Radiology	"String sign" and strictures	"Lead colon pipe"
Colon cancer risk	Small risk (1%–3%)	Large risk (25%)
Surgical intervention	Only for complications	Curative, colectomy → ileostomy/J-pouch
Medical intervention	5-ASA meds, steroids, biologics (infliximab, adalimumab)	5-ASA meds, steroids

5-ASA, 5-Aminosalicylic acid.

leads to dilation and further inflammation of the colon, resulting in abdominal distension, fever, and septic shock. UC also carries a greater risk of colorectal cancer relative to CD.

PPx: N/A

MoD: Continuous mucosal inflammation (no skip lesions) that begins at the rectum and ascends proximally.

Dx:

1. FOBT
2. Colonoscopy
3. Biopsy

Tx/Mgmt:

1. Initial treatment: For mild disease, oral/rectal 5-aminosalicylic acid (5-ASA) or sulfasalazine. For moderate to severe disease: Oral glucocorticoids.
2. Maintenance therapy: 5-ASA agent.

Disorders of the Oral Cavity

Dental Caries

Buzz Words: Pain with eating + prolonged bottle feeding + falling asleep with a nipple in the mouth

Clinical Presentation: Can be asymptomatic or cause transient pain with heat, cold, or sweet foods/drinks. Occurs more commonly in children with prolonged bottle feeding, or those that frequently fall asleep with a nipple in the mouth.

PPx: Oral hygiene, regular dental evaluation, do not allow children to take bottles to bed

MoD: Due to bacterial demineralization of tooth. *Streptococcus mutans* is the most common causative agent.

Dx:
1. Discoloration/cavitation of tooth

Tx/Mgmt:
1. Placement of dental filling/crowns

Teething Syndrome

Clinical Presentation: Eruption of teeth is usually symmetric with the mandibular central incisors being the first primary teeth to appear. This process typically begins between 6 and 10 months of age. Infants whose primary teeth are erupting tend to have gingival irritation, demonstrate fussiness, frequent chewing on objects, and excessive drooling. May be accompanied by systemic symptoms such as slightly increased temperature (no fever, temp below 100.4°F), runny nose, and diarrhea.

PPx: N/A

MoD: Eruption of teeth is usually symmetric with the mandibular central incisors being the first primary teeth to appear.

Dx:
1. Clinical

Tx/Mgmt:
1. A chilled teething device and acetaminophen

Disorders of the Stomach, Small intestine, and Colon

Appendicitis

Buzz Words: Acute periumbilical pain that migrates to RLQ + leukocytosis + peritoneal signs + fever + anorexia + increased white blood cells (WBCs) with leukocytosis

Clinical Presentation: Presents with constant dull periumbilical pain that localizes to McBurney's point (an area 2/3 from the umbilical to the anterior superior iliac spine). Also see fever, nausea, vomiting and anorexia. Rovsing sign, psoas sign, obturator sign, Dunphy sign may be present. Appendiceal diameter greater than 6 mm in imaging studies. Occurs more commonly in adults, but does occur in school-age children and adolescents. Involuntary guarding and rebound tenderness suggest peritonitis secondary to appendiceal perforation. High yield for Pediatrics subject exam.

PPx: N/A

MoD: Nonspecific obstruction of appendiceal lumen most commonly by fecalith, undigested food, or lymphoid hyperplasia. Once the lumen is obstructed, the appendiceal lumen becomes distended and ischemic, leading to release of inflammatory mediators. Without surgical intervention, it may perforate (most common after 72 hours)

Dx:

1. Physical exam.
2. Ultrasound = first-line imaging, if unable to visualize, can perform computed tomography (CT).
3. If female of reproductive age, must first obtain urine pregnancy test to rule out ectopic pregnancy (surgical emergency) and consider urine analysis to rule out UTI.

Tx/Mgmt:

1. Fluid resuscitation
2. Antibiotics
3. Appendectomy

Peptic Ulcer Disease

Buzz Words:

Epigastric pain **exacerbated** with eating → gastric ulcer

Epigastric pain **improved** with eating → duodenal ulcer

Clinical Presentation: Peptic ulcer disease (PUD) is characterized by gastric or duodenal ulcers, which are defects in the mucosa that extend into the deeper layers of the stomach or intestinal wall. Occurs less commonly in children than in adults, but should be considered in patients with long-term nonsteroidal anti-inflammatory drugs (NSAIDs) use or *Helicobacter pylori* infection.

Epigastric pain is the most prominent symptom in patients with peptic ulcers. With gastric ulcers, pain is exacerbated by eating due to release of gastric acids. Alternatively, pain caused by duodenal ulcers is relieved by eating, due to release of pancreatic bicarbonate secretions, which neutralizes the overall acidity of secretions. With posterior duodenal ulcers, must be concerned about perforation and injury to the gastroduodenal artery → patient will manifest with signs and symptoms of acute abdomen and upper GI bleed.

PPx: Minimize NSAID use or use celecoxib in place of NSAIDs

MoD: NSAIDs reduce production of prostaglandins, which protects the mucosal lining from injury by luminal acid. *H. pylori* leads to impaired mucosal defense and leads to hyper-secretion of gastric acids.

Dx:

1. Rule out *H. pylori* infection with urea breath test, blood antibodies to *H. pylori*, or detection of *H. pylori* in feces.
2. Endoscopy to confirm presence of ulcers.

Tx/Mgmt:

1. If *H. pylori* infection is present, eradicate via triple therapy (PPI, amoxicillin, clarithyromycin).
2. If NSAIDS-related ulcers, start PPIs and avoid/discontinue NSAIDS.

Hirschsprung Disease

Buzz Words: Neonate + failure to pass meconium + "squirt sign"

Clinical Presentation: Presents with symptoms of colonic obstruction, including bilious/feculent emesis, abdominal distension, and failure to pass meconium within 48 hours of birth. Increased incidence in trisomy 21. High yield for Pediatrics subject exam.

PPx: N/A

MoD: Caused by failure of ganglion cells to migrate caudally to the distal rectum during embryonic development.

Dx: Explosive expulsion of gas and stool ("squirt sign") on digital rectal examination. Suction rectal biopsy showing absence of ganglion cells is gold standard for diagnosis.

Tx/Mgmt: Resection of the affected segment with primary anastomosis of the bowel (Fig. 9.4).

Intussusception

Buzz Words: Colicky abdominal pain + 6–12 months old + "currant jelly" stools + sausage shaped mass in RUQ + bull's eye sign on ultrasound + drawing up legs toward the abdomen

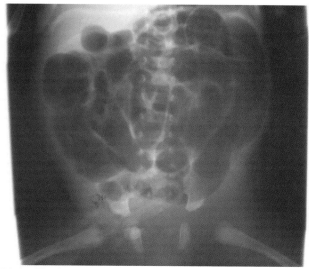

FIG. 9.4 Hirschsprung on radiography. (From Robb et al., *Hirschsprung's Disease, Surgery,* 2008, Elsevier.)

Clinical Presentation: Intussusception is a process in which part of the intestine telescopes into itself, which may lead to ischemia due to disrupted blood supply. Previously healthy infants or children present with intermittent abdominal pain, irritability, cramping, vomiting, and "currant jelly" stool (stool mixed with blood, mucus, and sloughed mucosa = late sign). During intervals between pain, observe periods of calm or normal behavior. Infants may draw up the legs toward the abdomen and cry when in pain.

PPx: N/A

MoD: Majority of cases are idiopathic, while the rest have an underlying cause that creates a lead point for intussusception. The most common cause of a lead point is intestinal infection with lymphadenopathy. Meckel diverticulum can also cause intussusception. The telescoping leads to occlusion of blood supply with ischemia and sloughing of mucosa leading to currant jelly stools.

Dx:

1. A "bull's eye" or "coiled spring" lesion on ultrasound, showing the telescoped intestinal layer
2. Resolution of symptoms with barium or air enema (both diagnostic and therapeutic)

Tx/Mgmt:

1. Barium or air anemia
2. If reduction not achieved with enema, surgery (Fig. 9.5)

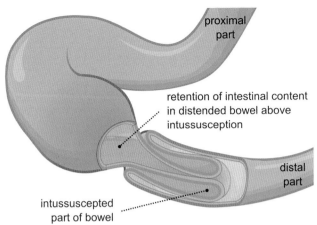

FIG. 9.5 Schematic for intussusception. (From Wikipedia.)

Functional Abdominal Pain

Buzz Words: Chronic abdominal pain that does not interfere with pleasurable activities or sleep

Clinical Presentation: This is the most common cause of chronic abdominal pain in children and adolescents. Chronic (>2 months) epigastric/periumbilical/infraumbilical pain, bloating, nausea, vomiting, early satiety with normal clinical findings. The pain does not interfere with pleasurable activities or sleep. May be exacerbated or triggered during times of stress. Functional abdominal pain disorder subtypes include functional dyspepsia, irritable bowel syndrome, and abdominal migraine.

PPx: N/A

MoD: Patient senses pain without an underlying organic cause. Risk factors include anxiety, life stressors, alcoholism, antisocial or conduct disorders, and family history of functional pain disorders.

Dx: See Rome diagnostic criteria

Tx/Mgmt:
1. Management of anxiety/stress through psychologic interventions (e.g., relaxation, distraction, SSRI).
2. Probiotics, water-soluble fiber, or peppermint oil.
3. Dietary restriction and antimotility agents are not recommended in children and adolescents, although used for adults.

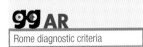
Rome diagnostic criteria

Necrotizing Enterocolitis

Buzz Words: Pneumatosis intestinalis and/or air in portal vein + premature/low-birth-weight newborn + bloody stools +feeding intolerance + abdominal distension. Any condition that predisposes to hypoperfusion of the bowel

Clinical Presentation: This is the one of the most common emergencies of the newborn.

Occurs in a premature or low-birth-weight newborn, usually within 30 days of birth. Presents with abdominal distension, abdominal tenderness, bloody stool, feeding intolerance. Breastfeeding reduces risk of necrotizing enterocolitis (NEC).

PPx: N/A

MoD: Although the exact cause is unknown, it is thought to be due to inadequate defenses of the bowel, leading to inflammation, bacterial invasion, and ischemic necrosis of the bowel mucosa.

Dx:

1. Clinical diagnosis.
2. Imaging may show pneumatosis intestinalis (air in the bowel wall), which is pathognomic for NEC. May also show air in portal vein, air-fluid levels, and thickened bowel walls.

Tx/Mgmt:

1. Medical management includes NPO, IV antibiotics, parenteral fluids and nutrition.
2. Proceed to surgical management if evidence of perforation (free air under the diaphragm or peritoneal signs) or clinical deterioration despite medical therapy. Involves exploratory laparotomy with resection of necrotic bowel segments.

Malrotation with Midgut Volvulus

Buzz Words: Small intestine with "corkscrew sign" + abnormal position of ligament of Treitz + emesis + neonate

Clinical Presentation: Intestinal malrotation occurs due to incomplete rotation of the embryonic gut. It is commonly seen with congenital diaphragmatic hernia, heterotaxy, and abdominal wall defects (i.e., omphalocele, gastroschisis, prune belly syndrome). Malrotation significantly increases the risk of the midgut to twist around itself and surrounding mesenteric vessels (i.e., volvulus), leading to obstruction and infarction of the bowel (surgical emergency).

Bilious or non-bilious emesis with abdominal discomfort. Signs of peritonitis, shock, and hematochezia suggest perforation and bowel ischemia. Onset can be insidious or sudden (insidious > sudden). Majority of children with malrotation present with volvulus

gg AR

Pneumatosis intestinalis

before 1 month of age, but can present in older children.

PPx: N/A

MoD: The intestines fail to undergo counter-clockwise rotation around the axis of the superior mesenteric artery after the 10th week of gestation. The end result is the cecum becomes abnormally attached to the right lateral abdominal wall by bands of peritoneum (Ladd bands), which can cross the bowel and cause obstruction.

Dx:

1. Contrast enema shows a high, medially directed cecum.
2. Upper GI imaging shows abnormal position of ligament of Treitz and "corkscrew sign" of the distal duodenum and proximal jejunum.

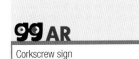
Corkscrew sign

Tx/Mgmt:

1. Ladd procedure, which involves division of Ladd bands and fixation of the cecum and colon in their correct anatomical location.

Milk Protein Allergy

Buzz Words: Healthy infant + **progressive** onset of vomiting, diarrhea, colicky abdominal pain, bloody stools

Clinical Presentation: Food protein-induced proctocolitis/enterocolitis (most commonly caused by milk-protein). This is a common phenomenon that occurs in an otherwise healthy young infant that typically resolves by 1 year of age.

Can present as an otherwise healthy young infant with progressive onset of diarrhea, severe vomiting, colicky abdominal pain, irritability, and blood-tinged stools with ingestion of cow's milk or soymilk (can occur with other dietary proteins). Chronic blood loss in stools can lead to anemia.

PPx: N/A

MoD: Non-IgE-mediated sensitivity to food proteins that results in inflammation of the colon or small bowel. Cow's milk and soy protein are the most common causes.

Dx:

1. Resolution of symptoms within a few weeks after elimination of the suspected protein from diet.

Tx/Mgmt:

1. For breast-fed infants, mother must remove all milk protein from her diet.
2. For formula-fed infants, must use elemental (hydrolyzed) formula.

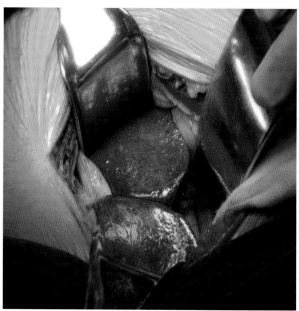

FIG. 9.6 Liver in Dubin-Johnson syndrome. (From Zhou et al., Dubin-Johnson syndrome with cholecystolithiasis and choledocholithiasis. *Intl J Surg Case Rep*, 2013, Elsevier.)

Disorders of Liver

Dubin-Johnson Syndrome

Buzz Words: Black liver + episodes of mild self-resolving jaundice + direct (conjugated) bilirubinemia (Fig. 9.6)

Clinical Presentation: Intermittent episodes of mild scleral icterus that may be accompanied by vague abdominal pain. Episodes are commonly triggered by illnesses, pregnancy, or use of oral contraceptives.

PPx: N/A

MoD: Defective canalicular excretion of conjugated bilirubin from the liver, resulting in leakage into the systemic circulation.

Dx:

1. Normal physical exam except for the scleral icterus.
2. Lab tests show conjugated hyperbilirubinemia with normal LFTs:
   - Differentiate from Rotor syndrome by urinary **coproporphyrin excretion** (normal in Dubin-Johnson, while elevated in Rotor syndrome) and liver biopsy (blackened appearance in Dubin-Johnson, normal in Rotor syndrome).

Tx/Mgmt:

1. Benign, no treatment required

Rotor Syndrome

Buzz Words: Absence of black liver + episodes of mild self-resolving jaundice + direct (conjugated) bilirubinemia

Clinical Presentation: Intermittent episodes of mild scleral icterus.

PPx: N/A

MoD: Defect in intrahepatic binding of direct bilirubin, leading to leakage of direct bilirubin into the circulation and subsequent direct hyperbilirubinemia. Genetics?

Dx:
1. Normal physical exam except for the scleral icterus.
2. Lab tests show conjugated hyperbilirubinemia with normal LFTs.
3. Elevated coproporphyrin and normal appearance on liver biopsy.

Tx/Mgmt:
1. Benign, no treatment required.

Gilbert Syndrome

Buzz Words: Jaundice in setting of stress + unconjugated hyperbilirubinemia

Clinical Presentation: Recurrent episodes of jaundice triggered by dehydration, fasting, overexertion, stress, and menstruation. Otherwise, patient is asymptomatic.

PPx: N/A

MoD: Decreased level of uridine diphosphoglucuronate-glucuronosyltransferase (UGT), which is a hepatic enzyme responsible for solubilization of bilirubin through conjugation. In periods of stress, bilirubin production is increased but unable to be compensated by UGT activity. The end result is increased serum levels of unconjugated bilirubin in times of stress. Genetics?

Dx:
1. Unconjugated (indirect) hyperbilirubinemia with normal LFTs.
2. Rifampin test: rise in unconjugated bilirubin upon administration of rifampin.

Tx/Mgmt:
1. Benign, no treatment required.

Crigler-Najjar

Buzz Words:
Severe jaundice/**kernicterus** in infant + indirect hyperbilirubinemia; Crigler-Najjar Type I
Severe/moderate jaundice responsive to phenobarbital + indirect hyperbilirubinemia; Crigler-Najjar Type II

QUICK TIPS
Crigler-Najjar Type I is worse than Type II.

QUICK TIPS
Cribler-Najjar I dies in infancy (<age **1**), while in a **crib**. Crigler-Najjar **II** lives longer (>age **2**, usually to adulthood).

Clinical Presentation: Persistent indirect (unconjugated) bilirubin within the few days after birth with normal liver function test. Two types of Crigler-Najjar exist: Type I is characterized by more severe hyperbilirubinemia (total bilirubin of 20–50 mg/dL) due to absent UGT activity. Kernicterus (deposition of bilirubin in basal ganglia) is present, resulting in opisthotonus, seizures, and **death in infancy.** Type II (total bilirubin <20 mg/dL) has reduced UGT activity and only rarely leads to kernicterus, patient usually **lives to adulthood** (Table 9.4).

PPx: N/A

MoD: Autosomal recessive inheritance: Absent/decreased UGT activity, leading to unconjugated hyperbilirubinemia.

Dx:

1. Liver panel shows very high total bilirubin and reduced fecal urobilinogen excretion due to significant reduction in the conjugated bilirubin (see bilirubin metabolism link):
   - Can be differentiated from other etiologies of jaundice due to its persistent nature and uniquely high level of total bilirubin.

Tx/Mgmt:

1. If type I, phototherapy and plasmapheresis: Liver transplant is the only cure.
2. If type II, phenobarbital or clofibrate.

Bilirbubin metabolism

TABLE 9.4 Congenital Hyperbilirubinemia

Syndrome	Inheritance	Abnormality	Clinical Features
Unconjugated Hyperbilirubinemia			
Gilbert's	Autosomal dominant	↓ Glucuronyl transferase	Intermittent mild jaundice (esp. with fasting)
Crigler-Najjar type I	Autosomal recessive	Absent glucuronyl transferase	Severe jaundice and kernicterus in neonate
Crigler-Najjar type II	Autosomal recessive	↓↓ Glucuronyl transferase	Severe/moderate jaundice in neonate
Conjugated Hyperbilirubinemia			
Dubin-Johnson	Autosomal recessive	↓ Canalicular excretion of bilirubin	Intermittent mild jaundice
Rotor's	Autosomal recessive	↓ Bilirubin uptake ↓ intrahepatic binding	Intermittent very mild jaundice

Congenital Disorders

Biliary Atresia

Buzz Words: Progressive onset of conjugated hyperbilirubinemia + neonate

Clinical Presentation: Newborn with progressive jaundice,
dark urine, pale stools, and hepatosplenomegaly.
Rapidly progresses to cirrhosis by 4 months of age
without intervention.

PPx: N/A

MoD: It is an idiopathic, obliterative disease of the extra-
hepatic biliary tree that presents with biliary obstruction. The causes of biliary atresia (BA) are unknown but
are thought to be multifactorial, involving infectious,
genetic, and immunologic mechanisms.

Dx:
1. Elevated conjugated bilirubin, LFTs, and gamma glu-
   tamyl transpeptidase (GGTP).
2. Cholangiogram is gold standard for confirmation.

Tx/Mgmt:
1. Kasai portoenterostomy (Roux-en-Y intestinal loop
   attached to the porta hepatis) is initial treatment of
   choice and will re-establish bile flow:
   • Younger age at the time the Kasai procedure is
     performed, better the outcome.
   • Most patients will eventually require liver transplan-
     tation, even with Kasai procedure.
   • BA is, in fact, the most common indication for liver
     transplantation in children.

Esophageal Atresia

Buzz Words:
Drooling + inability to pass oral gastric tube into stomach
  → Isolated esophageal atresia
Choking/coughing with first feeding + drooling +
  inability to pass oral gastric tube into stomach →
  Esophageal atresia (EA) with tracheoesophageal
  fistula (TEF)

Clinical Presentation: This is a common congenital defect of
the GI tract, in which the upper esophagus does not
connect with the lower esophagus/stomach. It most
commonly occurs with a distal TEF. Newborn with
excessive drooling. First feeding often produces coughing, respiratory distress, and choking. Polyhydramnios
is commonly present during gestation in isolated
esophageal atresia, due to inability to swallow amniotic

99 AR

Esophageal atresia types

fluid in utero. On the other hand, if TEF is present, polyhydramnios is absent as a result of fluid moving into the stomach through the fistula. EA is often seen as part of the VACTERL or CHARGE associations.

PPx: N/A

MoD: N/A

Dx:

1. If isolated EA, ultrasound reveals polyhydramnios in utero.
2. Failure to pass oral gastric tube into stomach.
3. TEF may be diagnosed with an upper GI series with water-soluble contrast agents.

Tx/Mgmt:

1. Surgical correction

Meckel Diverticulum

Buzz Words: **Painless** lower GI bleeding in an otherwise healthy child + ectopic gastric mucosa

Clinical Presentation: Meckel diverticulum is a true diverticulum that arises from an incomplete obliteration of the vitelline (omphalomesenteric) duct. One of the most high-yield diseases for the Pediatrics shelf.

Can present as painless lower GI bleeding during the first 2 years of life. May be seen with recurrent small bowel intussusception.

PPx: N/A

MoD: Meckel diverticulum is a vitelline duct remnant, which usually obliterates by the seventh week of embryonic development. The pouch may contain gastric mucosa that causes excess gastric secretions, leading to mucosal ulceration and bleeding.

Dx:

1. Technetium nuclear scan to identify gastric mucosa

Tx/Mgmt:

1. For symptomatic patients, fluid and electrolyte replenishment, PPIs to reduce gastric secretions, then surgical resection of the gastric mucosa.
2. For asymptomatic patients, observe.

Pyloric Stenosis

Buzz Words: Projectile, nonbilious emesis in an infant+ "olive-like" mass in RUQ

Clinical Presentation: Infant 3–6 weeks old presents with forceful, nonbilious emesis immediately after eating. Newborn remains hungry and eager to eat, but unable to keep the food down. A small "olive-like" mass may be palpated in the RUQ. There may also be signs of dehydration.

MoD: Idiopathic hypertrophy of the pyloric sphincter that develops over the first 3–6 weeks of life. Risk factors are being a first-born male and early administration of oral erythromycin. Persistent vomiting will result in hypokalemic, hypochloremic, metabolic alkalosis.

Dx:

1. Abdominal ultrasound is the diagnostic method of choice and shows thickened and elongated pylorus.
2. Barium swallow may show "string sign" (elongated, narrow pyloric lumen).

Tx/Mgmt:

1. Must first correct electrolyte abnormalities and dehydration, most often will see hypochloremic, hypokalemic metabolic alkalosis.
2. Once clinical status is stable, proceed with surgery (Ramstedt pyloromyotomy).

Duodenal Atresia

Buzz Words: Bilious/nonbilious vomiting in the first day of life + "double bubble sign" + polyhydramnios + trisomy 21

Clinical Presentation: Newborn presents with gastric distension and vomiting in the first day of life. Vomiting is often bilious but may be nonbilious due to being proximal to the ampulla of Vater. It is commonly associated with trisomy 21.

MoD: Failure to re-canalize the intestinal tract during 8 to 10 weeks of gestation, resulting in congenital absence of the duodenal lumen.

Dx:

1. Abdominal imaging shows "double bubble" sign due to air entrapment in the stomach and proximal duodenum.

Tx/Mgmt:

1. NG tube decompression and IV fluids
2. Surgery (duodenoduodenostomy)

Disorders of Jaundice

Physiologic Jaundice

Buzz Words: Indirect hyperbilirubinemia + within first week of life + adequate weight gain/maintenance + normal urine/stool output

Clinical Presentation: Jaundice in a healthy-appearing newborn with appropriate weight gain/maintenance during the first week of life. Typically resolves by the end of the first week of life in term infants, but can last a little longer in preterm infants.

MoD: Newborns have low levels of glucuronosyltransferase, which normally conjugates bilirubin. Additionally, there is an increased bilirubin load due to shorter life span of fetal red blood cells and decreased enterohepatic circulation.

Dx:

1. Clinical diagnosis + liver function panel (mild indirect hyperbilirubinemia)

Tx/Mgmt:

1. Benign, observe (Fig. 9.7)

Breastfeeding Jaundice

Buzz Words: Indirect hyperbilirubinemia + within the first week of life + jaundice + decreased urine/stool output

Clinical Presentation: Newborn less than 1 week of age presents with jaundice and weight loss. If not treated may lead to kernicterus.

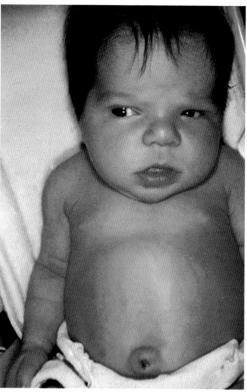

FIG. 9.7 Jaundice in newborn. (From Wikipedia.)

PPx: Monitoring and assessment of breastfeeding during the birth hospitalization: Postnatal education and support on breastfeeding

MoD: Failure to successfully initiate breastfeeding, resulting in inadequate nutrient intake, significant weight loss, and dehydration. This also results in decreased passage of stool and urine, which leads to decreased excretion of bilirubin.

Dx:
1. Clinical diagnosis
2. Liver function panel (indirect hyperbilirubinemia)

Tx/Mgmt:
1. Phototherapy may be required.
2. If infant has lost more than 7% of birth weight at 5 days of life, supplementation with banked human milk or formula milk is recommended:
   - Glucose water or sterile water should not be used.

Breast Milk Jaundice

Buzz Words: Indirect hyperbilirubinemia + after the first week of life + jaundice + adequate/excessive breast milk intake

Clinical Presentation: An otherwise healthy newborn presents with jaundice after the first week of life.

PPx: N/A

MoD: Total bilirubin levels are typically mildly elevated (>5 mg/dL) for several weeks following birth. Human milk contains beta-glucuronidase enzyme that deconjugates intestinal bilirubin, which is easily absorbed through enterohepatic circulation and leads to accumulation of indirect bilirubin in the systemic circulation.

Dx:
1. Clinical diagnosis
2. Liver function panel (mild indirect hyperbilirubinemia)

Tx/Mgmt:
1. Usually benign and self-limited.
2. If pathological (total bilirubin > 20), replace breast feeding with formula for 1–2 days ± phototherapy.

GUNNER PRACTICE

1. A 13-month-old male is brought to the Emergency Department by his mother. She states that for the past few hours, he has been having repeated 1–2-minute episodes of screaming and appearing confused. He was born without complication via spontaneous vaginal

delivery at 39 weeks and 3 days, and his remaining medical history is significant only for eczema and a single emergency department visit for bronchiolitis. His vital signs are T 99.1°F, BP 90/54, HR 125, RR 30, SpO$_2$ 98% on room air. On exam, he is a well-appearing, playful child with no detectable abnormalities. However, 15 minutes later, another "episode" is observed, during which an abdominal ultrasound yields the image below from the right upper quadrant. What is the most likely diagnosis?

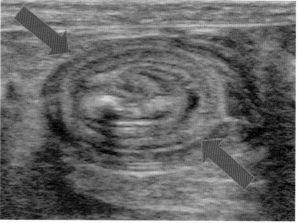

(Gore RM, Silvers RI, Thakrar KH, Wenzke DR, Mehta UK, Newmark GM, Berlin JW: Bowel obstruction. *Radiol Clin North Am* 53(6):1225–1240, 2015. Copyright © 2015 Elsevier Inc.)

- A. Viral gastroenteritis
- B. Intussusception
- C. Necrotizing enterocolitis
- D. Meckel diverticulum
- E. Volvulus due to malrotation

2. A 2-week-old female infant is brought to the pediatrician's office. Her mother complains that she is not eating and digesting well. The baby has appeared less and less interested in latching during the last week, and has had increasing emesis, sometimes dark green in color, after her small feeds. She was born at 37 weeks and 4 days without apparent complication, but failed to pass meconium for 51 hours after delivery. Since then, she has had five total bowel movements, each of which required digital stimulation of the rectum and resulted in "explosions" of gas and feces. Her family history is notable for hypertension on her mother's side and diabetes on her father's side. The infant's vital signs are T 98.3°F, HR 135, BP

82/46, RR 35, SpO$_2$ 98% on room air. Examination yields a calm infant with a mildly distended abdomen. Stool is palpated through the abdominal wall in the left lower quadrant, and rectal exam results in expulsion of stool. Of the following, which is the next best step in management?

A. Contrast enema
B. Abdominal CT scan
C. Emergent laparotomy
D. Colonoscopy
E. Reassurance and lactation consultation

3. A 15-year-old male is brought to the pediatric office by his father. He states that he has been having more than four painless bowel movements per day for the last 20 days. During the last 2 days, his stools have progressed from watery to frankly bloody, and have increased to 15 or more daily. He also notes fatigue, chills, and left knee pain. His past medical history is notable only for two episodes of back, hip, and knee discomfort accompanied by fatigue, both in the last 2 years. His vital signs are T 100.2°F, HR 103, BP 104/72, RR 18, SpO$_2$ 98% on room air. Examination yields conjunctival pallor, mild tenderness to palpation in both lower quadrants of the abdomen and a slightly swollen, tender, and warm left knee joint. Initial labs show WBC 12.1, Hgb 10.2, PLT 292, normal basic metabolic panel and liver function tests, albumin 3.3, CRP 15 and ESR 44. Stool cultures are negative. Of the following, what is the next best step in management?

A. Levofloxacin treatment
B. Colonoscopy
C. Schedule for colectomy
D. Infliximab and azathioprine treatment
E. Surgical consult for emergent laparotomy

ANSWERS: What Would Gunner Jess/Jim Do?

1. WWGJD? A 13-month-old male is brought to the Emergency Department by his mother. She states that for the past few hours, he has been having repeated 1–2 minute episodes of screaming and appearing confused. He was born without complication via spontaneous vaginal delivery at 39 weeks and 3 days, and his remaining medical history is significant only for eczema and a single emergency department visit for bronchiolitis. His vital signs are T 99.1°F, BP 90/54, HR 125, RR 30, SpO$_2$ 98% on room air. On exam, he is a well-appearing, playful child with no detectable abnormalities. However, 15 minutes later, another "episode" is observed, during which an abdominal ultrasound yields the image below from the right upper quadrant. What is the most likely diagnosis?

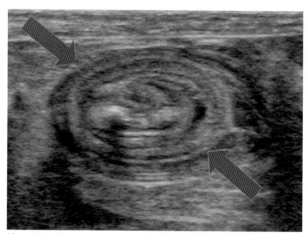

(Gore RM, Silvers RI, Thakrar KH, Wenzke DR, Mehta UK, Newmark GM, Berlin JW: Bowel obstruction. *Radiol Clin North Am* 53(6):1225–1240, 2015. Copyright © 2015 Elsevier Inc.)

Answer: B, Intussusception

Explanation: This question assesses for recognition of a serious medical condition, given nonspecific complaints and a classic image. This is a 13-month-old male child with intermittent screaming, concurrent with the above abdominal ultrasound finding. This finding, called the "target" sign, is the *en face* view of small intestine telescoping into small intestine. It typically occurs in children under 2 years old. There are multiple "lead points" that can cause the intestinal invagination in children, a common one being enlarged Peyer patches due to viral infection (or rotavirus vaccination). Symptoms can be nonspecific and include pain, screaming, and altered mental status, as well as vomiting (nonbilious progressing to bilious) and, classically, "currant jelly" stools (due to blood and mucus from ischemic bowel wall mixing with stool).

A. Viral gastroenteritis → Incorrect. This patient has had no vomiting or loose stools, and has no fever or other signs of infection.

C. Necrotizing enterocolitis → Incorrect. This is generally a disease of newborns, especially premature infants, involving ischemia of the bowel wall and invasion of bowel flora past the mucosal layer. Infants may present with bilious emesis, hematochezia, and exam findings consistent with an acute abdomen. Imaging of advanced cases will classically reveal pneumatosis intestinalis (air in the bowel wall), portal vein gas, and pneumoperitoneum.

D. Meckel diverticulum → Incorrect. The classic patient with a symptomatic Meckel diverticulum is a 2-year-old with painless hematochezia.

E. Small intestinal volvulus due to malrotation → Incorrect. Though this can present at any time, it is characterized by bilious emesis, hematochezia, abdominal distention, and/or peritonitis with imaging consistent with malrotation or midgut volvulus.

2. WWGJD? A 2-week-old female infant is brought to the pediatrician's office. Her mother complains that she is not eating and digesting well. The baby has appeared less and less interested in latching during the last week, and has had increasing emesis, sometimes dark green in color, after her small feeds. She was born at 37 weeks and 4 days without apparent complication, but failed to pass meconium for 51 hours after delivery. Since then, she has had five total bowel movements, each of which required digital stimulation of the rectum and resulted in "explosions" of gas and feces. Her family history is notable for hypertension on her mother's side and diabetes on her father's side. The infant's vital signs are T 98.3°F, HR 135, BP 82/46, RR 35, SpO_2 98% on room air. Examination yields a calm infant with a mildly distended abdomen. Stool is palpated through the abdominal wall in the left lower quadrant, and rectal exam results in expulsion of stool. Of the following, which is the next best step in management?

Answer: A, Contrast enema

Explanation: This question tests the ability to recognize a common congenital abnormality. This is a 2-week-old infant with a history of delayed meconium passage, constipation, distention, bilious emesis, and "explosions" of feces and gas with rectal stimulation (known as the "squirt sign"). This is a classic presentation of Hirschsprung disease (HD), a disorder in which at least a segment of colon is aganglionic and will not propel fecal matter appropriately. Reasonable approaches in infants include barium enema (looking for a "transition" between abnormal and normal colon), manometry (looking for abnormal motor responses of the colon), and rectal suction biopsy (looking for aganglionic colon). As contrast enema was the provided choice of these three, A is the solution. Of note, Hirschsprung disease is one of the two most common disorders associated with failure to pass meconium within 2 days (the other being cystic fibrosis, or CF), and is highly associated with multiple syndromes, including trisomy 21. When a newborn has delayed meconium passage, think CF or HD.

B. Abdominal CT scan → Incorrect. While abdominal CT scan may or may not reveal the defective segment of colon, it is neither the most efficacious nor the safest way to proceed. Remember, radiation from imaging is to be avoided whenever possible, especially in Pediatrics.

C. Emergent laparotomy → Incorrect. The infant is calm with normal vital signs, and there is nothing to suggest that there is an acute abdomen picture here. This is also not the appropriate management for suspected HD.

D. Colonoscopy → Incorrect. This neither addresses the question of whether HD is present nor provides a logistically feasible option. Again, tests with significant risk, including sedation requirements, are less favorable in pediatrics, and especially in infants.

E. Reassurance and lactation consultation → Incorrect. This is inappropriate, as there is concern for HD here.

3. WWGJD? A 15-year-old male is brought to the pediatric office by his father. He states that he has been having more than four painless bowel movements per day for the last 20 days. During the last 2 days, his stools have

progressed from watery to frankly bloody, and have increased to 15 or more daily. He also notes fatigue, chills, and left knee pain. His past medical history is notable only for two episodes of back, hip, and knee discomfort accompanied by fatigue, both in the last 2 years. His vital signs are T 100.2°F, HR 103, BP 104/72, RR 18, SpO$_2$ 98% on room air. Examination yields conjunctival pallor, mild tenderness to palpation in both lower quadrants of the abdomen and a slightly swollen, tender, and warm left knee joint. Initial labs show WBC 12.1, Hgb 10.2, PLT 292, normal basic metabolic panel and liver function tests, albumin 3.3, CRP 15 and ESR 44. Stool cultures are negative. Of the following, what is the next best step in management?

Answer: B, Colonoscopy

Explanation: This question tests recognition of a common disease and understanding of how it is to be formally diagnosed. This is an adolescent male with subacute, progressive, bloody diarrhea, arthritis, and systemic symptoms. Additionally, he is mildly anemic and hypoalbuminemic, with high levels of inflammation and a negative (albeit limited) evaluation for bacterial infection. This is a classic presentation of IBD. It is crucial to remember that IBD and treatments for it are differentiated based on whether the patient has UC or CD, and how severe the disease is at the time. Thus, when there is suspicion of IBD, as long as the patient is not in emergent danger, the key is to diagnose appropriately. For this, pathologic diagnosis (often supplemented by imaging) is required. As colonoscopy is the only suggested answer designed as a diagnostic intervention, it is the right answer.

A. Levofloxacin treatment → Incorrect. This patient has had a negative evaluation for bacterial infection so far and IBD is more likely based on the complaints and the chronicity of the symptoms.

C. Schedule for colectomy → Incorrect. This is extremely invasive and inappropriate. If the patient has CD, for example, a colectomy may not relieve his symptoms or inflammation.

D. Infliximab and azathioprine treatment → Incorrect. This is a combined biologic treatment given to certain patients with diagnosed IBD. This patient has not yet been diagnosed and it would be inappropriate to initiate treatment with such specific indications.

E. Surgical consult for emergent laparotomy →
    Incorrect. Though the patient likely has an IBD
    exacerbation, there is no information in the stem
    that would indicate that the patient is unstable or in
    an emergent situation (e.g., toxic megacolon). This
    could, however, be the appropriate management of
    a patient with toxic megacolon, intestinal perfora-
    tion, or acute abdomen.

Gynecologic Disorders

Hao-Hua Wu, Joanne M. Cyganowski, Leo Wang, and
Rebecca Tenney-Soeiro

Introduction

Gynecologic disorders may make up as many as five questions on exam day. These questions involve female patients, many of whom are teenagers, who present with issues concerning puberty, pregnancy and the menstrual cycle. All of the questions here overlap with Pediatrics content, but anything that affects a patient over the age of 18 will not be tested.

This chapter is organized into (1) Infectious, Immunologic and Inflammatory Disorders, (2) Menstrual and Endocrine Disorders, (3) Congenital Disorders, and (4) Gunner Practice.

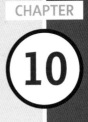

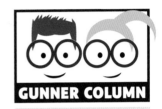

GUNNER COLUMN

Infectious, Immunologic and Inflammatory Disorders

Pelvic Inflammatory Disease

Buzz Words: Cervical motion tenderness

Clinical Presentation: Pelvic inflammatory disease (PID) occurs when an infection of the vagina ascends to the cervix, uterus, fallopian tubes, ovaries, or beyond. The most common causes are *Neisseria gonorrhea* and *Chlamydia trachomatis*. It is not uncommon to find more than one bacterial culprit. Women often complain of low abdominal pain, cramps, fever, and cervical motion tenderness on exam. Patients often have so much pain that they "jump to the chandelier" when performing a pelvic exam and touching the patient's cervix; this is known as the chandelier sign. Patients also can have adnexal tenderness. Because PID is often a sequela of untreated STIs, risk factors include having multiple sexual partners and not using a condom. Complications of untreated PID include adhesions causing infertility.

Prophylaxis (PPx): Decrease number of sexual partners, use condom, treat STIs before they progress to PID

Mechanism of Disease (MoD): STI with bacteria such as *Neisseria gonorrhea* or *Chlamydia trachomatis* ascends female reproductive tract into uterus, fallopian tubes, ovaries, or further into pelvis.

Diagnostic Steps (Dx):

1. Clinical diagnosis with constellation of symptoms and cervical motion tenderness or adnexal tenderness
2. Laparoscopy (definitive diagnosis)

Treatment and Management Steps (Tx/Mgmt):

1. Treatment is Ceftriaxone or Cefoxitin or Cefotetan plus Doxycycline, or Clindamycin plus Gentamycin.

Human Papillomavirus

Buzz Words: Genital wart + cervical dysplasia

Clinical Presentation: One of the most common STDs. Has multiple strains. Human papillomavirus (HPV) 6–11 is low risk and leads to condyloma acuminatum (genital warts). HPV 16–18, 31, 33, 45 are high-risk strains that can lead to cervical dysplasia and cancer.

PPx:

1. Gardasil: quadrivalent vaccine indicated for women 11–26 years old

MoD: Skin-skin contact

Dx:

1. Clinical

Tx/Mgmt:

1. Podophylin for genital warts

Toxic Shock Syndrome

Buzz Words: History of recent tampon use OR nasal packing + septic shock + scalded skin syndrome + no other plausible explanation → toxic shock syndrome 2/2 bacterial toxin transmitted by tampon

Septic shock + diffuse maculopapular rash + subsequent desquamation of hands and feet (scalded skin syndrome) + multisystem involvement (e.g., vomiting, diarrhea, myalgias, nonfocal neuro findings, strawberry tongue) → toxic shock syndrome

Clinical Presentation: Toxic shock syndrome refers to the devastating sequelae of infection by *Staphylococcus aureus* (principal cause) or *Streptococcus pyogenes* through an intramucosal nidus (e.g., tampon or nasal packing) and toxin-mediated over-activation of the immune system. **Nonmenstrual TSS** can occur in anyone with an identifiable focus of *S. aureus* or *S. pyogenes* infection. Learn the Buzz Words as well as the work-up/management of these types of patients well.

PPx: (1) Avoid prolonged use of same tampon or nasal packing. (2) Avoid food poisoning.

MoD: Caused by **toxins** released by *Staph aureus* or *Strep pyogenes*. Toxic shock syndrome toxin (TSST-1)

or exotoxin A (*Strep pyogenes*) bind to MHC II and T-cell receptor → activation of T-cell (cell-mediated immunity) → release of pyrogenic cytokines such as interleukin (IL)-1, IL-2 and tumor necrosis factor (TNF)-alpha → symptoms such as shock

Dx:
1. CBC
2. CMP
3. Liver panel (increased AST, ALT, bilirubin)
4. Cultures (blood, wound if appropriate)

Tx/Mgmt:
1. ABCs (e.g., fluids to stabilize pressure)
2. Antibiotics (broad spectrum or with beta-lactamase resistant antibiotics, e.g., nafcillin) or Vanco if MRSA prevalent area. Add Clinda to reduce toxin production
3. Inpatient admission

> **QUICK TIPS**
> Unlike Step 1, the Pediatrics subject exam will not test you directly on mechanism. However, learning the mechanism will help you understand and remember disease process.

Menstrual and Endocrine Disorders

Polycystic Ovarian Syndrome (aka Stein-Leventhal Syndrome)

Buzz Words: Hirsutism + acne + male patterned baldness + amenorrhea/oligorrhea + multiple cysts in ovaries + acanthosis → PCOS

Clinical Presentation: Polycystic ovarian syndrome (PCOS) is a disorder (common disorder of reproductive hormone dysfunction + metabolic abnormalities) of unknown etiology that is a common cause of secondary amenorrhea. It is diagnosed if patients meet two of three Rotterdam criteria: (1) laboratory or clinical signs (e.g., male-pattern baldness, acne, or hirsutism) if high serum androgen present; (2) amenorrhea or oligomenorrhea; (3) cystic ovaries seen on pelvic ultrasound (string of pearls). Because insulin resistance is a characteristic of PCOS, patients with PCOS are at increased risk of diabetes, dyslipidemia, cardiovascular disease, and metabolic syndrome. In addition, patients have increased risk of endometrial hyperplasia and endometrial cancer.

PPx:
1. None to prevent PCOS, but once patient has PCOS, PPx diabetes and cardiovascular disease

MoD: Unknown but associated with insulin resistance, cystic ovaries, and hyperandrogenism

Dx:
1. Clinical evaluation (Rotterdam criteria)
2. Pelvic ultrasound of ovaries
3. Testosterone (will be elevated)

4. FSH/LH (should be elevated, LH > FSH so higher LH:FSH ratios)
5. Glucose tolerance test (>140 2-hour GTT → insulin resistance; >200 2-hour GTT → diabetes mellitus)
6. Fasting lipid panel → for all newly diagnosed patients

Tx/Mgmt:
1. Metformin
2. Lifestyle/diet to control diabetes/weight
3. Clomiphene citrate
4. Ketoconazole
5. Spironolactone:
   - Metformin used for PCOS treatment because:
     Prevents T2DM
     Helps lose weight
     Helps induce ovulation in PCOS (mechanism unknown but likely by altering insulin levels to allow for more favorable ovulation)
     Suppresses androgen production by decreasing ovarian gluconeogenesis (helps correct hirsutism)
   - Clomiphene citrate used to induce ovulation; mechanism not elucidated but clomiphene citrate = estrogen analog that improves GnRH and FSH release

Mittelschmerz

Buzz Words: Teenager + mid-cycle unilateral/bilateral lower abdominal pain + normal ultrasound + normal H&P

Clinical Presentation: Mittelschmerz (German for "middle pain") is a phenomenon whereby patients experience pain halfway between their menstrual cycles due to normal follicular enlargement prior to ovulation. As long as the pelvic ultrasound is normal, reassurance is all that is needed for treatment.

PPx:
1. N/A

MoD: Pain from normal follicular enlargement prior to ovulation

Dx:
1. PE
2. Ultrasound

Tx/Mgmt:
1. Reassurance, no treatment needed
2. Can use Tylenol/Motrin prn pain
3. OCPs to prevent ovulation and midcycle pain

Ovarian/Adnexal Torsion

Buzz Words:

Acute intermittent abdominal pain + pelvic exam deferred for discomfort + **history of adnexal mass** + impaired ovarian blood flow → torsion of ovarian cyst

Sudden onset pelvic pain (usually R sided) + unilateral adnexal mass + N/V + low grade fever → ovarian/adnexal torsion

Sudden onset severe unilateral abdominal pain **following physical activity** + free fluid near ovarian cyst → ruptured ovarian cyst

Clinical Presentation:

Ovarian or adnexal torsion is a surgical emergency. This disorder must be ruled out before more benign causes of pelvic pain (e.g., Mittelschmerz) can be considered. Patients with masses in the ovary or fallopian tube are more likely to suffer from torsion.

In addition, make sure to rule out ovarian cyst rupture, which occurs in the setting of **physical activity.** Ovarian/adnexal torsion, on the other hand, can occur without physical activity on the exam.

PPx: N/A

MoD: Partial or complete torsion of the ovary around the infundibulopelvic (suspensory) ligament of the ovary and the utero-ovarian ligaments:

- More commonly right-sided because left rectosigmoid colon occupies space around the left ovary:
  - **Ovarian torsion** = partial or complete rotation of the ovary around the infundibulopelvic (suspensory) ligament of the ovary and utero-ovarian ligaments
  - **Adnexal torsion** = fallopian tube also twisting along with the ovary

Dx:

1. PE
2. Beta-hCG to exclude ectopic pregnancy
3. Ultrasound (shows edematous ovary and **impaired ovarian blood flow**)
4. CBC/BMP

Tx/Mgmt:

1. Laparoscopic surgery for detorsion
2. Salpingo-oophorectomy for obvious adnexal necrosis or suspected ovarian malignancy

Ectopic Pregnancy

Buzz Words:

Abdominal pain + amenorrhea + vaginal bleeding + palpable adnexal mass → ectopic pregnancy

Abdominal pain + amenorrhea + vaginal bleeding + orthostatic changes + hypovolemic shock → ruptured ectopic pregnancy

Beta hCG >2000 + **thin endometrial stripe** + "no adnexal masses" + no fetal pole in uterus → ectopic pregnancy

Clinical Presentation: Ectopic pregnancy is a condition in which the fertilized egg matures outside of the uterus (e.g., in the fallopian tube). It can present as lower quadrant abdominal pain and be mistaken for a gastrointestinal (GI) disorder (e.g., appendicitis). Patients with hypotension or vital signs that suggest hypovolemic shock likely have ruptured ectopic pregnancy, and require admission and surgery. The first test to be ordered is beta-hCG, which would show lower than expected levels. Diagnosis is confirmed with ultrasound. Patients with a history of previous pelvic/tubal surgery, pelvic inflammatory disorder, IUD use, multiple sexual partners, infertility, and in utero DES exposure are more at risk for ectopic pregnancy.

PPx: Avoid risk factors such as (1) previous ectopic/pelvic/tubal surgery, (2) in utero DES exposure, (3) infertility treatment, (4) IUD use, (5) PID, (6) multiple sexual partners.

MoD: Ectopic pregnancy is caused by failure of a fertilized egg to implant in the endometrium. Most often occurs in the ampulla of the fallopian tube

Dx:
1. Pelvic exam
2. Beta-hCG
3. Pelvic ultrasound

Tx/Mgmt:
1. If stable, methotrexate
2. Surgery for hemodynamically unstable patients

Congenital Disorders

Müllerian Agenesis (aka Mayer-Rokitansky-Küster-Hauser Syndrome)

Buzz Words: Primary amenorrhea + normal secondary sex characteristics + normal 46XX karyotype

Clinical Presentation: The müllerian (paramesonephric) ducts normally develop into the fallopian tubes, uterus, cervix, and superior vagina. Agenesis of the ducts naturally results in deficiencies in these structures; however, müllerian agenesis is a broad term that encompasses several different manifestations or classes. For example, class I patients lack a vagina and uterus but have normal functioning fallopian tubes and ovaries. While the specific classes are beyond the scope of your exam, it will serve you well to note that variations may be presented on your exam. Müllerian agenesis is associated with intrauterine exposure to teratogens, for example, DES, thalidomide.

PPx: N/A
MoD: Multifactorial effect on embryogenesis
Dx: Pelvic ultrasound
Tx/Mgmt:
1. Retroperitoneal ultrasound for additional abnormalities with urinary or genital tract
2. Optional: Surgical elongation of vagina

Bicornuate Uterus, Uterine Didelphys

Buzz Words: Two uteri/cervixes/vaginas + dysmenorrhea + miscarriage + preterm labor + tampon not working

Clinical Presentation: The uterus, cervix, and upper vagina are formed by the fusion of the paramesonephric ducts in utero. Incomplete fusion may lead to a bicornuate uterus or uterine didelphys. Bicornuate uterus often manifests with a single vagina and cervix but a split or two-horned uterus. Further lack of fusion leads to uterine didelphys, which has two uteri, two cervixes, and possibly two vaginas. These are two distinguishable pathologies but lay on the same spectrum, derived from the same pathology. Thus, they are presented together. The most common chief complaint is amenorrhea or two uteri on vaginal exam. It is associated with preterm labor, recurrent miscarriage, renal anomaly.

PPx: N/A
MoD: Müllerian ducts fail to fuse in utero → two functional uteri each leading to one ovary
Dx: Transvaginal ultrasound or hysterosalpingogram (HSG):
- Must distinguish bicornuate uterus from septate uterus, which is associated with increased risk of infertility.

Tx/Mgmt:
1. Uteroplasty/hysteroplasty/metroplasty if recurrent miscarriages

GUNNER PRACTICE

1. A 14-year-old girl with no past medical history comes into the emergency department after she was found to be unresponsive at home. Patient does not take any medications, and her parents deny any medications or known drug use. She met all of her developmental milestones growing up and was found to be of average weight and height for her age group at her last doctor's visit. She also recently began having her menstrual period. At school, she performs well in class and plays for the marching band. Her vital signs are 60/40 mm Hg,

110 bpm, 101°F, and 24 RR. On exam, she is febrile and disoriented, with a maculopapular rash on her abdomen, back and lower extremities. She is noted to have a reddish bumpy tongue. A pelvic exam reveals the presence of a tampon. She is given fluids and admitted to the hospital from the emergency room. A urine drug screen is negative. Her blood glucose is normal. What is the mechanism of her most likely diagnosis?

A. Overdose on ethanol
B. Bleeding superficial to the dura mater
C. Bleeding deep to the dura mater
D. Toxin-mediated immunogenic response
E. Inflammation of meninges

2. A 17-year-old girl comes to the physician for concern of amenorrhea. She states that her last menstrual period was 2 months ago. She had started menses at the age of 12 and her menstrual cycle ranges from 26 to 28 days. The only medication she takes is a topical antibiotic for acne. She played soccer and softball last year but has since quit to join the school's debate team. The patient denies smoking or using any drugs. She states that she is worried about her weight at times, but mostly eats what she wants. College entrance exams are coming up and she really wants to get into a good college. Her vitals are BP 120/80, HR 80 bpm, T 98.6°F, and RR12. No abnormalities are found on her physical exam. What is the most appropriate next step in diagnosis?

A. Reassurance
B. Urine pregnancy test
C. Basic metabolic panel
D. Follicle stimulating hormone levels
E. Transvaginal ultrasound

Notes

ANSWERS: What Would Gunner Jess/Jim Do?

1. WWGJD? A 14-year-old girl with no past medical history comes into the emergency department after she was found to be unresponsive at home. Patient does not take any medications, and her parents deny any medications or known drug use. She met all of her developmental milestones growing up and was found to be of average weight and height for her age group at her last doctor's visit. She also recently began having her menstrual period. At school, she performs well in class and plays for the marching band. Her vital signs are 60/40 mm Hg, 110 bpm, 101°F, and 24 RR. On exam, she is febrile and disoriented, with a maculopapular rash on her abdomen, back and lower extremities. She is noted to have a reddish bumpy tongue. A pelvic exam reveals the presence of a tampon. She is given fluids and admitted to the hospital from the emergency room. A urine drug screen is negative. Her blood glucose is normal.

   What is the mechanism of her most likely diagnosis?

   Answer: D, Toxin-mediated immunogenic response

   Explanation: This patient has toxic shock syndrome, which is an over activation of the immune system mediated by a toxin released by *Staph aureus* (or *Strep pyogenes*—especially if you mention strawberry tongue above). The giveaway is the presence of an old tampon. Nasal packing can also have the same effect.

   A. Overdose on ethanol → Incorrect. Symptoms are not consistent with alcohol intoxication, which would present as altered mental status, ophthalmoplegia, and ataxia (AOA) from thiamine deficiency; what is AOA? Is it related to adolescents? or more of an adult phenomenon?).

   B. Bleeding superficial to the dura mater → Incorrect. Symptoms are not consistent with epidural hematoma, since there was no evidence of trauma. Patients with epidural hematoma have a lucid interval before losing consciousness and deteriorating rapidly.

   C. Bleeding deep to the dura mater → Incorrect. Symptoms are not consistent with a subdural hematoma, which would lead to gradually worsening headache and a CT scan suggestive of subdural bleed.

   E. Inflammation of meninges → Incorrect. Meningitis should be on the differential for a patient who is febrile with altered mental status and signs of sepsis. However, the combination of rash, hypotension, and tampon use is more indicative of toxic shock syndrome.

2. WWGJD? A 17-year-old girl presents with concern of amenorrhea. She states that her last menstrual period was 2 months ago. She had started menses at the age of 12 and her menstrual cycle ranges from 26 to 28 days. The only medications she takes is a topical antibiotic for acne. She played soccer and softball last year but has since quit to join the school's debate team. The patient denies smoking or using any drugs. She states that she is worried about her weight at times, but mostly eats what she wants. College entrance exams are coming up and she really wants to get into a good college. Her vitals are BP 120/80, HR 80 bpm, T 98.6°F, and RR 12. No abnormalities are found on her physical exam. What is the most appropriate next step in diagnosis?

Answer: B, Urine pregnancy test

Explanation: A urine pregnancy test as the first step. Even if patient has signs or symptoms females of reproductive age presenting with amenorrhea should be worked-suggestive of something else, this test should always be performed on a teenager with new onset of amenorrhea.

A. Reassurance → Incorrect. Pregnancy test is needed before reassuring patient.

C. Basic metabolic panel → Incorrect. Electrolyte imbalance could be suggestive of an eating disorder such as anorexia. Eating disorders can lead to secondary amenorrhea but unlikely in this patient.

D. Follicle stimulating hormone levels → Incorrect. High FSH may be indicative of ovarian dysfunction (e.g., amenorrhea 2/2 Turner syndrome). However, again this is not the next best step.

E. Transvaginal ultrasound → Incorrect. TVUS would help confirm pregnancy but should not be done before beta-hCG levels are tested.

CHAPTER

11

Renal, Urinary, and Male Reproductive System

Leo Wang, Jacques Greenberg, Hao-Hua Wu, Diana Kim,
Eloise Salmon, and Rebecca Tenney-Soeiro

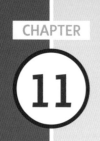

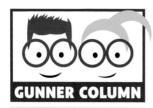

GUNNER COLUMN

Introduction

The Pediatrics exam will focus heavily on diseases of the renal, urinary, and male reproductive system. This section will make up 10–15 questions of your clinical subject exam, so knowing these topics will be incredibly important to doing well. The following sections are included in this chapter: (1) Embryonic Development, Fetal Maturation, and Perinatal Changes; (2) Infectious Disorders of Kidney, Urinary Tract, and Male Reproductive System; (3) Glomerular Disorders; (4) Malignant Neoplasms; (5) Congenital Disorders of the Kidney; (6) Traumatic/Mechanical Disorders; (7) Complications of Circumcision; (8) Congenital Disorders of the Male Reproductive System; (9) Channelopathies in the Kidney; and (10) Gunner Practice. The most important sections are **infectious disorders, congenital disorders of the kidney,** and **malignant neoplasms.** Focus on these sections if pressed for time.

One of the most common diseases that is tested on the Pediatrics exam is hemolytic uremic syndrome. It is only tangentially related to the kidneys, and is further expounded upon in other chapters. Hemolytic uremic syndrome (HUS) is a disease characterized by hemolytic anemia with kidney failure and low platelet count that occurs after food-borne illness, with the most common causative agents being *Escherichia coli* O157:H7, *Shigella*, and *Campylobacter*. One of the hallmarks is a microangiopathy that destructs platelets and red blood cell counts (RBCs). Treatment is typically supportive and antibiotics should **NOT** be given. This is one of the single most commonly tested diseases on any subject exam.

As usual, the four physician tasks are going to be tested heavily in this section, which include Prophylaxis (PPx), Mechanism of Disease (MoD), Diagnostic Steps (Dx), and Treatment and Management Steps (Tx/Mgmt). Use the Buzz Words to help hone in on a disease, and focus specifically on Dx and Tx/Mgmt for the diseases in this section. A basic overview of nephrogenesis is included in the first section, which can be used to help explain the MoD for many congenital malformations, but is not necessary for succeeding on the Pediatrics exam.

Embryonic Development, Fetal Maturation, and Perinatal Changes

Kidney development is also known as **nephrogenesis**. The development occurs through three stages in formation of the pronephros, mesonephros, and metanephros:

1. The pronephros develops from mesoderm in the cranial/cervical region of the embryo around day 20. They form a series of tubules that then join with the **pronephric duct.**

2. Proceeding inferiorly toward the caudal direction, the pronephros and pronephric duct induces the formation of **mesonephric tubules.** These tubules form a capsule around distal branches coming from the aorta, leading to the functional equivalent of a glomerulus. Filtrate can then come through the newly formed mesonephric tubules into the former pronephric duct, which is now called the **mesonephric** or wolffian duct.

3. During the fifth week of gestation, the mesonephric duct pinches out a ureteric bud which grows cranially. This ureteric bud eventually becomes the ureters and major and minor calyces, which interact with the intermediate mesoderm to form renal tubules.

Renal agenesis occurs when the ureteric bud fails to form. If both kidneys fail to form, then a patient is diagnosed with **Potter syndrome.** This is a pathology in strictly neonatal populations, as the resulting oligohydraminos (secondary to anuria) leads to fetal compression, limb and facial deformities, and a pulmonary hypoplasia that is usually fatal. Retinoic acid plays a significant role in the development of the kidney. Any signaling interruption throughout the renal organogenesis, especially those involving perturbations in retinoic acid, may thus lead to renal abnormalities, including renal hypoplasia and agenesis. **Vesicoureteral reflux**, in a similar but unrelated etiology, may arise from defects in the mesothelial-to-epithelial transformation process—this is a major cause of urinary tract infections in young children (Fig. 11.1).

Infectious Disorders of Kidney, Urinary Tract, and Male Reproductive System

Infectious disorders are the most high-yield topic in this section and include infections of the kidney/urinary tract system and infections of the male reproductive system (most sexually transmitted). Know how to recognize these

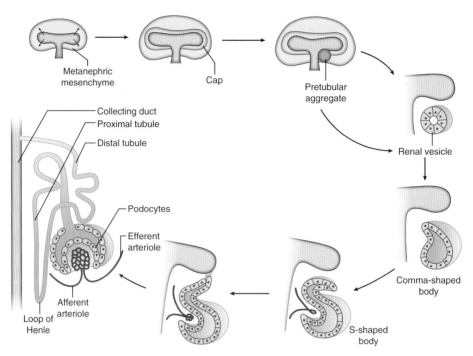

FIG. 11.1 Kidney development. (Reprinted with permission from Moritz KM, Wintour EM, Black MJ, et al: Factors influencing mammalian kidney development: implications for health in adult life. *Adv Anat Embryol Cell Biol* 196:1–78, 2008; and modified by Justin Hewlett, Multimedia Services, Monash University.)

diseases from the Buzz Words. As a rule, a urinalysis and urine culture should always be ordered here. Treatment/management is usually with antibiotics.

Urinary Tract Infection (Cystitis/Pyelonephritis)

Buzz Words: Fever + pain during urination + cloudy/foul-smelling urine + frequent urination or wetting bed + vomiting

Clinical Presentation: Urinary tract infections (UTIs) are a common problem in young children, with girls getting them more commonly than boys (10:1). Most are not serious, but can lead to complications and kidney damage. Many UTIs are caused by vesicoureteral reflux. Uncircumcised boys are also at greater risk of UTIs. Infection may be limited to bladder (**cystitis**) or kidney (**pyelonephritis**). UTIs in infants can be the first sign of an obstructive anomaly or severe vesicoureteral reflux.

PPx: Circumcision in boys

MoD: Ascent from fecal flora in older children, younger children can get UTIs from bacteremia

Dx:

1. UA
2. UCx

3. Renal bladder ultrasound for all children younger than 24 months with fever or recurrent UTI
4. Voiding cystourethrogram (VCUG) if abnormal RBUS or second febrile UTI
5. Dimercaptosuccinic acid scan of kidney

Tx/Mgmt:
Cystitis: (1) Amoxicillin or trimethoprim/sulfamethozaxole for older children.
Pyelonephritis: (1) Cefixime/cefotaxime. (2) Ampicillin + gentamicin.

Urethritis

Buzz Words: Painful urination in children
Clinical Presentation: While urethritis is another type of urinary tract infection, it is specifically localized to the urethra and is typically caused by either gonorrhea (gonococcal urethritis) or chlamydia (chlamydial urethritis). Other causes are less important for the pediatric exam, but include *E. coli*, adenoviruses, CMV, HSV, GBS, MRSA, or trichomonas.
PPx: Proper perineal hygiene, barrier contraception
MoD: Perianal spread as well as sexually transmitted
Dx:
1. UA
2. UCx

Tx/Mgmt:
1. Antibiotic treatment for gonorrhea (ceftriaxone) or chlamydia (azithromycin, doxycycline)

Chancroid (*Haemophilus ducreyi*)

Buzz Words: Painful chancre + inguinal lymphadenopathy, "school of fish" on Gram stain + formation of swollen inflamed lymph node (bubo) with pus inside
Clinical Presentation: Patient has painful genital area 2–10 days after sexual contact.
PPx: (1) Barrier contraception. (2) Test partner.
MoD: Infection caused by *H. ducreyi*, G-bacillus with rounded ends
Dx:
1. Clinical diagnosis
2. Culture (difficult to culture) or polymerase chain reaction (PCR)
3. HIV/syphilis test

Tx/Mgmt:
1. Azithromycin
2. Ceftriaxone
3. Aspirate buboes

FOR THE WARDS

Outpatient management of UTIs in children

99 AR

Treatment of urinary tract infections in children

QUICK TIPS

Some children will present with idiopathic urethritis. It is thought to be an autoimmune phenomenon and can be treated with steroids.

QUICK TIPS

Can differentiate chancroid from lymphogranuloma venereum (LGV) because chancroid buboes are **painful** while LGV buboes are **painless.**

MNEMONIC

Chancroid is painful because patients with *H. ducreyi* "do cry."

Genital Herpes

Buzz Words: Painful ulcer + solitary/grouped **vesicles** on erythematous base + inguinal **adenopathy** + can evolve to **shallow**, punched-out ulcerations/erosions

URI 10 days ago + vulvar burning, irritation + new sexual partner/no barrier contraception + no painful lesions → HSV Prodrome

Clinical Presentation: Painful recurrent oral and genital vesicles with the potential to rupture. Dissemination may occur, especially in pregnant women and the immunocompromised:

1. HSV-1 typically on oropharynx, though can infect genitals:
   a. Associated with Bell palsy
   b. Associated with gingivostomatitis in young children
2. HSV-2 typically on genitals, though can infect oropharynx

PPx: (1) Avoid routes of transmission (e.g., kissing, sexual contact). (2) Avoid vaginal delivery of baby if mother has active HSV lesions (C-section instead to avoid spread of herpes). (3) Acyclovir.

MoD: Replication in dermis/epidermis before retrograde travel to dorsal root ganglia → remains latent until activated by event (e.g., stress, immunodeficiency)

Dx:

1. Clinical
2. Tzanck is quickest (uses Wright stain). Multinucleated giant cells are characteristic of herpes and varicella; if cultures negative → PCR

Tx/Mgmt:

1. Acyclovir, valacyclovir, foscarnet
2. Increased risk of contracting HIV

Human Papillomavirus Infection

Buzz Words: Genital wart + cervical dysplasia

Clinical Presentation: This is the most common STD in adolescents and children and is high yield for the Pediatrics exam:

HPV 6–11: low-risk strains of condyloma acuminatum (genital warts)

HPV 16–18/31/33/45: high-risk strains for cervical dysplasia and cancer

PPx: Gardasil: quadrivalent vaccine indicated for women 11–26 years old and men 11–21 years old

MoD: Skin-skin contact

Dx: Clinical

Tx/Mgmt:

1. *Podophylin* for genital warts

Neisseria Gonorrhoeae (Gonorrheal Urethritis)

Buzz Words: Yellow endocervical discharge (Mucopurulent discharge) + Gram positive

Clinical Presentation: Gonorrhea is a one of the most common STIs in the world and is spread through unprotected sexual intercourse. It is extremely high yield on the Pediatrics exam. Many patients are asymptomatic or may present with abnormal discharge. However, it is very important to treat gonorrhea to avoid important sequelae such as pelvic inflammatory disease and **Fitz-Hugh-Curtis syndrome.** One of the only infections (other being chlamydia) where treatment is given **before** definitive diagnosis is made. Since gonorrhea and chlamydia are so common and can be treated fairly easily, definitive treatment is provided before diagnostic tests are complete. Patients with gonorrhea may often be coinfected (46%) with chlamydia—therefore, the treatment of choice should always be dual treatment for gonorrhea (ceftriaxone) and chlamydia (azithromycin/doxycycline). Untreated gonorrhea or chlamydia can lead to pelvic inflammatory disease and infertility.

PPx: (1) Barrier contraception. (2) Screen from when patient begins being sexually active until 25 years old. (3) Ceftriaxone if sexual partner has gonorrhea.

MoD: Transmission/infection through sexual contact (vaginal, oral, anal)

Dx:

1. Gram stain positive
2. Nucleic acid amplification test
3. Test for syphilis and HIV

Tx/Mgmt:

1. Ceftriaxone + azithromycin/doxycycline (given rates of coinfection with chlamydia)

Chlamydia Trachomatis (Chlamydial Urethritis)

Buzz Words: Yellow endocervical discharge (mucopurulent discharge) + Gram negative → chlamydia in females
Epididymitis + Gram negative → chlamydia in males

Clinical Presentation: Chlamydia is the most common STI in the world and is spread through unprotected sexual intercourse. It is extremely high yield on the Pediatrics exam. Many patients are asymptomatic or may present with abnormal discharge. However, it is very important

99 AR

Fitz-Hugh-Curtis Syndrome is inflammation of liver as a result of gonococcal/chlamydial infection. Suspect in adolescent female with RUQ with history of STI.

to treat chlamydia to avoid important sequelae such as pelvic inflammatory disease and Fitz-Hugh-Curtis syndrome. Like gonorrhea, chlamydia is treated **before** definitive diagnosis is made. Since gonorrhea and chlamydia are so common and can be treated fairly easily, definitive treatment is provided before diagnostic tests are complete.

PPx: (1) Barrier contraception. (2) Screen from when patient begins being sexually active until 25 years old.

MoD: Transmission/infection through sexual contact (vaginal, oral, anal). *Chlamydia trachomatis* serovars L1–L3 can lead to lymphogranuloma venereum (LGV); but these strains of chlamydia are not the same as the one that causes chlamydia transmission/infection through sexual contact (vaginal, oral, anal)

Dx:
1. Gram stain negative
2. Nucleic acid amplification test (aka DNA probe test)
3. Test for syphilis and HIV

Tx/Mgmt:
1. Azithromycin + ceftriaxone (concomitant treatment for gonorrhea)
2. Cefotetan or cefoxitin + doxy or clindamycin + gentamicin for inpatient IV treatment

Syphilis (Primary and Congenital)

Buzz Words: Newborn + **Rhinitis** + hepatosplenomegaly + skin lesions + interstitial keratitis + Hutchinson teeth (smaller teeth, widely spaced, with notches on biting surfaces) + saddle nose + saber shins + deafness → Syphilis (Congenital)

Sexually active + **painless papule** + lymphadenopathy + RPR/VDRL positive → Syphilis (primary)

Clinical Presentation: Syphilis is the highest yield STI and one of the most commonly tested topics, and thus high yield on the Pediatrics exam because it can present in either a congenital or primary fashion in the pediatrics population. Very rarely will you see secondary syphilis in a pediatric population, but this will be characterized by systemic constitutional signs/symptoms and is characterized by rashes on the palms and soles. Tertiary syphilis will never appear on the Pediatrics exam. The key to the Pediatrics exam is to recognize Buzz Words and how to differentiate syphilis from diseases with similar presentations (e.g., vs. granuloma inguinale and LGV for painless ulcers; vs. Rocky Mountain spotted fever and hand-foot-mouth disease from Coxsackie A virus for rash on palms/soles of foot). In addition, know that definitive diagnosis is made by dark-field microscopy and penicillin is used for treatment.

PPx: (1) Barrier contraception. (2) Test for concomitant HIV, gonorrhea, chlamydia (+HBV if newborn).

MoD: Syphilis is an infection caused by *Treponema pallidum*, a spirochete that disseminates infection widely throughout the body. Transmission through sexual contact or maternal → fetal spread.

Dx:
1. RPR
2. VDRL (may be false-positive with lupus, rheumatic fever, and viral infections)
3. If positive at 1:4 → progress on to FTA-A
4. Fluorescent treponemal antibody absorption test
5. Dark-field microscopy → definitive diagnosis

Tx/Mgmt:
1. Penicillin; if allergic, desensitize by incremental doses of PO penicillin V

Balanitis

Buzz Words: Uncircumcised boy <4 years old + painful penis/redness + inability to retract foreskin

Clinical Presentation: Balanitis refers to inflammation of the glans penis. It is usually secondary to poor hygiene of the foreskin. If recurrent, can lead to pathologic **phimosis**, which is the inability to retract the foreskin. These conditions can lead to meatal obstruction. Low yield for the Pediatrics exam.

PPx: Hygiene

MoD: Poor hygiene → infection and inflammation, may also occur from allergy/irritants

Dx:
1. Foreskin swab
2. UA/UCx

Tx/Mgmt:
1. Steroid cream to treat phimosis/antibiotic ointment for balanitis

Epididymitis

Buzz Words: Fever, pyuria + tender spermatic cord + pain with urination + pain/swelling in testicles, sexually transmitted in teenage boys

Clinical Presentation: While epididymitis does not threaten the testicle, testicular torsion must be ruled out emergently. Therefore, one must obtain a diagnostic ultrasound immediately. Once torsion has been excluded, diagnostic tests for epididymitis may be run.

PPx: N/A

MoD: *E. coli* infection from perianal spread or STI from gonorrhea/chlamydia

Dx:
1. Physical exam
2. Ultrasound

Tx/Mgmt:
1. Antibiotic treatment (Ceftriaxone/Azithromycin/Doxycycline for gonorrhea/chlamydia/urethritis); quinolones if enteric organisms, often rest and pain management for pre-pubertal boys

Orchitis

Buzz Words: Testicular pain + parotitis + no MMR vaccination

Clinical Presentation: Orchitis refers to infection of the testicle. It is most commonly tested in the setting of a mumps infection (10% of boys with mumps will get orchitis). Understand that this is preventable with appropriate vaccination and can accompany a parotitis. In children, mumps orchitis can lead to infertility. Bacterial infections are less likely to lead to an orchitis. Orchitis often occurs in conjunction with epididymitis.

PPx: MMR vaccination

MoD: Mumps infection of the testicle, can be idiopathic

Dx:
1. PE
2. Ultrasound

Tx/Mgmt:
1. Conservative for mumps orchitis:
   a. Analgesia, bedrest
2. Antibiotics for bacterial orchitis

Glomerular Disorders

Glomerular disorders can present as nephrotic or nephritic syndrome and are an important part of pediatric nephrology. A general overview of nephrotic versus nephritic syndrome is in Fig. 11.2, although specific pathologies relevant to pediatrics are presented below:

Alport Syndrome (Hereditary Nephritis)

Buzz Words: Nephritic and nephrotic syndrome, hematuria + deafness, ocular defects

Clinical Presentation: Nephritic or nephrotic syndrome in patients with deafness, blindness, nerve disorders, light microscopy-split glomerular basement membrane (LM-split GBM), family history. Most males and 20% of females

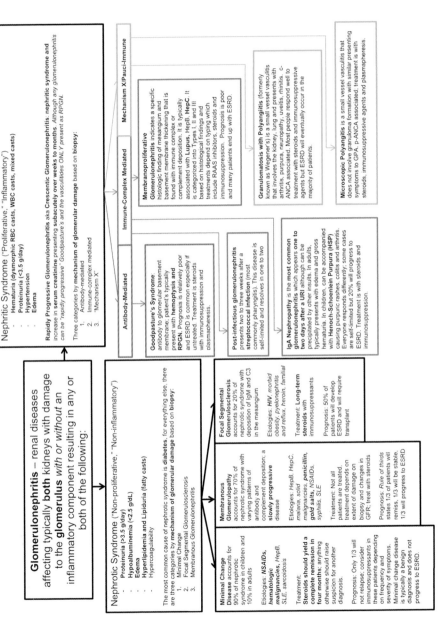

Glomerulonephritis – renal diseases affecting typically **both** kidneys with damage to the **glomerulus** *with or without* an inflammatory component resulting in any or both of the following:

Nephritic Syndrome ("Proliferative," "Inflammatory")
- Hematuria (dysmorphic RBC casts, WBC casts, mixed casts)
- Proteinuria (<3.5 g/day)
- Hypertension
- Edema

Rapidly Progressive Glomerulonephritis aka **Crescentic Glomerulonephritis: nephritic syndrome and** increase in **serum creatinine** presenting **subacutely over weeks to months**. *Although any glomerulonephritis can be "rapidly progressive" Goodpasture's and the vasculitides ONLY present as RPGN.*

Three categories by **mechanism of glomerular damage** based on **biopsy**:
1. Antibody-mediated
2. Immune-complex mediated
3. "Mechanism X"

Antibody-Mediated

Goodpasture's Syndrome: antibody to glomerular basement membrane; patient's typically present with **hemoptysis and RPGN.** Prognosis is relatively poor and ESRD is common especially if untreated. Treatment is steroids with immunosuppression and plasmapheresis.

Immune-Complex Mediated

Post-infectious glomerulonephritis presents two to three weeks after a **streptococcal infection** (most commonly pharyngitis). This disease is self-limited and resolves in one to two

IgA Nephropathy is the **most common glomerulonephritis** which appears **one to two days after a URI** although can be precipitated by other insults. In adults, typically presents with edema and gross hematuria. In children, can be accompanied with **Henoch-Schoenlein Purpura (HSP)** causing purpuric rashes, colitis and arthritis. Everyone responds differently; some cases are self-limited but 20% will progress to ESRD. Treatment is with steroids and immunosuppression.

Mechanism X/Pauci-Immune

Membranoproliferative Glomerulonephritis indicates a specific histologic finding of mesangium and basement membrane thickening that is found with immune complex or complement deposition. It is typically associated with **Lupus, HepB. HepC.** It is categorized into Types I, II and III based on histological findings and treatments depend on typing which include RAAS inhibitors, steroids and immunosuppression. Prognosis is poor and many patients end up with ESRD.

Granulomatosis with Polyangitis (formerly known as Wegener's) is a small vessel vasculitis that involves the kidney, lung and presents with arthritis, purpura, neuropathy, uveitis, rhinitis, c-ANCA associated. Most people respond well to treatment with steroids and immunosuppressive agents but ESRD will eventually occur in the majority of patients.

Microscopic Polyangitis is a small vessel vasculitis that does not involve granuloma formation with similar presenting symptoms to GPA. p-ANCA associated; treatment is with steroids, immunosuppressive agents and plasmapheresis.

Nephrotic Syndrome ("Non-proliferative," "Non-inflammatory")
- Proteinuria (>3.5 g/day)
- Hypoalbuminemia (<2.5 g/dL)
- Edema
- Hyperlipidemia and Lipiduria (fatty casts)
- Hypercoagulability

The most common cause of nephrotic syndrome is **diabetes**, for everything else, there are three categories by **mechanism of glomerular damage** based on **biopsy**:
1. Minimal Change
2. Focal Segmental Glomerulosclerosis
3. Membranous Glomerulonephritis

Minimal Change Disease accounts for 90% of nephrotic syndrome in children and 10% in adults.

Etiologies: *NSAIDs, hematologic malignancies, HepB, SLE, sarcoidosis.*

Treatment: **Steroids should yield a complete remission in four months**; anything otherwise should raise suspicion for another diagnosis.

Prognosis: Only 1/3 will not relapse; consider immunosuppressants in these patients depending on frequency and severity of symptoms. Minimal change disease is typically a benign diagnosis and does not progress to ESRD.

Membranous Glomerulopathy accounts for 70% of nephrotic syndrome with varying patterns of antibody and complement deposition; a **slowly progressive** disease

Etiologies: *HepB, HepC, malaria, solid malignancies, penicillin, gold salts, NSAIDs, syphilis, SLE.*

Treatment: Not all patients are treated, treatment depends on extent of damage on biopsy and changes in GFR; treat with steroids

Prognosis: *Rule of thirds* states 1/3 will remiss, 1/3 will be stable, 1/3 will progress to ESRD

Focal Segmental Glomerulosclerosis accounts for 20% of nephrotic syndrome with deposition of IgM and C3 in the mesangium

Etiologies: *HIV, morbid obesity, pyelonephritis and reflux, heroin, familial*

Treatment: **Long-term steroids** with immunosuppressants

Prognosis: 50% of patients will develop ESRD and will require transplant

FIG. 11.2

will progress to renal failure by adulthood. This disease is extremely high yield for the Pediatrics shelf.

PPx: Genetic counseling

MoD: X-linked recessive change in type IV collagen or autosomal-dominant

Dx:

1. UA
2. BMP
3. Biopsy
4. Genetic testing

Tx/Mgmt:

1. Renal transplantation

Post-Infectious (aka Post-Streptococcal) Glomerulonephritis

Buzz Words: Cola-colored urine + periorbital edema + recent strep throat or cellulitis +LM-"lumpy bumpy" + antigen-antibody complexes with subendothelial immunoglobulin (Ig)G and IgM deposition + elevated ASO + decreased complement + usually occurs 7–14 days after infection

Clinical Presentation: Nephritic syndrome 7–14 days after impetigo or URI. This is one of the most commonly tested concepts on any subject exam, including the Pediatrics exam.

PPx: NA

MoD: Antigen-antibody complex with sub-epithelial deposition of IgG, IgM, and C3 leading to "lumpy bumpy" appearance on light microscope

Dx:

1. UA
2. BMP
3. Biopsy (rarely in kids, more common in adults)

Tx/Mgmt:

1. Controversial use of antibiotics, but Abx treatment if active infection.
2. Supportive measures such as fluid restriction.

Immunoglobulin A Nephropathy

Buzz Words: Recurrent hematuria 1 day after respiratory/ gastrointestinal (GI) infections + Henoch-Schonlein purpura + LM-mesangial deposits + immunofluorescence (IF)-IgA stain

Clinical Presentation: Associated with glomerular hematuria, HSP, nephritic syndrome after URI or gastroenteritis. Frequent past medical history of URI, gastroenteritis, Henoch-Schonlein purpura. Can see increased IgA in serum.

PPx: N/A
MoD: Mesangial deposition of IgA and C3
Dx:
1. UA
2. BMP
3. Biopsy
Tx/Mgmt:
1. Steroids only questionably beneficial

Minimal Change Disease

Buzz Words: Foot process effacement + swollen face/extremities + ascites
Clinical Presentation: Nephrotic syndrome in children, often co-morbid with viral syndrome, Hodgkin disease, non-Hodgkin lymphoma. Extremely high yield on the Pediatrics exam.
PPx: NA
MoD: Systemic T cell dysfunction
Dx:
1. UA
2. BMP
3. No need for biopsy
Tx/Mgmt:
1. Steroids

Malignant Neoplasms

Wilms Tumor

Buzz Words: Childhood renal tumor 3–5 years old, unilateral flank mass + constipation + hematuria → Wilms tumor OR unilateral flank mass + aniridia + retardation → Wilms tumor in setting of WAGR syndrome (Wilms tumor, Aniridia, Genitourinary lesion, mental Retardation)
Clinical Presentation: Presents as a renal mass/abdominal pain in child. Most common renal neoplasm in *children*. This disease is extremely high yield on the Pediatrics exam. Look for WAGR syndrome (deletion of short arm of chromosome 11), Beckwith-Wiedemann syndrome (Wilms, hemihypertrophy, adrenal cytomegaly).
PPx: N/A
MoD: Loss of Wilms tumor suppressor gene (WT1), thought to occur through the two-hit hypothesis
Dx:
1. Abdominal ultrasound
2. Abdominal computed tomography (CT)
3. Biopsy → microscopic pattern resembling fetal kidney nephrogenic zone
4. Staging from exploratory laparotomy

QUICK TIPS

Unlike neuroblastoma (the other most common abdominal tumor in children), Wilms tumor DOES NOT cross the midline. Neuroblastoma does.

MNEMONIC

WAGR
Wilms tumor
Aniridia
Genitourinary abnormalities
Retardation (mental)

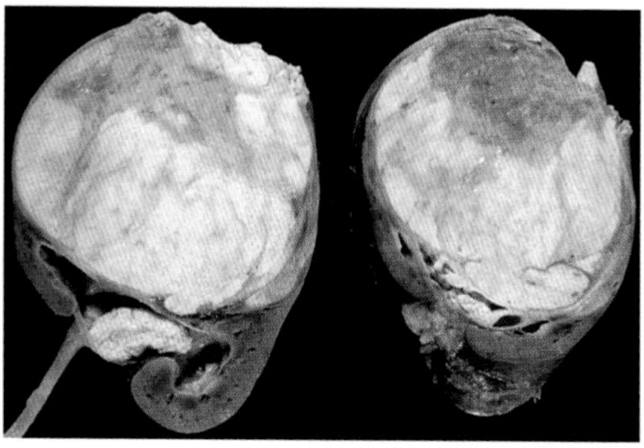

FIG. 11.3 Wilms tumor. (https://en.wikipedia.org/wiki/Wilms%27_tumor.)

QUICK TIPS

Unlike most tumors, in Wilms the histology is actually more important than staging in determining a patient's prognosis.

Tx/Mgmt: Surgery, chemo, and radiation lead to high cure rate; unilateral → immediate resection (Fig. 11.3)

Renal Cell Carcinoma

Buzz Words: Adolescent age 15–19 + renal mass

Clinical Presentation: Very rare in children, includes papillary renal cell carcinoma, renal medullary carcinoma, and oncocytic renal cell carcinoma following neuroblastoma.

PPx: N/A

MoD: Most are related to translocations in XP11, renal medullary carcinoma associated with sickle cell

Dx:

1. Ultrasound
2. CT
3. Biopsy

Tx/Mgmt:

1. Surgical resection + chemo/radiation therapy

Renal Tumors Associated With Congenital/Hereditary Conditions

Disease/Syndrome	**Associated Renal Tumor**
Tuberous sclerosis	Renal angiomyolipoma
Von-Hippel-Lindau	**Bilateral** renal cell carcinoma
Wilms tumor-Aniridia syndrome	Wilms tumor
Frasier syndrome	Wilms tumor
Hereditary leiomyomatosis	Renal cell carcinoma
Denys-Drash syndrome	Wilms tumor
Beckwith-Wiedemann syndrome	Wilms tumor
Hereditary papillary renal cell carcinoma	Renal cell carcinoma

Congenital Disorders of the Kidney

Congenital disorders in the kidney are some of the most commonly tested pathologies on the exam. Horseshoe kidney is extremely high yield on every standardized exam, as are autosomal dominant polycystic kidney disease (ADPKD) and autosomal recessive polycystic kidney disease (ARPKD). Focus on these diseases if pressed on time.

Double Ureters/Ureteral Duplication/Double Collecting System

Buzz Words: Hydronephrosis + vesicoureteric reflux + recurrent UTIs in young infant

Clinical Presentation: Spectrum ranges from double ureter to complete duplication, usually asymptomatic, but occasionally can cause hydronephrosis, comorbid with Fanconi anemia.

PPx: N/A

MoD: Premature division of the ureteric bud prior to penetration of the metanephros

Dx:
1. Ultrasound

Tx/Mgmt:
1. Manage associated conditions, including vesicoureteric reflux or hydronephrosis

Horseshoe Kidney

Buzz Words: Inferior mesenteric artery + Turner syndrome + pyelonephritis + stones + hydronephrosis + Trisomy 18

Clinical Presentation: This is a congenital disease leading to increased risk of pyelonephritis and kidney stone formation that is especially prominent in those with Turner syndrome. Highly coincident with Fanconi anemia. Prognosis is usually good with treatment.

PPx: N/A

MoD: Kidneys initially form near the tail of the embryo. The growth of the embryo in a caudal-rostral direction leads to renal "ascension." Horseshoe kidney arises during ventral fusion with subsequent entrapment below the inferior mesenteric artery.

Dx:
1. In utero ultrasound

Tx/Mgmt:
1. Tx UTI/hydronephrosis with antibiotics (Fig. 11.4)

Renal Agenesis

Buzz Words: Newborn is missing one or both kidneys + high blood pressure + proteinuria/hematuria + swelling

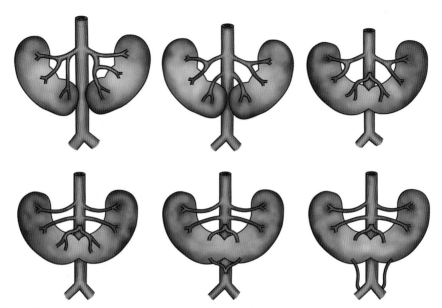

FIG. 11.4 Horseshoe kidney and vascular supply. (From Taghavi et al: *J Pediatr Urol*, 2016, Elsevier.)

Clinical Presentation: Both kidneys failing (bilateral agenesis) to develop during gestation can cause **Potter sequence** and oligohydramnios, leading to further malformations. Males are more commonly affected and if born alive, do not live long because oligohydramnios prevents development of lungs. Some with bilateral renal agenesis (BRA) can have dialysis for extended periods of time. Unilateral agenesis is asymptomatic but can cause hypertension and is associated with infertility.

PPx: Young maternal age, alcohol, diabetes → renal agenesis, born with unilateral → avoid contact sports

MoD: Gene mutations in RET or UPK3A

Dx:

1. Prenatal ultrasound
2. Prenatal magnetic resonance imaging (MRI)

Tx/Mgmt:

1. Conservative:
   a. Frequent BP, UA, and BMP for kidney function
2. Dialysis if needed

Renal Hypoplasia

Buzz Words: Failure of full kidney development in utero + small kidney + recurrent UTI, hydronephrosis

Clinical Presentation: Unilateral hypoplasia is asymptomatic, no management. Bilateral hypoplasia is more serious and requires recurrent checkups as may lead to chronic kidney disease.

QUICK TIPS

Herlyn-Werner-Wunderlich syndrome is unilateral renal agenesis + blind hemivagina + ureteral didelphys (Fig. 11.5).

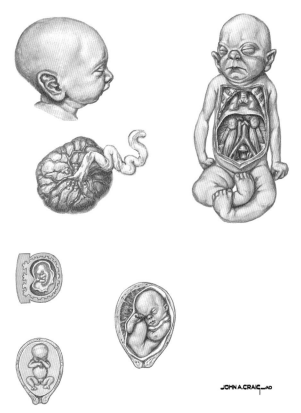

FIG. 11.5 Potter sequence. (Netter medical illustration used with permission of Elsevier. All rights reserved.)

PPx: N/A
MoD: Idiopathic
Dx:
1. Antenatal ultrasound, ultrasound after birth
Tx/Mgmt:
1. UA/BMP
2. Ultrasound
3. Dialysis if renal failure

Renal Dysplasia

Buzz Words: Abnormal kidney development in utero + dysfunctional, if bilateral + recurrent UTI, hydronephrosis

Clinical Presentation: Occurs in 1 in 4000 babies and can occur in one or both kidneys. May lead to recurrent UTIs, hydronephrosis, high BP, and increased risk of cancer. Unilateral dysplasia usually has good prognosis. Renal aplasia and dysplasia are very similar, but have different etiologies. Aplasia is a failure in development altogether (quantitative defect), whereas dysplasia is inappropriate development (qualitative defect). There is nothing wrong with the way a kidney develops in aplasia, it is just not developing enough and will not reach the right size. In dysplasia, it is not developing the right way (though it may reach the right size).

PPx: Avoid antiepileptics or cocaine use in mother

MoD: Combination of genetics + antiepileptics/hypertensives or cocaine in mother

Dx:
1. Ultrasound
2. UA/BMP/BP

Tx/Mgmt:
1. BP/BMP frequent measurements
2. UA
3. Ultrasound
4. Dialysis/transplant

Autosomal Dominant Polycystic Kidney Disease

Buzz Words: Berry aneurysm, HTN, liver cysts, parathyroid hyperplasia in adulthood, most common cause of chronic kidney disease, usually presents with hematuria, HTN, palpable kidneys, pyelonephritis

Clinical Presentation: Most common inherited cause of chronic kidney disease, but because few clinical presentations in adolescence; not commonly tested on pediatric exam. Renal failure in 50% of patients, most commonly from recurrent pyelonephritis or nephrolithiasis. Patients may have associated endocrine abnormalities due to the kidney's inability to produce vitamin D or to properly excrete phosphate. Secondary hyperparathyroidism may occur.

PPx: NA

MoD: Autosomal dominant transmission with polycystin-1 and polycystin-2 gene mutation found in renal tubules

Dx:
1. Renal ultrasound showing cysts that envelope the entire kidney

Tx/Mgmt:
1. Treat symptomatically
2. Anti-hypertensives
3. Antibiotics for infections
4. Cyst drainage *only* if symptomatic

Autosomal Recessive Polycystic Kidney Disease

Buzz Words: Cysts in renal collecting ducts + hepatic fibrosis → portal hypertension (HTN) and cholangitis, Potter sequence

Clinical Presentation: Bilateral, symmetrically enlarged kidneys in utero with renal failure at birth; neither parent is usually affected given autosomal recessive inheritance pattern. Despite being rarer than ADPKD due to its inheritance pattern, this disease actually is higher yield on the Pediatrics exam.

PPx: NA

MoD: PKHD1 gene mutation that encodes for the fibrocystin in the kidney, liver, and pancreas

Dx: Neonatal or prenatal ultrasound showing renal cysts with hepatomegaly

Tx/Mgmt: MCC of death is pulmonary disease (hypoplasia) because of enlarged kidneys. Treat with renal replacement and respiratory support.

Traumatic and Mechanical Disorders

The most important diseases in this section are differentiating between varicocele/hydrocele/spermatocele. Being able to manage testicular/penile trauma will not be frequently tested on the Pediatrics exam, but a basic understanding is high yield for many of the subject exams.

Testicular Torsion

Buzz Words: Boy age 12–16 + sudden severe scrotal pain + painful urination

Clinical Presentation: May occur secondary to epididymitis and history of previous testicular torsion or family history. Can lead to infertility or testicular infarction. This is a medical emergency!

PPx: N/A

MoD: Testicle rotates, twists spermatic cord, thus cutting off blood flow to scrotum → pain and swelling

Dx:
1. Physical exam
2. UA/UCx
3. Scrotal ultrasound
4. Exploratory surgery

Tx/Mgmt:
1. Surgical reduction

Penile Trauma (Blast Injuries, Burns, Penile Fracture, Urethral Injury)

Buzz Words: "Eggplant penis" + acute pain + erection

Clinical Presentation: Acute onset of pain following injury to erect penis. Penile fracture is most commonly tested. Complications include erectile dysfunction and urethral injury.

PPx: N/A

QUICK TIPS

Differentiate testicular torsion with cremasteric reflex, if missing → torsion

MoD: Fracture of the tunica albuginea surrounding the corpus cavernosa

Dx:

1. Clinical, but may also perform diagnostic cavernography or MRI

Tx/Mgmt:

1. Surgical repair of tunica albuginea

Varicocele/Hydrocele/Spermatocele

Disease	Buzz Words	PPx	MoD	Dx	Tx/Mgmt
Hydrocele (very common in male infants)	Painless swelling, not reducible, transilluminant + no cough impulse	N/A	Idiopathic or indicative of underlying pathology	1. PE 2. Ultrasound	1. Lord's operation 2. Jaboulay's operation
Varicocele	"Bag of worms," reducible swelling when lying down	N/A	Idiopathic absence of valves in testicular vein	1. PE 2. Ultrasound	Varicocelectomy, risk of infertility
Spermatocele	Palpable testis + Chinese lantern appearance, "third testis"	Tx epididymitis	Degeneration of epididymis	1. PE 2. Ultrasound	1. Conservative 2. Excision

Complications of Circumcision

Buzz Words: Bleeding/infection after circumcision

Clinical Presentation: Circumcision is the surgical removal of the penile foreskin. Debate exists over the utility of circumcision, although recently the AAP stated the health benefits (decreased risk of STI, UTI, penile cancer, phimosis) outweighed the costs, but the decision is left to parents. This being said, circumcision is **the single most common surgical procedure** performed in the United States. Greater than 70% of US-born men are circumcised compared to less than 50% of non-US born men. You will not be responsible for recommending for or against circumcision in any instance on the exam, but be peripherally aware of complications. Prophylaxis against complications includes meticulous attention to anatomy and correct use of surgical equipment. These complications are rare (2–5 per 1000 circumcisions). For the curious (but low-yield for subject exams), the following is a list of complications:

1. Bleeding/hematoma
2. Infection

3. Ischemia/necrosis
4. Phimosis/inadequate tissue loss
5. Urinary retention

PPx: Surgical expertise

MoD: See above

Dx:

1. Clinical

Tx/Mgmt:

1. Based on complication, most commonly hemorrhage →
   local pressure application

Congenital Disorders of the Male Reproductive System

There are very few congenital disorders of the male reproductive system on the Pediatrics exam. The most important is Klinefelter syndrome, a pathology caused by XXY nondisjunction or translocation—this is a high-yield topic on the Pediatrics exam and you should know everything from Buzz Words to Tx/Mgmt. Two other important pathologies are hypospadias and cryptorchidism.

Hypospadias

Buzz Words: Urethral opening on ventral penis

Clinical Presentation: The external genitalia arise from proliferation of mesoderm and ectoderm around a primordial cloacal membrane. This produces the primordial external genital tissues of both sexes: the genital tubercle, genital folds, and genital swellings. Abnormal development of the urogenital folds around the urogenital sinus potentially leads to a high-yield pathology: hypospadias. Increased risk of UTI. These patients should NOT be circumcised, as urology may use the foreskin to repair the defect. Circumcision should also be avoided in patients with a spiral raphe.

PPx: N/A

MoD: Improper formation of the penile raphe due to incomplete fusion of the urogenital fold around the urogenital sinus

Dx: Clinical

Tx/Mgmt:

1. Avoid circumcision

Klinefelter Syndrome

Buzz Words: Male gynecomastia + atrophic testis + azoospermia + long extremities + testicular neoplasm

Clinical Presentation: The mesonephric (wolffian) ducts ultimately give rise to the male genital ducts. The

QUICK TIPS

Epispadias is an opening on the upper aspect, dorsum of penis. Know that epispadias is associated with exstrophy of the bladder!

development of exclusively the male reproductive system will be discussed here. While the female reproductive system will largely be reviewed elsewhere, a brief review of the differentiation between the two is necessary. Differentiation is determined by the presence of the SRY gene on the Y chromosome. The SRY gene will induce the primitive gonad to develop into the testis, which is composed of spermatogonia, Leydig cells, and Sertoli cells. Leydig cells produce testosterone. Sertoli cells produce anti-müllerian hormone, which will lead to the regression of the paramesonephric duct (female reproductive system). Both Sertoli cells and Leydig cells function improperly in the commonly tested pathology, Klinefelter syndrome. Some of the common presenting features include hypogonadism, long extremities, female hair distribution, gynecomastia, azoospermia, testicular atrophy.

PPx: N/A

MoD:

1. 47 XXY from nondisjunction or translocation:
   a. loss of Sertoli cells and dysgenesis of seminiferous tubules:
      i. Sertoli cells produce inhibin. Loss of inhibin leads to an increase in FSH, which upregulates aromatase (converts testosterone to estrogen).
   b. Leydig cell dysfunction:
      i. Decreased testosterone
      ii. Elevated LH (loss of negative feedback)

Dx:

1. Chromosomal analysis

Tx/Mgmt:

1. Depending on pathology, monitor for testicular neoplasms

Cryptorchidism

Buzz Words: Undescended testicles

Clinical Presentation: Cryptorchidism is the failure of one or both testes to descend into the scrotum and is the most common birth defect of male genitals. Increased risk of testicular cancer and decreased fertility. Can also be associated with testicular torsion and inguinal hernias.

PPx: Diabetes/obesity in mother can increase risk of cryptorchidism, prevent exposure to phthalate, and analgesics (ibuprofen, acetaminophen)

MoD: Idiopathic cause, elevated temperature of undescended testicle → defective spermatogenesis

Dx:

1. Physical exam (distinguish from retractile testis)
2. Pelvic ultrasound/MRI

Tx/Mgmt:

1. Conservative, may descend later
2. Orchiopexy until puberty, then orchiectomy due to risk
   for cancer
3. HCG hormone therapy

Channelopathies in the Kidney

Channelopathies refer to problems with ion channels in the nephron itself—they are infrequently tested on the Pediatrics exam as they are most often managed by specialists. However, there are a few channelopathies that are important to recognize only because of their prevalence on exams that range from pediatrics to medicine to USMLE Step I/2. The three most common to know and understand are Bartter, Gitelman, and Liddle syndrome. For these, recognize only the clinical features and treatment. The diagnosis will ALWAYS be made based on a BMP and UA. There is no prophylaxis of inheritable disorders.

Syndrome	Buzz Words	PPx	MoD	Dx	Tx/Mgmt
Bartter	Polyuria, metabolic alkalosis, hypokalemia, PGE, urine Ca	N/A	Inactivating mutation in NKCC, AR inheritance	BMP/UA	K+ supplements, spironolactone, NSAIDs, ACEI, indomethacin
Gitelman	Metabolic alkalosis, hypokalemia, hypocalciuria, hypotension		Inactivating mutation in NCC, AR inheritance		K+ supplements, spirinolactone
Liddle	Hypertension, low renin, low aldosterone		Activating mutation in ENAC, AD		Amiloride, Na restriction
Pseudohypoaldosteronism I	Salt wasting, hypotension, hyperkalemia, high aldosterone, high renin		Inactivating mutation in ENAC, AD/AR		Amiloride, Na restriction
Pseudohypoaldosteronism II (Gordon's)	Opposite of Gitelman, hypertension, hyperkalemia		Activation mutation in NCC, AD		Diuretic use

TABLE 11.1 Outpatient Management of Pediatric Urinary Tract Infections (Oral Therapy)[a]

Common Pathogens	Type of Infection	Drug	Dosage	Min Length of Therapy (Days)
Escherichia coli; Enterobacter, Klebsiella, Proteus sp.; group B streptococcus (neonates)	Cystitis	Amoxicillin	<3 months: 20–30 mg/ kg per day bid ≥3 months: 25–50 mg/ kg per day bid Adolescents: 250 mg tid or 500 mg bid	3–7
		Amoxicillin-clavulanate[b]	<3 months: 30 mg/kg per day bid ≥3 months: 25–45 mg/ kg per day bid Adolescents: 875/125 mg bid	
		Cefixime	16 mg/kg per day bid × 1 day then 8 mg/kg per day bid thereafter	
		Cephalexin	25–50 mg/kg per day qid (max: 4 g)	
		TMP-SMX[c]	≥2 months: 8–10 mg/kg per day bid Adolescents: 160 mg bid	
	Acute pyelonephritis	Recommended therapy for cystitis	See above OR	10
		Ciprofloxacin	Infants >1 year: 20–30 mg/kg per day bid (max: 1.5 g/day)	

[a]All dosages are suggestions only. Some antibiotics will require adjustment in the presence of renal impairment. For pregnant adolescents, clinicians should review pregnancy risk factors prior to administration. All patients should be screened for drug allergies.
[b]Amoxicillin-clavulanate dose is based on the amoxicillin component.
[c]TMP-SMX dose is based on the trimethoprim component. Not recommended for patients ≤2 months or patients who have renal insufficiency. Empiric use of TMP-SMX is not recommended if regional resistance to E. coli is ≥20%.
max, Maximum; min, minimum; sp., species; TMP-SMX, trimethoprim/sulfamethoxazole; UTI, urinary tract infection.

GUNNER PRACTICE

1. A 4-year-old boy presents to your clinic with his mother for hematuria. Recently, his mother has noticed blood in his urine and the boy has had a decline in appetite over the past month. On physical exam, you note a left abdominal mass; there is no pain or tenderness to palpation. The mother tells you his grandfather had an "abdominal mass" removed as a child but cannot tell you specifics. Which of the following is the most appropriate next step in diagnosis?

A. Abdominal ultrasound

B. Exploratory laparotomy

 C. Urinalysis
 D. Urine culture
 E. Digital rectal exam
2. A 3-year-old child presents to your office with his father for a follow-up after orchiopexy for cryptorchidism. The surgical site has healed well with no signs of infection. Despite surgical correction, which of the following is this child still most at risk for?
 A. Urinary tract infection
 B. Spermatocele
 C. Testicular torsion
 D. Testicular cancer
 E. Epididymitis
3. A previously healthy 8-year-old boy is brought to your office due to a rash on his arms over the past 4 days. Physical exam shows a crusted, excoriated rash over his forearms and lower arm. The remainder of the exam is within normal limits, although his mother says his eyes are "more swollen than usual." His blood pressure is 155/80. Urinalysis shows 3+ protein, 30–50 RBCs and 10–20 WBCs. Which of the following is the most appropriate next step in management?
 A. Antibiotics
 B. Steroids
 C. NSAIDs
 D. Nephrectomy
 E. Foley catheter placement

ANSWERS: What Would Gunner Jess/Jim Do?

1. WWGJD? A 4-year-old boy presents to your clinic with his mother for hematuria. Recently, his mother has noticed blood in his urine and the boy has had a decline in appetite over the past month. On physical exam, you note a left abdominal mass; there is no pain or tenderness to palpation. The mother tells you his grandfather had an "abdominal mass" removed as a child but cannot tell you specifics. Which of the following is the most appropriate next step in diagnosis?

Answer: A, Abdominal ultrasound

Explanation: A patient between 3 and 5 years of age presenting with an abdominal mass should always be suspected of Wilms tumor or other kidney tumor, especially in setting of hematuria and a family history of a potential tumor. Abdominal ultrasound is always the first step in diagnosis.

B. Exploratory laparotomy → Incorrect. This is important in staging Wilms tumor, but cannot be used until a diagnosis has been made already.

C. Urinalysis → Incorrect. May help you refine your diagnosis, but is not specific or sensitive enough to diagnose Wilm's.

D. Urine culture → Incorrect. Would be indicated for suspected infection but there are no presenting features, including fever. UTI would also not usually cause hematuria.

E. Digital rectal exam → Incorrect. Would be indicated in *E. coli* prostatitis if boy were presenting with fever and back pain but unnecessary in this case.

2. WWGJD? A 3-year-old child presents to your office with his father for a follow-up after orchiopexy for cryptorchidism. The surgical site has healed well with no signs of infection. Despite surgical correction, which of the following is this child still most at risk for?

Answer: D, Testicular cancer

Explanation: Although cryptorchidism will lead to increased rates of testicular cancers, orchiopexy is not completely curative as cancer can still occur in the contralateral testicle. This has been postulated to be due to hypergonadotrophism.

A. Urinary tract infection → Incorrect. Not associated with orchiopexy.

B. Spermatocele → Incorrect. Not associated with orchiopexy.

C. Testicular torsion → Incorrect. not associated with orchiopexy.

E. Epididymitis → Incorrect. Not associated with orchiopexy.

3. WWGJD? A previously healthy 8-year-old boy is brought to your office due to a rash on his arms over the past 4 days. Physical exam shows a crusted, excoriated rash over his forearms and lower arm. The remainder of the exam is within normal limits, although his mother says his eyes are "more swollen than usual." His blood pressure is 155/80. Urinalysis shows 3+ protein, 30–50 RBCs and 10–20 WBCs. Which of the following is the most appropriate next step in management?

Answer: A, Antibiotics

Explanation: This is a typical case of postinfectious glomerulonephritis secondary to impetigo infection. The most important feature is the acute presentation of this that coincides with high blood pressure and high urine protein. There is heavy debate over the use of antibiotics in the treatment of post-strep glomerulonephritis EXCEPT in obvious cases where there is clear evidence of infection. If this patient's infection had subsided, treatment would be conservative.

B. Steroids → Incorrect. Not indicated for post-strep glomerulonephritis; indicated for other, more chronic glomerular pathologies.

C. NSAIDs → Incorrect. Not indicated for post-strep glomerulonephritis and may precipitate interstitial nephropathy.

D. Nephrectomy → Incorrect. Not indicated for post-strep glomerulonephritis.

E. Foley catheter placement → Incorrect. Not indicated for post-strep glomerulonephritis, used for bladder incontinence.

12

Disorders of Pregnancy, Childbirth, and Puerperium

Hao-Hua Wu, Daniel Gromer, Morgan Brown, Leo Wang, and Rebecca Tenney-Soeiro

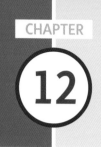

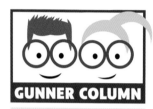

GUNNER COLUMN

Introduction

The NBME states that "Disorders of Pregnancy, Childbirth and Puerperium" comprises 1–5 questions. What they mean are disorders of the newborn not otherwise covered. You will not need to know conditions that affect only the mother during or after childbirth, such as endometritis or postpartum hemorrhage. Instead, focus on high-yield disorders encountered in neonatalogy such as androgen insensitivity syndrome (AIS), TORCH infections, Kallman syndrome, and 22q11.2 deletion syndrome (formerly known as DiGeorge's).

This chapter is organized into (1) Disorders of Ambiguous Genitalia, (2) Aneuploidy Disorders, (3) Congenital Infection, (4) Miscellaneous Disorders of the Newborn, and (5) Gunner Practice.

Disorders of Ambiguous Genitalia

For the Pediatrics exam, be sure to know the differential of patients with ambiguous genitalia at birth. Notably, these patients may present as adolescents in the question stem (e.g., ambiguous genitalia at birth, present as teenagers because of infertility).

Androgen Insensitivity Syndrome

Buzz Words: No hair + female phenotype + no uterus/fallopian tube/ovary + b/l inguinal masses + blind vaginal pouch + 46XY + primary amenorrhea + breast development with no hair

Clinical Presentation: AIS has end-organ resistance to androgens because of a mutated androgen receptor. Patients have functioning testes that secrete anti-müllerian hormone, which is why there are no müllerian structures (e.g., no uterus, fallopian tube, or ovary; regression of upper genital tract). However, there is a blind vaginal pouch because of no androgen stimulation. The most important Buzz Words for AIS are patients with **no hair** and **XY chromosome**.

Prophylaxis (PPx): N/A

Mechanism of Disease (MoD): Dysfunction of androgen receptors → inability to respond to testosterone → free floating testosterone converted to estrogen → feminization of external genitalia and breast development

Diagnostic Steps (Dx):

1. PE (shows no pubic or axillary hair, no penis/scrotum but may have testes palpable in inguinal canal/labio-scrotal folds)
2. Karyotype analysis
3. Abdominal ultrasound (finds **cryptorchid testes**)

Treatment and Management Steps (Tx/Mgmt):

1. Gonadectomy **after puberty** to reduce chance of testicular carcinoma but allow breast development.
2. Estrogen therapy after removal of gonads.

5-Alpha Reductase Deficiency

Buzz Words: 46XY + Amenorrhea + **ambiguous external genitalia until puberty** + male internal genitalia (seminal vesicles, epididymis, ejaculatory duct, ductus deferens) → 5-alpha reductase deficiency

Clinical Presentation: 5-Alpha reductase converts testosterone to dihydrotestosterone (DHT). Patients who have a deficiency of 5-alpha reductase cannot produce DHT, leading to disruption in the formation of the male external genitalia. The result is ambiguous genitalia or even female phenotype. The hallmark of this disease is that male sexual characteristics start to develop during puberty, coinciding with a normal surge of hormone production. However, no DHT-dependent secondary sexual characteristics will develop (no acne, body/facial hair).

PPx: N/A

MoD: Mutation of *SRD5A2* gene for 5-alpha reductase deficiency

Dx:

1. PE
2. Karyotype analysis
3. Abdominal ultrasound

Tx/Mgmt:

1. Hormone replacement therapy
2. Gonadectomy if female gender assignment

Aromatase Deficiency

Buzz Words: 46XX + normal internal genitalia (uterus, fallopian tube, ovary) + **ambiguous external genitalia** + primary amenorrhea + **clitoromegaly** + sexual infantilism + high testosterone/androstendione + high FSH/LH + low estrogen/estradiol levels + **multiple ovarian cysts (e.g., multicystic ovaries, most often after puberty)** → Aromatase deficiency

Masculinization of mother during pregnancy + masculinization resolves with delivery → aromatase deficiency of baby

Clinical Presentation: Aromatase converts testosterone into estrogen. Folks with aromatase deficiency can be either XX or XY. You will get one of two chief complaints: (1) newborn with ambiguous genitalia with eventual primary amenorrhea and multiple ovarian cysts, or (2) a mother who experiences virilization during pregnancy. In both cases, the symptoms are caused by high testosterone levels. Treatment for 46XX patients is hormone therapy to replace the missing estrogen.

PPx: N/A

MoD: Mutation of *CYP919A1* gene → deficiency of aromatase

Dx:
1. FSH/LH (high)
2. Estrogen and estradiol (low)
3. Testosterone and androstenedione concentrations (high)
4. Ultrasound → Ovarian cysts

Tx/Mgmt:
1. Estrogen replacement

Congenital Adrenal Hyperplasia

Buzz Words:

46XX + Ambiguous genitalia or phallus/scrotum present + virilization + hypotension + hyperaldosterone + increased sex steroid → 21-alpha hydroxylase

46XX + delayed puberty, no ambiguous genitalia + hypertension → 17-alpha hydroxylase deficiency

46XX + ambiguous genitalia + virilization + high levels of sex hormones + hypertension → 11-beta hydroxylase

Clinical Presentation: Congenital adrenal hyperplasia (CAH) consists of three types of disorders that do not make cortisol, which is what induces the hyperplasia of the adrenal glands. Depending on the enzyme deficiency, however, different steroids are high or low.

21-alpha hydroxylase deficiency = decreased mineralocorticoid → hypotension + ambiguous genitalia:
- Can be salt wasting (e.g., no aldosterone, no salt retention → hyponatremia and hyperkalemia) or virilizing (aldosterone is present; only cortisol synthesis impaired)

17-hydroxylase deficiency = mineralocorticoid producing → hypertension + delayed puberty + androgens not elevated so no ambiguous genitalia

11-beta hydroxylase deficiency = mineralocorticoid producing (11-deoxycorticosterone) → hypertension + ambiguous genitalia

PPx: N/A

MoD: For 21-hydroxylase deficiency, no conversion of progesterone to deoxycorticosterone (intermediates on aldosterone pathway) and 17-hydroxyprogesterone to 11-deoxycortisol (on the cortisol pathway) → buildup of hormone precursors that are converted to androgens → ambiguous genitalia for 46XX

For 17-hydroxylase deficiency → progesterone and pregnenolone are not converted to 17-hydroxyprogesterone and 17-hydroxypregnenolone, respectively → no production of cortisol and buildup of aldosterone/androgen

For 11-beta hydroxylase deficiency → penultimate step of aldosterone (deoxycorticosterone to corticosterone) and terminal step of cortisol (11-deoxycortisol → cortisol) pathways are inhibited → even though no aldosterone, 11-deoxycortisol acts as weak mineralocorticoid → shunts hormones to androgens → ambiguous genitalia

Dx:
1. PE
2. Ultrasound to identify internal genitalia
3. Labs for sex steroids (e.g., elevated androgens in 21- and 11-hydroxylase deficiency)
4. Karyotype (essential part of evaluation)

Tx/Mgmt:
1. Glucocorticoids for all types of CAH
2. If 21-alpha hydroxylase deficiency → mineralocorticoid
3. If 17-hydroxylase → sex steroids (estrogen)

XY Gonadal Dysgenesis (aka Swyer Syndrome)

Buzz Words: 46XY + internal/external female genitalia + nonfunctional ovaries + failure of breast development/menarche + axillary/pubic hair present

Clinical Presentation: XY gonadal dysgenesis (aka Swyer syndrome) is the only disorder that has a 46XY karyotype and **both** internal and external female reproductive structures. This is because of a defect in *SRY* gene, thus stunting testicular formation.

PPx: N/A

MoD: *SRY* gene defect in Y chromosome → no testicular formation → no testosterone or anti-müllerian hormone produced → wolffian ducts fail to develop and müllerian ducts take its place

> **QUICK TIPS**
> Do not confuse XY gonadal dysgenesis with XY disorder of sex development (DSD), which is a 46XX individual with male external genitalia 2/2 excessive exposure to androgens as a neonate. Congenital adrenal hyperplasia is an example of XY DSD.

Dx:

1. FSH/LH (high, no estrogen downregulating them)
2. Karyotype

Tx/Mgmt:

1. **Immediate** removal of gonads (don't wait until puberty)
2. Hormone replacement (estrogen for breast development; progestin for periods)
3. Embryo transfer if patient wishes to be pregnant

QUICK TIPS

Swyer syndrome requires immediate removal of gonads because risk of cancer is much higher than in AIS, which can have gonads removed after puberty.

Aneuploidy Disorders

Unlike the Ob/Gyn exam, you will not be expected to know granular details about Quad screen results (e.g., inhibin A, hCG, AFP, and estriol) on the Pediatrics exam. However, it is important to know that mothers with alpha-fetoprotein (AFP) tested in the first/second trimester are likely to be carrying a fetus with a neural tube defect. On the other hand, low AFP may be indicative Down syndrome.

Trisomy 21

Buzz Words: Newborn **+ sandal gap toes** + hypotonia + flat facies/flattened nasal bridge + small, rotated cup-shaped ears + small size + **Simian creases** + epicanthic folds + oblique/up-slanting palpebral fissures

Clinical Presentation: Trisomy 21 is the constellation of signs and symptoms that occur secondary to presence of three copies of chromosome 21. The most high-yield Buzz Words are sandal gap toes and simian crease of the hands. This is very frequently tested on the exam and is seen in Ob/Gyn, Medicine, Surgery, Neurology, and Psychiatry. For the Pediatrics exam, just be able to identify the newborn Buzz Words. You may also be tested on the medical complications of Trisomy 21 that affect the pediatric population, such as increased risk of ALL, atlantoaxial instability, hypothyroidism, as well as **cardiac** and **GI** complications that can present at birth:

1. Endocardial cushion defects:
   - Ventricular septal defect (e.g., "holosystolic murmur")
   - Atrial septal defect (e.g., "fixed split S2" and "low-grade diastolic murmur")
2. Patent ductus arteriosus
3. Hirschsprung disease (e.g., "failure to pass meconium")
4. Intestinal atresia (most commonly duodenal atresia)
5. Annular pancreas
6. Imperforate anus

PPx: **More likely tested on Ob/Gyn instead of Pediatrics shelf, but good to know for the wards.** (1) First trimester: Pregnancy-associated protein A (PAPP-A) and free beta hCG (known as the combined test) = screening for trisomy 21; positive if **high hCG** and **low PAPP-A.** (2) First trimester: Nuchal translucency and presence/absence of nasal bone on ultrasound = screening for trisomy 21. (3) Second semester: Quad screening test. (4) Higher risk if advanced maternal age when pregnant.

MoD: Nondisjunction of chromosome 21 (or more rarely translocation)

Dx:
1. Karyotype analysis with amniocentesis if quad screening shows decreased AFP/estriol and increased hCG and inhibin A
2. Echo for cardiac defects
3. Abdominal ultrasound for abdominal defects

Tx/Mgmt:
1. Supportive
2. Surgery to repair cardiac or abdominal defects

Trisomy 18 (Edwards Syndrome)

Buzz Words: Rockerbottom feet + VSD + clenched hand and overlapping flexed fingers + horseshoe kidney

Clinical Presentation: Trisomy 18 is aneuploidy of chromosome 18 that causes rockerbottom feet, horseshoe kidney, and VSD. Other heart defects include ASD, PDA. Can also be associated with microcephaly, cleft lip/palate.

PPx:
1. Quad screen test (all components low)

MoD: Nondisjunction of chromosome 18

Dx:
1. If Quad screen positive, karyotype with amniocentesis

Tx/Mgmt:
1. Surgery for VSD
2. Ten percent survival at 1 year

Trisomy 13 (Patau Syndrome)

Buzz Words: Newborn + cleft lip/palate + polydactyly

Clinical Presentation: Trisomy 13 is aneuploidy of chromosome 13 that causes cleft lip/palate and polydactyly of the newborn. Most often associated with midline defects (e.g., microcephaly, holoprosencephaly, omphalocele).

PPx: N/A

MoD: Nondisjunction (or translocation) of chromosome 13

99 AR

Peyton Manning mnemonic for Trisomy 18

99 AR

Buzz Word mnemonic for Trisomy 13

Dx:
1. If quad screen positive, karyotype with amniocentesis
Tx/Mgmt:
1. Surgery to correct cleft palate
2. Death often before 6 months of age

Turner Syndrome

Buzz Words: Amenorrhea + infertility + streak ovaries + short stature + coarctation of aorta (differences in BP among extremities) + bicuspid aortic valve + generalized edema (hydrops)/lymphedema + webbed neck + cubitus valgus (when forearm is angled away from body to greater degree than normal when fully extended) + horseshoe kidney + low hairline (where hair starts growing is too close to eyebrows) + **osteoporosis** (2/2 ovarian dysgenesis)

Clinical Presentation: Turner syndrome is a genetic disorder that is high yield on the Pediatrics exam. It affects only females (XO on chromosomal analysis can present in many different ways: newborns may be found to have lower than normal blood pressure in their lower extremities [coarctation of aorta]; infants/toddlers may be found to have a webbed neck, nuchal folds, lymphedema, and growth failure; and adults may have cardiovascular problems due to a bicuspid aortic valve). Patients with Turner syndrome have **normal cognitive abilities.** Make sure to learn the Buzz Words, MoD, Dx and Tx/Mgmt of this disease well as it can also appear on your Ob/Gyn, Psychiatry, and Medicine shelf.

PPx:
1. None
MoD:
1. XO genotype
   - Rib notching 2/2 development of collateral vessels that develop to bypass coarctation of aorta
   - Lymphedema occurs 2/2 dysgenesis of the lymphatic network

Dx:
1. FSH levels (likely will have high FSH and LH because of ovarian dysgenesis and no negative feedback)
2. Inhibin levels (will likely be low because inhibin → measure of ovarian function)
3. Estrogen/testosterone → lower estrogen and normal testosterone
4. **Karyotype analysis for definitive diagnosis**
5. ECG and Echo to screen for cardiac abnormalities
6. BMP to look at renal function
7. RBUS to evaluate horseshoe kidney

Tx/Mgmt:
1. Treatment for coarctation of aorta (e.g., prostaglandins and surgical repair) and bicuspid aortic valve (e.g., valvular replacement)
2. Recombinant human growth hormone

Congenital Infection

You may be asked to identify a congenital infection on the Pediatrics exam (Table 12.1). Below are the 7 most commonly tested infections. Be sure to know the difference between early and late congenital syphilis (<2 years old vs. ≥2 years old) as well as what periventricular versus intracranial calcifications mean (periVentricular= congenital CMV; intracranial = congenital Toxoplasmosis).

TABLE 12.1 Congenital Infections

Buzz Words	Infection
Newborn + failure to thrive + lymphadenopathy + hepatosplenomegaly + thrush + maternal IV drug use + recurrent infections	Congenital HIV
Newborn + IUGR + microcephaly + sensorineural hearing loss + patent ductus arteriosus murmur + cataracts (leukocoria) or glaucoma + hepatosplenomegaly + thrombocytopenic purpura (**blueberry muffin rash**) + anemia + leukopenia	Congenital rubella
Newborn + IUGR + microcephaly + sensorineural hearing loss + no heart abnormality + **periventricular** calcifications + hepatosplenomegaly + chorioretinitis	Congenital CMV
≥2 years old + **sensorineural hearing loss** + no heart abnormality + saber shins + snuffles+ frontal bossing + **interstitial keratitis** + **Hutchinson incisors** + bulldog facies 2/2 maldevelopment of maxilla + gummatous ulcers of nose and hard palate	Late congenital syphilis (≥2 years old)
<2 year old + runny nose + copper colored macular rash on palms and soles + vesiculobullous eruptions + hepatosplenomegaly + neutropenia/ thrombocytopenia	Early congenital syphilis (<2 years old)
Newborn + microcephaly + limb hypoplasia + intrauterine growth restriction + cataracts + chorioretinitis + mother with pruritic vesicular rash	Congenital varicella syndrome
Newborn + **intracranial** calcifications + chorioretinitis + hydrocephalus + hepatosplenomegaly + jaundice	Congenital toxoplasmosis

Miscellaneous Disorders of the Newborn

Gastroschisis and Omphalocele

Buzz Words: Newborn + abdominal organs with no covering → gastroschisis

Newborn + abdominal organs with covering membrane → omphalocele

Clinical Presentation: Gastroschisis and omphalocele are abdominal wall defects that are seen at birth. Gastroschisis has no abdominal membrane covering (**fascial defect** usually just to the right of the umbilical cord), while an omphalocele has a covering (**central defect with an intact membranous sac**). On the shelf, only the Buzz Words will be tested.

PPx: N/A

MoD: N/A

Dx:

1. PE
2. Ultrasound

Tx/Mgmt:

1. Surgery

Fetal Alcohol Syndrome

Buzz Words: Smooth philtrum + ADHD-like symptoms + microcephaly + growth retardation + mental retardation (most common acquired cause)

Clinical Presentation: Fetal alcohol syndrome (FAS) is the constellation of signs and symptoms that occur in the fetus 2/2 alcohol use during pregnancy. The most characteristic Buzz Word for FAS is smooth philtrum of the upper lip. The mechanism is unknown and treatment is supportive.

PPx: Avoid alcohol during pregnancy

MoD: Unknown

Dx:

1. Diagnosis of exclusion
   - Requires history of maternal alcohol use + growth restriction + CNS involvement + facial abnormalities

Tx/Mgmt:

1. Supportive
2. Counseling

22q11.2 Deletion Syndrome (aka DiGeorge Syndrome, aka Velocardiofacial Syndrome, aka Conotruncal Anomaly Face Syndrome)

Buzz Words: Conotruncal cardiac defects (cyanotic disorders such as truncus arteriosus and tetralogy of Fallot) + Abnormal facies (low set ears and micrognathia) + **T**hymic aplasia/hypoplasia + **C**left palate + **H**ypocalcemia (seizures, QT prolongation)

Clinical Presentation: 22q11.2 deletion syndrome is a genetic disorder that describes the phenotypical traits of a patient with a deletion at 22q11.2, which is the most common microdeletion in humans. This was formerly known as DiGeorge syndrome, Velo-cardio-facial syndrome, or conotruncal anomaly face syndrome, but was changed into a unifying name once it was clear the genetic abnormality was the same. Since many of the exam questions were written a while ago, you may still see the terms DiGeorge syndrome or velo-cardio-facial syndrome pop up. Just be sure to know the distinguishing features of this syndrome: low set ears, micrognathia, conotruncal abnormalities (e.g., tetralogy of Fallot, truncus arteriosus), immunodeficiency, thymic aplasia/hypoplasia, cleft palate, and hypocalcemia.

One thing to be aware of is that the exam presentation of 22q11.2 deletion syndrome could be very different from what you see clinically. Many patients with 22q11.2 deletion syndrome are now living into adulthood and have been found to suffer from concomitant psychiatric disease (e.g., schizophrenia), intellectual disability, autoimmune disorders, hypothyroidism, Parkinson disease, and neurodegenerative disease. These manifestations have not been classically seen on the exam as Buzz Words for 22q11.2 deletion syndrome (aka DiGeorge aka velo-cardio-facial syndrome). However, as questions get updated, these adult manifestations may begin to appear as well (Fig. 12.1).

PPx:
1. Avoid live vaccines such as rotavirus, yellow fever, polio because of thymic aplasia → immunodeficiency; inactivated or killed vaccines are OK

MoD: Chromosome 22q11.2 deletion → defective development of third and fourth pharyngeal pouches resulting in hypoplasia or absence of parathyroid glands and thymus.
- Hypocalcemia 2/2 hypoplasia of parathyroid glands + cleft palate + congenital heart disease (truncus arteriosus) + immunodeficiency 2/2 thymic aplasia/hypoplasia and resultant T-cell deficiency

Dx:
1. BMP to assess for life-threatening hypocalcemia
2. Chest x-ray (CXR) will show absent thymus
3. ECG and echo to assess cardiac defects
4. Chromosomal analysis

MNEMONIC

CATCH DiGeorge if you can (**C**onotruncal cardiac defects, **A**bnormal facies, **T**hymic aplasia/hypoplasia, **C**left palate, **H**ypocalcemia)

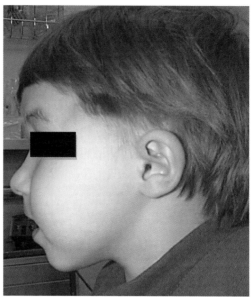

FIG. 12.1 Characteristic facies of 22q11.2 deletion syndrome including micrognathia and low set ears.

Tx/Mgmt:
1. Replete calcium if hypocalcemic
2. Surgical correction of conotruncal cardiac defects
3. Surgical correction of cleft palate
4. Genetic counseling

GUNNER PRACTICE

1. A newborn female is brought to the neonatal intensive care unit for jaundice. During gestation, she was repeatedly noted to be small for gestational age, but her delivery was otherwise unremarkable, as is her family history. Her vital signs are T 97.3°F, HR 140, RR 40, SpO$_2$ 98% in room air. Physical examination reveals a comfortable, jaundiced newborn with diffuse petechiae and purpura. Fundoscopy reveals bilateral cataracts, and initial labs reveal PLT 47 and ALT 69. Two days after delivery, cardiac auscultation yields a constant, machinery-like murmur heard best 2 cm to the left of the left upper sternal border. The infant also fails her audiology screening assessment at that time. What is the most likely diagnosis?
A. Congenital syphilis infection
B. Galactosemia
C. Congenital rubella infection
D. HIV infection
E. Congenital parvovirus infection

2. A 3-month-old male infant is brought to the Emergency Department by his mother for not waking up to feed. She reports that the child was irritable earlier in the day, but his behavior has become more concerning since that time. His birth history is notable for shoulder dystocia, but interim examinations by his pediatrician have not revealed evidence of anoxic brain injury or developmental delay. His single older sister has autism spectrum disorder. The infant's vital signs are T 97.4°F, HR 79, and SpO_2 is 98%. The child subsequently has a 2-minute tonic-clonic seizure. After stabilization of the patient, skin examination reveals erythema on both buttocks and symmetrically around both arms. Of the following, what is the next best step in management?

A. Electroencephalogram

B. Fundoscopy

C. Echocardiogram

D. MRI brain

E. Vancomycin and ceftriaxone administration

ANSWERS: What Would Gunner Jess/Jim Do?

1. WWGJD? A newborn female is brought to the neonatal intensive care unit for jaundice. During gestation, she was repeatedly noted to be small for gestational age, but her delivery was otherwise unremarkable, as is her family history. Her vital signs are T 97.3°F, HR 140, RR 40, SpO$_2$ 98% on room air. Physical examination reveals a comfortable, jaundiced newborn with diffuse petechiae and purpura. Fundoscopy reveals bilateral cataracts, and initial labs reveal PLT 47 and ALT 69. Two days after delivery, cardiac auscultation yields a constant, machinery-like murmur heard best 2 cm to the left of the left upper sternal border. The infant also fails her audiology screening assessment at that time. What is the most likely diagnosis?

Answer: C, Congenital rubella infection

Explanation: This question assesses your understanding of presentations of TORCH infections. This is a newborn infant with jaundice, purpura, thrombocytopenia, hepatitis, cataracts, patent ductus arteriosus, and auditory dysfunction, a classic presentation of congenital rubella infection. The jaundice and purpura cause these patients to be referred to as "blueberry muffin" babies.

A. Congenital syphilis infection → Incorrect. These patients have a myriad of manifestations, including nasal discharge ("snuffles"), lymphadenopathy, and bony anomalies.

B. Galactosemia → Incorrect. These patients may exhibit jaundice, liver abnormalities, and cataracts, as well as other manifestations, but they are less likely to have cardiac defects and auditory dysfunction (and likely to be more ill than this comfortable patient after 2 weeks of feeds, as well as less obviously ill at birth).

D. HIV infection → Incorrect. This is diagnosed via HIV testing of infant, and is not indicated by these symptoms and signs.

E. Congenital parvovirus infection → Incorrect. Congenital parvovirus infection can cause hydrops fetalis or transient effusions in the fetus, but is unlikely to cause the constellation of symptoms seen in this patient.

2. WWGJD? A 3-month-old male infant is brought to the Emergency Department by his mother for not waking up to feed. She reports that the child was irritable earlier

in the day, but his behavior has become more concerning since. His birth history is notable for shoulder dystocia, but interim examinations by his pediatricians have not revealed evidence of anoxic brain injury or developmental delay. His single older sister has Autism Spectrum Disorder. The infant's vital signs are T 97.4°F, HR 79, and SpO$_2$ is 98%. The child subsequently has a 2-minute tonic-clonic seizure. After stabilization of the patient, skin examination reveals erythema on both buttocks and symmetrically around both arms. Of the following, what is the next best step in management?

Answer: B, Fundoscopy

Explanation: This question is designed to test your recognition of the nonspecific symptoms and signs of a common and important diagnosis. The patient is an infant with bradycardia, apneic events, altered mental status, and seizure, as well as symmetrical skin markings on odd and concerning body surfaces. This constellation of symptoms should raise your concern for non-accidental trauma, or NAT. The symptoms leading to this diagnosis can be variable and nonspecific, so a high level of suspicion is important. Frequently, questions will assert that an infant was injured while achieving a milestone that they should not be capable of (like a 2-month-old crawling). This patient should be evaluated with fundoscopy (looking for retinal hemorrhages, a common finding in these infants with head trauma or shaken baby syndrome) and a head CT (looking for cranial and intracranial injuries). Additionally, the proper authorities and entities within the hospital should be contacted.

A. Electroencephalogram → Incorrect. EEG is not an appropriate next step toward diagnosis. Suspicion for a seizure disorder is low in this child with no relevant past medical history (except for the shoulder dystocia) and with findings concerning for cranial injuries.

C. Echocardiogram → Incorrect. While apnea, bradycardia, and altered mental status can certainly be indicative of a cardiac condition disorder in an infant, this child has signs and symptoms more indicative of NAT.

D. MRI brain → Incorrect. This patient should receive a head CT, which is faster, reliably detects intracranial hemorrhage, and should not require the sedation that might be required in an infant for

MRI. Additionally, it is reasonable to argue that, if the patient is stable, the physical exam maneuver (fundoscopy) should precede advanced imaging techniques if suspicion is heightened or the diagnosis confirmed.

E. Vancomycin and ceftriaxone administration → Incorrect. This patient is less likely to have bacterial meningitis and more likely to have NAT.

Disorders of the Skin and Subcutaneous Tissues

Kishore Jayakumar, Nina Fainberg, Hao-Hua Wu,
Leo Wang, and Rebecca Tenney-Soeiro

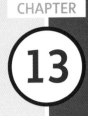

Dermatologic problems are common complaints in pediatrics, making up approximately 10% of visits to general pediatricians and family physicians. This chapter focuses on the most common (and most commonly tested) primary diseases of the integumentary system, which includes the skin, hair, and nails. The vast range of disorders affecting the skin allows examiners to pose questions relating to infectious diseases, immunology, rheumatology, congenital anomalies, and more. On the other hand, none of these diseases will be examined in detail, so you may best prepare for the Pediatrics exam by understanding the basic features of each disorder.

Questions about skin topics on the exam will focus on the textbook description of a disease, often with an accompanying photograph. As such, you should strive for the following: (1) know the classic "Buzz Word" descriptors that commonly appear in the question stem and (2) be familiar with the appearance of the skin disease, to allow for recognition of a photograph if provided.

This chapter is divided into several sections, including (1) Infectious Disorders and Infestations, (2) Immunologic and Inflammatory Disorders, (3) Disorders of the Hair and Hair Follicles, (4) Disorders of Sweat and Sebaceous Glands, (5) Congenital Disorders, and (6) Gunner Practice (application of the material learned). As always, each disease process is sorted into the four physician tasks on which you will be tested: (1) Prophylactic (PPx) management, (2) Mechanism of Disease (MoD), (3) Diagnostic Steps (Dx), and (4) Treatment/Management (Tx/Mgmt).

Infectious Disorders and Infestations

Cellulitis

Buzz Words: **Poorly demarcated, nonelevated** area of skin erythema + swelling, warmth, tenderness + lower extremity > upper extremity + unilateral > bilateral

Clinical Presentation: The most common chief complaint is a painful red rash. Systemic symptoms may occur. Patient may report previously injured skin (trauma,

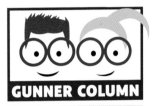

GUNNER COLUMN

insect bites, inflammation, preexisting infection, venous insufficiency) and diabetes.

PPx: Antibiotics for patients with recurrent cellulitis with predisposing conditions

MoD: Bacterial entry via disruption to skin barrier. Beta-hemolytic streptococci and *Staphylococcus aureus* are most common.

Dx:

1. Clinical
2. Ultrasound with Gram stain and culture of expressed fluid if underlying abscess

Tx/Mgmt:

1. Elevation
2. Antibiotics (for nonpurulent cellulitis, first-generation cephalosporin empirically covers beta-hemolytic strep and methicillin-sensitive S. *aureus* [MSSA]; for purulent cellulitis, clindamycin, trimethoprim-sulfamethoxazole [TMP-SMX], or doxycycline empirically covers methicillin-resistant S. *aureus* [MRSA])

Erysipelas

Buzz Words: Sharply demarcated + elevated area of skin erythema + swelling + warmth + tenderness + frequent facial involvement (butterfly) and involvement of ear (Milian sign) + lower extremity > upper extremity + unilateral > bilateral

Clinical Presentation: Patients present with a painful red rash and more frequently have systemic symptoms than patients with cellulitis. Patient may have previously injured skin (trauma, insect bites, inflammation, preexisting infection, venous insufficiency) and diabetes.

PPx: N/A

MoD: Group A streptococci

Dx:

1. Clinical
2. Ultrasound with Gram stain and culture of expressed fluid if underlying abscess

Tx/Mgmt:

1. Antibiotics, often IV, especially if systemic manifestations are present (ceftriaxone, cefazolin)

Impetigo

Buzz Words: Contagious superficial bacterial infection + papules + vesicles + pustules, **honey-colored crusts** + nonbullous > bullous

Clinical Presentation: Most common in ages 2–5. Presents as sores or blisters on face, neck, and hands. More likely in warm conditions. Transmitted among individuals in close contact.

PPx: N/A

MoD: Bullous (*S. aureus*); nonbullous (*S. aureus* > group A strep)

Dx:
1. Clinical
2. Gram stain and wound culture

Tx/Mgmt:
1. Topical antibiotics (mupirocin)
2. Oral antibiotics if topical therapy fails or if extensive disease (cephalexin)

Staphylococcal Scalded Skin Syndrome

Buzz Words: Systemic exotoxin-mediated **exfoliative disease** + flaccid blisters (positive Nikolsky sign) + **mucous membrane involvement absent**

Clinical Presentation: Chief complaint of desquamation of skin caused by exotoxin

PPx: N/A

MoD: Exotoxin causing cleavage of desmoglein-1 (desmosome protein) at stratum granulosum

Dx:
1. Clinical
2. Culture focus of suspected infection

Tx/Mgmt:
1. Hospitalization
2. IV antibiotics (nafcillin or oxacillin, or vancomycin if high prevalence of MRSA)
3. Emollients
4. Fluid and electrolyte repletion

Leprosy

Buzz Words: **Hypopigmented, well-demarcated patch with anesthesia/hypoesthesia** → tuberculoid
disfiguring **papules and nodules** → lepromatous

Clinical Presentation: Bimodal age distribution (10–15 years, 35–45 years)
Presents as hypopigmented skin patches. Early nerve involvement (diminished or loss of sensation) is very common. Can be seen in immigrants, patients in developing countries, immunocompromised individuals.

PPx: Bacille Calmette-Guérin (BCG) vaccination is partially protective.

> **QUICK TIPS**
> Post-streptococcal glomerulonephritis is a potential complication occurring 1–2 weeks following infection.

> **QUICK TIPS**
> Remember, there is no mucous membrane involvement with staphylococcal scalded skin syndrome (in contrast to SJS/TEN).

MoD: *Mycobacterium leprae* infection of the skin and peripheral nerves; spreads by respiratory route

Dx:

1. Biopsy (demonstrating acid-fast bacilli)

Tx/Mgmt:

1. Multiple drug regimen (dapsone and rifampicin; add clofazimine for lepromatous disease)

Scarlet Fever

Buzz Words: Sandpaper-like blanching erythroderma, **Pastia lines** (linear petechiae in flexural areas), **circumoral pallor** with sparing of the nasolabial area, **desquamation**

Clinical Presentation: Most commonly associated with strep throat

PPx: N/A

MoD: Erythrotoxin produced by group A strep

Dx:

1. Clinical
2. Rapid strep test, throat culture

Tx/Mgmt:

1. Antibiotic (oral penicillin V, amoxicillin)

Herpes Simplex Virus Type 1

Buzz Words: Viral eruption of **grouped, painful, tingling, burning vesicles on an erythematous base** + orolabial region ("cold sores")

Clinical Presentation: Genital and disseminated infections can occur. **Eczema herpeticum** (severe herpes infection in a patient with primary skin disease, especially **atopic dermatitis**) is associated. Nearly everyone is inoculated by age 40. Presents as a painful skin lesion. Fever and malaise may be present, especially in the setting of primary infection.

PPx: (1) Condoms

MoD: Primary infection involves herpes simplex virus (HSV) type 1 inoculation into skin and nerve endings. Remains latent in ganglion neurons and can produce recurrent infection with reactivation symptoms.

Dx:

1. Viral culture
2. Serology (anti-HSV antibodies)
3. Polymerase chain reaction (PCR)
4. Tzanck prep

Tx/Mgmt:

1. Acyclovir, valacyclovir (for acute symptoms and for chronic suppressive therapy for patients with frequent recurrences)

Herpes Simplex Virus Type 2

Buzz Words: Sexually active adolescent + viral eruption of grouped, painful, tingling, burning vesicles on an erythematous base, usually found in the genital region

Clinical Presentation: Presents as a painful skin lesion. Fever and malaise may be present, especially in the setting of primary infection. Patient is usually sexually active. Patient can be immunocompetent or immunocompromised with disrupted skin barrier (HIV, organ transplant, atopic dermatitis).

PPx: (1) Condoms

MoD: Primary infection involves HSV-2 inoculation into skin and nerve endings. Remains latent in ganglion neurons and can produce recurrent infection with reactivation symptoms.

Dx:
1. Viral culture
2. Serology (anti-HSV antibodies)
3. PCR
4. Tzanck prep

Tx/Mgmt:
1. Acyclovir, valacyclovir (for acute symptoms and for chronic suppressive therapy for patients with frequent recurrences)

Molluscum Contagiosum

Buzz Words: Firm flesh-colored, dome-shaped, umbilicated papule + face or anogenital region

Clinical Presentation: Common disease in young children. Immunocompromised patients (especially with HIV) may have severe disease.

PPx: N/A

MoD: Poxvirus

Dx:
1. Clinical
2. Biopsy demonstrating pathognomonic eosinophilic cytoplasmic inclusions (Henderson-Patterson bodies)

Tx/Mgmt:
1. Cryotherapy
2. Cantharadin
3. Curettage
4. Covering of lesion (to reduce transmission risk)

Hand, Foot, and Mouth Disease

Buzz Words: Painful vesicles of the oral cavity + macular, maculopapular, or nontender vesicles of the hands, feet, and buttocks

QUICK TIPS
Genital herpes in children is highly suggestive of sexual abuse.

MNEMONIC
MolluscUM is UMbilicated.

Clinical Presentation: Seen in young children who present with skin and oral mucosa lesions, mouth and throat pain, and refusal to eat.

PPx: N/A

MoD: Enteroviruses (especially Coxsackievirus A16, Enterovirus A71)

Dx:

1. Clinical

Tx/Mgmt:

1. Supportive therapy (self-limited disease)

Herpangina

Buzz Words: Yellow-white papulovesiclular lesions on tonsils and soft palate + high fever + vomiting + neck stiffness + dysphagia + headache

Clinical Presentation: Seen in young children with oral lesions and systemic symptoms

PPx: N/A

MoD: Enteroviruses (especially Coxsackievirus A1–A6, A8, A10)

Dx:

1. Clinical

Tx/Mgmt:

1. Supportive therapy (self-limited disease)

Erythema Infectiosum (Fifth Disease)

Buzz Words: Prodrome (fever, headache, sore throat, arthralgias) + erythematous malar rash with circumoral pallor ("slapped cheeks" + reticular ("lace-like") rash on extremities

Clinical Presentation: Higher risk in sickle cell patients. Also, older patients with this disease experience more joint pain.

PPx: N/A

MoD: Parvovirus B19

Dx:

1. Clinical

Tx/Mgmt:

1. Supportive therapy (self-limited disease)

Chickenpox (Varicella)

Buzz Words: Pruritic, successive crops of lesions appearing first on face before spreading to trunk and extremities + lesions simultaneously in different stages of evolution (papules, vesicles, pustules, crusting)

QUICK TIPS

Herpangina is associated with febrile seizures.

QUICK TIPS

Anemia with LOW reticulocyte count, leukopenia, and/or thrombocytopenia is associated with fifth disease.

Clinical Presentation: Children with chickenpox often have a prodrome (fever, malaise, anorexia). Seen in patients who are unvaccinated or immunocompromised.

PPx: (1) Varicella vaccine (live attenuated)

MoD: Varicella zoster virus (VZV), transmitted by droplets

Dx:
1. Clinical
2. Serology (anti-VZV antibodies)
3. PCR

Tx/Mgmt:
1. Supportive therapy (self-limited disease)
2. Oral acyclovir, valacyclovir (for immunocompetent patients >12 years of age)
3. IV acyclovir (for children at risk for complications and immunocompromised patients)

Rubella

Buzz Words: Prodrome (fever, malaise, **posterior auricular and suboccipital lymphadenopathy**, conjunctivitis) + **pinpoint, pink + morbilliform papule + 3-day rash** appearing first on face before spreading caudally

Clinical Presentation: Seen in unvaccinated patients

PPx: Measles/mumps/rubella (MMR) vaccine

MoD: Rubella virus (Togavirus), transmitted by droplets

Dx:
1. Clinical
2. Serology (IgM antirubella antibodies)

Tx/Mgmt:
1. Supportive therapy (no specific treatment)

Measles

Buzz Words: Prodrome (fever with **3 Cs—cough, conjunctivitis, coryza**) + white spots on buccal mucosa (**Koplik spots**) + **erythematous, morbilliform, maculopapular exanthem that later turns brown**

Clinical Presentation: Rash appears first on face before spreading to trunk and extremities. Seen in unvaccinated children.

PPx: MMR vaccine

MoD: Measles virus, transmitted by droplets (highly contagious)

Dx:
1. Clinical
2. Serology (IgM antimeasles antibodies)
3. PCR

QUICK TIPS
Newborns may be at risk of congenital rubella if mom is affected during pregnancy. Congenital rubella is covered in Chapter 12.

QUICK TIPS
Think of rubella as a mild form of measles; the rash is shorter and lighter-colored, and the systemic symptoms are less severe.

QUICK TIPS
Mumps is covered in Chapter 9.

Tx/Mgmt:

1. Measles immune globulin (for individuals at increased risk for complications)
2. Vitamin A

Roseola (Sixth Disease, Exanthem Subitum)

Buzz Words: Prodrome (3–5 days of high fever, lymphadenopathy, followed by erythematous, blanching, macular rash spreading from face to trunk and extremities)

Clinical Presentation: Seen in patients younger than 2 years of age (peak prevalence 7–13 months). Other features include **erythematous papules on the soft palate and uvula (Nagayama spots),** erythematous tympanic membranes, respiratory symptoms, irritability, anorexia.

PPx: N/A

MoD: HHV-6 (most common), HHV-7

Dx:

1. Clinical

Tx/Mgmt:

1. Supportive therapy (self-limited disease)

Verruca Vulgaris (Common Warts)

Buzz Words: Tender, flesh-colored, cauliflower-like papules often present at sites of pressure (hands, fingers, joints)

Clinical Presentation: Associated with atopic dermatitis, immunocompromised, meat handling

PPx: (1) Human papilloma virus (HPV) vaccine (for genital warts)

MoD: HPV

Dx:

1. Clinical

Tx/Mgmt:

1. No intervention (self-limited)
2. Topical salicylic acid
3. Cryotherapy (avoided in young children due to associated pain)
4. Topical immunomodulators for refractory warts, though evidence limited (5-FU, imiquod, bleomycin, dinitrochlorobenzene)

Cutaneous Candidiasis

Buzz Words: Beefy red, confluent erythema involving the inguinal folds ("intertrigo," "diaper dermatitis") with fine peripheral scaling + satellite lesions

Clinical Presentation: Balanitis can be seen in male infants. Rash is pruritic and associated with skin friction and moisture, recent broad-spectrum antibiotic use, diabetes mellitus, obesity, immunosuppression, chronic mucocutaneous candidiasis.

PPx: N/A

MoD: Infection with *Candida* species (most commonly *Candida albicans*)

Dx:
1. Clinical
2. KOH preparation
3. Culture of skin scrapings

Tx/Mgmt:
1. Topical antifungal agents (nystatin, clotrimazole, ketoconazole)
2. Oral antifungal agents for severe or refractory cases (fluconazole, itraconazole)

Dermatophytosis (Tinea Infections)

Buzz Words: Tinea corporis, on the body ("ringworm"): pruritic, annular scaling patch with central clearing

Tinea cruris, on the groin ("jock itch"): erythematous patch with central clearing, often appearing first on inner thigh

Tinea pedis, on the foot ("athlete's foot"): pruritic, scaly erosions often in interdigital spaces

Tinea capitis, on the scalp: scaly patches with alopecia and black dots

Clinical Presentation: Superficial fungal infections, multiple subtypes:
- Tinea capitis more common in prepubertal children
- Tinea pedis more common in adolescence, associated with being barefoot in locker rooms or near swimming pools
- Tinea cruris: obesity, diabetes mellitus
- Tinea corporis: wrestlers, contact with infected children or animals

PPx: N/A

MoD: *Tricophyton, Microsporum, Epidermophyton* genera

Dx:
1. Clinical
2. KOH preparation
3. Fungal culture

Tx/Mgmt:
1. Tinea corporis, cruris, and pedis: Topical antifugal agent (clotrimazole, ketoconazole)
2. Tinea capitis, oral antifungal agent (terbinafine, griseofulvin, itraconazole, fluconazole)

Tinea Versicolor (Pityriasis Versicolor)

Buzz Words: **Hypopigmented, hyperpigmented,** or **erythematous macules** on trunk and upper extremities

Clinical Presentation: Most common in adolescents in tropical climates, who present with hypo/hyperpigmented skin macules

PMH/PSuH/PFH/PSoH: Tropical climates

PPx: N/A

MoD: *Malassezia* infection

Dx:

1. Clinical
2. KOH preparation (demonstrating hyphae and yeast, appearing as "**spaghetti and meatballs**")

Tx/Mgmt:

1. Topical antifungal agents (azoles, terbinafine, selenium sulfide)
2. Oral azoles for refractory or widespread disease

Diaper Dermatitis

Buzz Words: **Irritant contact dermatitis** in the **diaper area** + **scattered erythematous patches and papules**

Clinical Presentation: Diaper rash is the chief complaint and is associated with infrequent diaper changes, infants with diarrhea, excessive cleansing.

PPx: N/A

MoD: Excessive moisture and friction disrupt the skin barrier, leading to irritation

Dx:

1. Clinical

Tx/Mgmt:

1. Barrier ointments (preparations of petroleum plus zinc oxide, such as Desitin)
2. Low-potency topical steroids (hydrocortisone)

QUICK TIPS

Diaper dermatitis is **NON**-infectious, but can become secondarily infected if left untreated.

Cutaneous Larva Migrans

Buzz Words: Papule that develops into migrating, **intensely pruritic, elevated, serpiginous, linear, reddish-brown migrating cutaneous track** (produced by larval migration)

Clinical Presentation: Commonly on the **foot**. Shows up more commonly in children than adults.

PPx: N/A

MoD: Eggs of *Ancylostoma caninum*, *Ancylostoma braziliense* shed in dog and cat feces, which penetrate bare skin

Dx:

1. Clinical
2. CBC (eosinophilia)
3. IgE titer (elevated)

Tx/Mgmt:
1. Oral antihelminthics are first-line (albendazole, mebandazole, ivermectin)
2. Topical antihelminthics (thiabendazole)

Hymenoptera (Bees, Hornets, Wasps, Fire Ants) Stings and Bites

Buzz Words: Bee sting + painful swelling at sting site ± anaphylactic reaction

Clinical Presentation: Local redness and **painful swelling** at site of sting or bite. May enlarge over several days. **Anaphylaxis** in allergic individuals.

PPx: N/A

MoD: Stinging apparatus lodges in the skin and releases venom, causing an inflammatory response.

Dx:
1. Clinical

Tx/Mgmt:
1. Cold compresses
2. Elevation of affected area
3. Systemic steroids (if significant spread of initial lesion)
4. Epinephrine in patients with anaphylaxis

Scabies

Buzz Words: **Severely pruritic** erythematous papules and burrows

Clinical Presentation: Typically involves the **interdigital spaces**, wrists, axillae, **penis, scrotum**, and buttocks. Neonates, on the other hand, have lesions where they came in contact with care provider. Chief complaint of pruritis and bumps.

PPx: N/A

MoD: *Sarcoptes scabiei* infestation, transmitted by person-to-person contact or through fomites

Dx:
1. Skin scraping (demonstrating mites, eggs, and feces)

Tx/Mgmt:
1. Topical permethrin (applied from the neck down)
2. Oral ivermectin

Lice

Buzz Words: Scalp or neck pruritus

Clinical Presentation: Very common in school-age children. Make sure to know treatment and management.

PPx: N/A

MoD: *Pediculus humanus capitis* (head louse)

Dx:
1. Visual examination of hair (demonstrating lice and eggs)

> **QUICK TIPS**
> The picture in your mind is all in the name—"larvae migrating cutaneously."

> **QUICK TIPS**
> Penile or scrotal itching is scabies until proven otherwise.

Tx/Mgmt:
1. Topical neurotoxins (pyrethroids, permethrin, malathion, ivermectin)
2. Oral ivermectin in refractory cases
3. Treat individuals who share bedding prophylactically

Immunologic and Inflammatory Disorders

Atopic Dermatitis (Eczema)

Buzz Words: Facial and extensor area + scaly, excoriated, erythematous papulovesicles in infants and young children + flexural lichenification (skin thickening) in older children

Clinical Presentation: Chronic, relapsing, pruritic, inflammatory disorder. Most manifest in infancy, and almost all by age 5. May have personal or family history of atopy (atopic dermatitis, allergic rhinitis, asthma).

PPx: N/A

MoD: Disruption of skin barrier (*filaggrin* gene mutation) and disordered immune response

Dx:
1. Clinical
2. Elevated IgE supports diagnosis

Tx/Mgmt:
1. Trigger avoidance (heat, low humidity)
2. Emollient moisturizers (such as petroleum jellies); topical steroids
3. Topical calcineurin inhibitors (tacrolimus)

> **MNEMONIC**
> Remember the triad of "A"s that go together: atopic dermatitis, asthma, allergies.

Pityriasis Rosea

Buzz Words: Herald patch + salmon-colored scaly papules and plaques + "Christmas tree" distribution

Clinical Presentation: Eruption of **ovoid, salmon-colored scaly papules and plaques** over the trunk and back in a **Christmas tree distribution**. Often begins with a **"herald" patch** (larger than the succeeding lesions).

PPx: N/A

MoD: Viral (hypothesized)

Dx:
1. Clinical
2. Rapid plasma regain (RPR) (if needed to exclude secondary syphilis as they appear similar)

Tx/Mgmt:
1. Supportive (self-limited disease)

Urticaria (Hives)

Buzz Words: Pruritic wheals + circumscribed, raised, erythematous plaques

Clinical Presentation: Usually **transient** (resolving within 24–48 hours), but can be chronic. Associated with upper respiratory infections, recently started medications (penicillin and cephalosporin antibiotics, nonsteroidal anti-inflammatory drugs, allopurinol, anticonvulsants, antipsychotics chemotherapeutics).

PPx: N/A

MoD: Dermal edema secondary to histamine-mediated increased vascular permeability

Dx:

1. Clinical

Tx/Mgmt:

1. Discontinue suspected offending drugs
2. Antihistamines (loratadine, hydroxyzine)
3. Oral prednisone

Erythema Multiforme

Buzz Words: Erythematous circular plaques + **target lesions** (with three zones of color) + distributed over the extremities > trunk; often with **mucous membrane involvement**

Clinical Presentation: Often with **mucous membrane involvement**. Seen in older children. Infections account for most cases—think HSV and *Mycoplasma.*

PPx: N/A

MoD: Immunologic reaction triggered by deposition of circulating immune complexes

Dx:

1. Clinical
2. Skin biopsy to exclude other disorders if diagnosis in question

Tx/Mgmt:

1. Treat underlying infection (macrolide for *Mycoplasma*, acyclovir or valacyclovir for HSV)
2. Discontinue suspected offending drug
3. Oral prednisone for extensive disease

Stevens–Johnson Syndrome/Toxic Epidermal Necrolysis

Buzz Words: Desquamation + involvement of mucous membranes + recently started medication

Clinical Presentation: Prodrome (high fever, flu-like symptoms), **erythematous macules** evolving into **bullae with large areas of desquamation and sloughing** present (Stevens–Johnson syndrome [SJS] <10% body surface area; toxic epidermal necrolysis [TEN] >30% body surface area). **Mucous membranes**

> **QUICK TIPS**
> When you see hives, you should think, "virus or drug?"

> **QUICK TIPS**
> The target is "multiforme"—with three different colors.

are involved. Seen in patients with recently started medications (allopurinol, anticonvulsants, antipsychotics, sulfonamide antibiotics are most common), *Mycoplasma*, cytomegalovirus.

PPx: N/A

MoD: Poorly understood; may be related to cytotoxic T cells

Dx:
1. Clinical

Tx/Mgmt:
1. Admit to hospital
2. Withdraw all potentially offending medications
3. Supportive therapy (fluid and electrolyte repletion, nutrition, pain control)
4. Systemic steroids (controversial)
5. Intravenous immunoglobulin (IVIG) (controversial)

QUICK TIPS
SJS/TEN is a life-threatening, dermatologic emergency.

Vitiligo

Buzz Words: Sharply demarcated, **nonscaling, completely depigmented** macules + face and extensor surfaces

Clinical Presentation: Chief complaint of white spots. May have history of autoimmune disease.

PPx: N/A

MoD: Autoimmune destruction of melanocytes

Dx:
1. Clinical (sometimes aided by Wood lamp)
2. Biopsy revealing loss of melanocytes

Tx/Mgmt:
1. Cosmetics (to make depigmented areas less conspicuous)
2. Topical steroids (clobetasol)
3. Ultraviolet B (UVB) light

QUICK TIPS
Contrast the complete depigmentation in vitiligo with the partial depigmentation in tinea versicolor.

Disorders of the Hair and Hair Follicles
Seborrheic Dermatitis

Buzz Words: Infant + yellow greasy scale + erythematous plaques

Clinical Presentation: Erythematous plaques with **yellow, greasy scale** present in areas rich in sebaceous glands (scalp, eyebrows, face). **Dandruff** when on scalp. **"Cradle cap"** in infants.

PPx: N/A

MoD: Poorly understood; possible role of *Malassezia* yeast

Dx:
1. Clinical

Tx/Mgmt:
1. Shampoos (selenium sulfide, zinc pyrithione)
2. Topical steroid (hydrocortisone)
3. Ketoconazole

Infectious Folliculitis

Buzz Words: Multiple **pruritic** papules and pustules **centered around hair follicles**

Clinical Presentation: Presents as multiple papules and pustules on the face, trunk, buttocks, and legs. Patient may have history of atopic dermatitis, exposure of hair follicles to friction (e.g., shaving), exposure to hot tubs.

PPx: N/A

MoD: Most commonly bacterial; *S. aureus* (most common cause); *Pseudomonas aeruginosa* ("hot tub folliculitis")

Dx:
1. Clinical
2. Gram stain and culture of expressed fluid

Tx/Mgmt:
1. Topical antibiotics (mupirocin, clindamycin)
2. Oral antibiotics (cephalexin, clindamycin)

Disorders of Sweat and Sebaceous Glands

Acne Vulgaris

Buzz Words: Teenager + blackheads/whiteheads + pustules + erythema + scarring

Clinical Presentation: Two types lesions: noninflammatory lesions characterized by **comedones** ("blackheads" and "whiteheads") and inflammatory lesions characterized by **pustules and nodules.** Distributed over face and upper trunk. Scarring and **postinflammatory hyperpigmentation occur.** May be associated with androgen or steroid excess, polycystic ovarian syndrome, stress, family history of acne.

PPx: N/A

MoD: Multifactorial disorder of the pilosebaceous follicles: androgen-induced sebum production, follicular hyperkeratinization, bacteria (*Propionibacterium acnes*), and inflammation

Dx:
1. Clinical
2. Evaluation of associated disorders (polycystic ovarian syndrome [PCOS], hyperandrogenism, Cushing disease)

Tx/Mgmt:
1. Topical agents (retinoids, benzoyl peroxide, azelaic acid, clindamycin)

2. Systemic agents (doxycycline for moderate to severe inflammatory acne, oral contraceptives for women, isotretinoin for severe cases)

Hidradenitis Suppurativa (Acne Inversa)

Buzz Words: Painful nodule + recurrent + armpit, groin or perineum

Clinical Presentation: Recurrent, painful nodules and abscesses located in the **intertriginous** areas (axillae, inguinal area, perineum), causing foul **odor and drainage.** **Sinus tracts** and **scarring** in chronic disease. Associated with family history of hidradenitis suppurativa, metabolic syndrome (obesity, dyslipidemia, diabetes), smoking.

PPx: N/A

MoD: Chronic occlusion of the folliculopilosebaceous unit

Dx:

1. Clinical

Tx/Mgmt:

1. Weight reduction
2. Smoking cessation
3. Skin hygiene
4. Topical clindamycin
5. Systemic antibiotics (doxycycline, clindamycin, minocycline)
6. Intralesional corticosteroids

Hyperhidrosis

Buzz Words: Excessive visible sweating + uncontrollable + social anxiety

Clinical Presentation: Excessive, **visible sweating** usually in a focal region (axillary, palmar, plantar), often with social or professional consequences. Easy to identify in question stem so most likely tested on Tx/Mgmt.

PPx: N/A

MoD: Exaggerated sympathetic stress response; usually idiopathic

Dx:

1. Clinical

Tx/Mgmt:

1. Topical antiperspirants (aluminum chloride)
2. Botulinum toxin
3. Sympathectomy

Ichthyosis Vulgaris

Buzz Words: White, "fish-like," "horny plate"; white to gray scaling of the abdomen and extensor surfaces of extremities + sparing of the face and flexural areas

Clinical Presentation: Seen in early childhood and associated with family history of ichthyosis vulgaris (**autosomal dominant**).

PPx: N/A

MoD: Loss-of-function mutation in *filaggrin* gene, causing abnormal epidermal cornification

Dx:
1. Clinical

Tx/Mgmt:
1. Emollients and humectants
2. Alpha hydroxyl acids (lactic and glycolic acid)

Congenital Disorders

Xeroderma Pigmentosum

Buzz Words: Melanoma early in childhood + extreme sunburn

Clinical Presentation: **Extreme sun sensitivity** with sunburn after first sunlight exposure. Development of basal cell carcinomas, squamous cell carcinomas, and melanomas early in childhood. Associated with **ocular and neurologic abnormalities.**

PPx: Sunscreen

MoD: Recessive mutations in nucleotide excision repair genes

Dx:
1. Clinical
2. Specialized laboratory testing (demonstrating cellular hypersensitivity to ultraviolet [UV] light)
3. Genetic testing

Tx/Mgmt:
1. Avoidance of sunlight
2. Sunscreen

Congenital Melanocytic Nevus

Buzz Words: Tan-to-black mole **present at birth or early in life**

Clinical Presentation: Can have irregular borders and increased hair density

PMH/PSuH/PFH/PSoH: N/A

PPx: N/A

MoD: Hamartomas composed of proliferation of benign melanocytes

Dx:
1. Clinical

Tx/Mgmt:
1. Follow over time
2. Surgical removal (for large nevi, because size is correlated with the risk of melanoma)

QUICK TIPS

Remember, not every skin change is a medical problem (Table 13.1).

TABLE 13.1 Benign Neonatal Skin Conditions

Condition	Etiology	Appearance
Milia	Maternal andro-gen exposure	1-2 mm yellow-white papules on face
Sebaceous hyperplasia	Maternal andro-gen exposure	Larger yellow-white papules
Erythema toxicum neonatorum	Unknown	Erythematous macules and papules on face or trunk
Congenital dermal melanocytosis (formerly "Mongolian spots")	Melanocytes entrapped during migration	Blue or blue-gray pigmented patch in the sacral or gluteal region (more common in African American, Hispanic, and Asian neonates)
Transient neonatal pustular melanosis	Unknown	Small fragile pustules on a nonerythematous base; they rupture easily to leave a collarette of scale

GUNNER PRACTICE

1. A 17-year-old Caucasian boy comes to clinic because he is concerned about "light spots" on his chest and back that he first noticed the day before. He states that he has spent a lot of time in the sun recently. He has a history of well-controlled acne. His pulse is 75/min, respirations 16/min, and blood pressure 110/75. Physical exam reveals prominent tan lines and multiple scaly hypopigmented macules scattered on his upper chest and back. Which of the following is the most likely diagnosis?
   A. Tinea versicolor
   B. Vitiligo
   C. Tinea corporis
   D. Psoriasis
   E. Leprosy

2. A 16-year-old girl presents to the emergency department for a burning rash on her face. For the last 2 days, she has been sick with a fever, sore throat, and chills. Her past medical history is notable for frequent urinary tract infections, for which she was recently prescribed trimethoprim-sulfamethoxazole. Her pulse 95/min, blood pressure 100/60, respirations 20/min, and

temperature 102°F. Examination shows several bullae located on the face and neck as well as desquamation of some parts of the skin. Her conjunctivae are inflamed, and there is sloughing of the tongue and oral mucosa. Which of the following is most likely responsible for this patient's symptoms?

A. Erythema multiforme
B. Stevens–Johnson syndrome
C. Staphylococcal scaled skin syndrome
D. Bullous pemphigoid
E. Scarlet fever

3. A 13-year-old girl comes to the office for "red spots" on her face. She states that she feels embarrassed around her friends because of the rash. She has no significant past medical history. Physical examination shows multiple red hair follicles with black and white centers. She denies alcohol, tobacco, and recreational drug use. Her pulse is 80/min, respirations 14/min, and blood pressure 108/72. What is the next best step in the management of this patient's condition?

A. Oral doxycycline
B. Isotretinoin
C. Cryotherapy
D. Avoiding spicy foods
E. Topical retinoid

ANSWER: What Would Gunner Jess/Jim Do?

1. WWGJD? A 17-year-old Caucasian boy comes to clinic because he is concerned about "light spots" on his chest and back that he first noticed the day before. He states that he has spent a lot of time in the sun recently. He has a history of well-controlled acne. His pulse is 75/min, respirations 16/min, and blood pressure 110/75. Physical exam reveals prominent tan lines and multiple scaly hypopigmented macules scattered on his upper chest and back. Which of the following is the most likely diagnosis?

Answer: A, Tinea versicolor

   Explanation: This adolescent patient is complaining of scattered hypopigmented macules consistent with tinea versicolor, a superficial fungal infection most commonly presenting on the trunk and upper extremities, which can become more noticeable after tanning.

   B. Vitiligo → Incorrect. First, vitiligo results in a complete depigmentation, not a partial loss of pigmentation. Second, it is not associated with scaling. Third, it typically presents on the face and extensor surfaces.

   C. Tinea corporis → Incorrect. Tinea corporis is a dermatophyte infection characterized by a scaly annular plaque with centrifugal spread and central clearing. It would not cause hypopigmentation.

   D. Psoriasis → Incorrect. Psoriasis is a chronic inflammatory disorder characterized by silvery-white scales over salmon-colored plaques. It does not cause hypopigmentation.

   E. Leprosy → Incorrect. Although leprosy can cause hypopigmentation, it is accompanied by loss of sensation and would be exceedingly rare in a patient without exposure to an endemic area.

2. WWGJD? A 16-year-old girl presents to the emergency department for a burning rash on her face. For the last 2 days, she has been sick with a fever, sore throat, and chills. Her past medical history is notable for frequent urinary tract infections, for which she was recently prescribed trimethoprim-sulfamethoxazole. Her pulse 95/min, blood pressure 100/60, respirations 20/min, and temperature 102°F. Examination shows several bullae located on the face and neck as well as desquamation of some parts of the skin. Her conjunctivae are inflamed,

and there is sloughing of the tongue and oral mucosa. Which of the following is most likely responsible for this patient's symptoms?

Answer: B, Stevens–Johnson syndrome

Explanation: This patient, who recently completed a course of the sulfonamide antibiotic TMP-SMX, is suffering from Stevens-Johnson syndrome (which is most commonly a drug reaction). The mucosal involvement and prodrome of flu-like symptoms is consistent with her condition.

A. Erythema multiforme → Incorrect. Erythema multiforme is characterized by prominent target lesions on the extremities and trunk. It is most commonly associated with EBV, HSV, and other viral infections and would not cause this clinical picture.

C. Staphylococcal scaled skin syndrome → Incorrect. Staphylococcal scaled skin syndrome is an exfoliative disease that can resemble SJS but lacks mucous membrane involvement.

D. Bullous pemphigoid → Incorrect. Bullous pemphigoid is an autoimmune blistering disease that occurs in elderly adults. It would be extremely rare in a 16-year-old patient.

E. Scarlet fever → Incorrect. Scarlet fever is a complication of a group A strep infection. Although flu-like symptoms and desquamation may be present in scarlet fever, mucous membranes would not be affected and bullae would not be present.

3. WWGJD? A 13-year-old girl comes to the office for "red spots" on her face. She states that she feels embarrassed around her friends because of the rash. She has no significant past medical history. Physical examination shows multiple red hair follicles with black and white centers. She denies alcohol, tobacco, and recreational drug use. Her pulse is 80/min, respirations 14/min, and blood pressure 108/72. What is the next best step in the management of this patient's condition?

Answer: E, Topical retinoid

Explanation: This adolescent patient has acne, a common skin disease among teenagers. The black and white centers of the hair follicles noted are consistent with open and closed comedones, respectively. Her embarrassment is a common response among teenage patients. The first-line treatment for noninflammatory (comedonal) acne is a topical retinoid.

A. Oral doxycycline → Incorrect. Oral antibiotics are used for moderate-to-severe inflammatory acne and would not be an appropriate first-line therapy for this patient.

B. Isotretinoin → Incorrect. Isotretinoin is an oral retinoid that is highly effective in treating nodular (inflammatory) acne. However, it is a therapy reserved for severe refractory cases because of its side effect profile.

C. Cryotherapy → Incorrect. Cryotherapy is effective in treating a variety of skin conditions including warts, skin tags, and seborrheic keratoses, but it would not be used to treat acne.

D. Avoiding spicy foods → Incorrect. Avoiding spicy foods may help to reduce the frequency of rosacea episodes but would be ineffective in treating or preventing acne.

Diseases of the Musculoskeletal System and Connective Tissue

*Rafael Madero-Marroquin, Atu Agawu, Daniel Gromer,
Hao-Hua Wu, Leo Wang, and Rebecca Tenney-Soeiro*

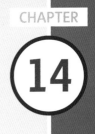

14

Introduction

This topic encompasses 10%–15% of the National Board of Medical Examiners (NBME) Pediatrics exam content, in which the most important task is to establish a diagnosis. In order to do this, it is important to know the basic anatomy of the joints and the classic clinical presentation of these disorders, including the findings on physical examination, imaging, and lab testing.

The ability to diagnose these disorders correctly is key to providing adequate treatment to the patients, which is of extreme importance with musculoskeletal disorders, since a delayed diagnosis can lead to permanent damage to the child's joints and an incorrect diagnosis can lead to an unnecessary surgical intervention.

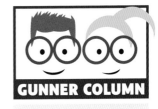

GUNNER COLUMN

99 AR

High-yield Pediatric Orthopedics video

Embryonic Development, Fetal Maturation, and Perinatal Changes

You do not have to memorize this subsection for the Pediatrics exam. However, an understanding of embryonic development may help you see how congenital disorders of the musculoskeletal system occur.

Skeletal tissue arises from the mesenchyme of the mesoderm or the neural crest. Mononuclear myoblasts fuse to form primary multinucleated myotubes, while secondary myotubes form around them and require innervation to mature into skeletal muscle fibers. Skeletal muscles of the limbs and trunk arise from the somites.

Each somite forms a sclerotome and a dermamyotome. Sclerotomes form the axial skeleton, while dermatomyotomes form the dermis of the back trunk, the musculature of the limbs; the myotome forms the muscles of the trunk. The lateral plate mesoderm forms the sternum and bones that form the limbs.

Myotomes split into an epimere and hypomere shortly after they form. The epimere forms the muscles of the back, whereas the hypomere forms the muscles of the ventral trunk. The vertebral column is formed by resegmentation of sclerotomes and myotomes into caudal and cranial segments; each of these segments then joins the adjacent cranial or caudal segment to form the vertebrae.

The Hox genes are a family of transcription factors that, when mutated, can cause limb alterations such as synpolydactyly. This is because Hox gene expression is essential for craniocaudal positioning of the limb buds and limb patterning.

Somite patterns video

Autoimmune Disorders

Juvenile Dermatomyositis

Buzz Words: Proximal muscle weakness + Gower sign + heliotrope rash (juvenile dermatomyositis [JDM]) + Gottron papules (JDM)

Clinical Presentation: Since JDM predominantly affects proximal muscles, the patient might have trouble climbing stairs or lifting his hands over his head. Dermatomyositis also presents with skin alterations, like periorbital violaceous heliotrope rash and erythematous and hypertrophic skin over metacarpal and proximal interphalangeal (PIP) joints (Gottron papules). May present with constitutional symptoms like weight loss, fever, fatigue, or headache. Unlike adult dermatomyositis, JDM is **not associated with malignancy.**

Prophylactic (PPx): (1) Vitamin D and calcium to prevent osteoporosis. (2) Sunscreen to prevent flare from sun exposure.

Mechanism of Disease (MoD): JDM is primarily a capillary vasculopathy, similar to that seen in adult polymyositis. HLA B8/DR3 and HLA DQalpha*0501 are associated with a higher risk of JDM; it is also sometimes associated with a viral illness.

Diagnostic Steps (Dx):

1. PE
2. Muscle strength testing
3. Labs to show increased muscle enzymes (creatine phosphokinase [CPK], lactate dehydrogenase [LDH], alanine aminotransferase [ALT], aspartate aminotransferase [AST], aldolase)
4. Muscle biopsy
5. Electromyography (EMG) and muscle biopsy should be used only when the diagnosis remains uncertain

Treatment and Management Steps (Tx/Mgmt):

1. Corticosteroids
2. Immunosuppressive agents (methotrexate, intravenous immunoglobulin [IVIG], cyclosporine, cyclophosphamide) for severe muscle disease

3. Physical therapy.
   - Treatment response is determined by a decrease in muscle enzymes and clinical symptoms.

Seronegative Spondyloarthropathies

Ankylosing Spondylitis

Buzz Words: Young male + HLA-B27 + back pain worse in the morning, better with activity + family history of spondyloarthritis

Clinical Presentation: Arthritis that affects the lower extremities and axial skeleton (frequent hip involvement). Limited lumbar spine range of motion and limitation of chest expansion. Pain has good response to nonsteroidal anti-inflammatory drugs (NSAIDs). Contrary to adult-onset ankylosing spondylitis (AS), enthesitis (inflammation of the tendinous insertions on the bone) and peripheral arthritis are more common in children at disease onset. Patients with late-onset pauciarticular juvenile rheumatoid arthritis (JRA) are at high risk of developing this syndrome as adults. Elevated erythrocyte sedimentation rate [ESR] or C-reactive protein (CRP) on lab exams.

PPx: N/A

MoD: A strong association with HLA-B27 and infectious etiology has been suggested but not proven.

Dx:
1. PE
2. Pelvic and lumbosacral x-ray (XR).
   - Clinical diagnosis based on evidence of bilateral sacroiliitis on imaging (or severe unilateral sacroiliitis), back pain, and features of spondyloarthritis (enthesitis, uveitis, dactylitis, etc.).
   - Juvenile AS refers to AS that occurs before the age of 16.

Tx/Mgmt:
1. NSAIDs to control pain
2. Physical therapy
3. Glucocorticoids if NSAIDs fail
4. Disease-modifying antirheumatic drugs (DMARDs; e.g., azathioprine) to prevent joint damage

Reactive Arthritis (Formerly Reiter Syndrome)

Buzz Words: Sexually active adolescent + unprotected sex + acute onset of conjunctivitis, urethritis, and arthritis → reactive arthritis

Clinical Presentation: Typically presents as oligoarticular arthritis of the lower extremities. Dactylitis and enthesitis may occur. Dermatologic manifestations like circinate

QUICK TIPS

Seronegative because rheumatoid factor and antinuclear antibody are typically negative in these diseases.

MNEMONIC

Seronegative spondyloarthropathies = PAIR (Psoriatic Arthritis, Ankylosing spondylitis, Inflammatory Bowel disease, Reactive arthritis)

99 AR

Seronegative arthritis video

MNEMONIC

Reiter's disease: Can't see (conjunctivitis), can't pee (urethritis), can't climb a tree (arthritis).

balanitis and keratoderma blennorrhagica may occur. Reiter syndrome is defined by the classic triad of arthritis, urethritis, and conjunctivitis, but it is relatively uncommon in children. Typically preceded by gastrointestinal/genitourinary (GI/GU) infection by 2–4 weeks (not always remembered).

PPx: Safe-sex and good food hygiene

MoD: Arthritis associated with a coexisting or recent extra-articular infection, typically an enteric (*Shigella, Yersinia, Salmonella, Escherichia coli*) or sexually transmitted (*Chlamydia trachomatis*) pathogen.

Dx:

1. PE
2. XR based on painful joint(s)
3. Ophthalmologic exam

Tx/Mgmt:

1. Antibiotics (if current infection suspected)
2. NSAIDs
3. Glucocorticoids

Juvenile Idiopathic Arthritis

Buzz Words: Articular pain for >3 months + morning stiffness that improves throughout the day

Clinical Presentation: This is an umbrella term that includes different causes of chronic arthritis. Clinical presentation varies by subtype; see Table 14.1.

PPx: N/A

MoD: Unclear. Alterations in both humoral and cell-mediated immunity. Th1 lymphocytes play a central role (tumor necrosis factor [TNF]-alpha), although B-cell activation, immune complex formation, and complement activation also promote inflammation.

Dx:

1. PE
2. XR of joint (osteopenia and subchondral sclerosis around involved joints)
3. Lab tests. Depending on the subtype, the patient might be antinuclear antibody (ANA) + rheumatoid factor (RF) + or have an ↑ ESR, but these tests are not diagnostic

Tx/Mgmt:

1. Goal is to prevent joint damage and induce disease remission. Treatment plan tailored to the specific subtype of juvenile idiopathic arthritis (JIA).
   - NSAIDs
   - Steroids
   - Disease-modifying antirheumatic drugs (DMARDs)

TABLE 14.1 Juvenile Idiopathic Arthritis Subtypes

Subtype	Clinical Presentation
Oligoarthritis	• ≤4 joints within first 6 months • Predominantly large joints and lower extremities • Persistent oligoarticular if ≤4 joints across disease course • Extended oligoarticular if >4 joints are eventually affected; worse prognosis • 30% have uveitis or iridocyclitis • Most cases resolve in less than 6 months
Polyarthritis	• ≥5 joints in both upper and lower extremities • RF-positive polyarthritis, resembling adult rheumatoid arthritis with rheumatoid nodules on extensor surfaces • Micrognathia, reflecting chronic temporomandibular joint disease • 60% enter remission within 15 years • Worse prognosis with older onset
Systemic (**Still disease**)	• Arthritis • Fever: spiking daily or twice-daily, ≥39°C (102.2°F) • Rash: **salmon-colored, trunk** and proximal extremities, evanescent • Hepatosplenomegaly, generalized lymphadenopathy, serositis • Variable course, 50% eventually achieve remission

Inflammatory Disorders

Osteochondritis Dissecans

Buzz Words: Young male athlete + deep knee pain that is worsened by exercise + magnetic resonance imaging (MRI) shows lesion in bone beneath cartilage

Clinical Presentation: Patients typically present with vague or deep knee pain that may localize along the medial or lateral joint line. If the fragment of dead bone with overlying cartilage becomes unstable, there may be locking of the joint. Boys are more commonly affected than girls. The knee is the most commonly affected joint, followed by the elbow and ankle.

PPx: N/A

MoD: Exact cause unclear, hypothesis: repetitive microtrauma leading to subchondral pathology (+ cartilage damage)

Dx:

1. Plain radiograph shows a subchondral bone fragment surrounded by a crescent-shaped radiolucency; however, radiographs can be normal.

2. MRI is used if plain radiography is normal and there is persistence of clinical symptoms.

Tx/Mgmt:

1. No weight bearing and immobilization
2. Physical therapy (PT)
3. Surgery
   - Skeletal immaturity, smaller lesion size, and absence of mechanical symptoms or pain have been associated with a higher likelihood of healing with nonoperative treatment.
   - Unstable lesions will not usually heal with conservative treatment.

Transient Synovitis (Toxic Synovitis)

Buzz Words: Six-year-old boy + hip/groin pain + history of upper respiratory infection 1–2 weeks prior to presentation

Clinical Presentation: Transient synovitis is inflammation of the synovium of the hip joint capsule due to viral infection. Patients experience acute onset of pain in the groin, anterior thigh, or knee and can present with a painful, limping gait. Often **afebrile**, contrary to septic arthritis.

PPx: N/A

MoD: Unclea; possibilities include posttraumatic, allergic, and infectious causes

Dx:

1. PE
2. Complete blood count (CBC)
3. ESR/CRP
4. XR (frog-leg view)
5. Ultrasound of joint
6. If unsure, rule out septic arthritis with blood cultures and aspiration of the joint, as the consequences of misdiagnosed septic arthritis can be serious:
   - White blood cells (WBCs) and ESR are normal or slightly elevated

Tx/Mgmt:

1. NSAIDs, bed rest, and observation. Most children recover completely within 3–6 weeks.

Septic Arthritis

Buzz Words: Acute onset of fever + exquisite joint tenderness with micromotion + swelling → septic arthritis

Clinical Presentation: Septic arthritis is infection of a joint and requires emergent treatment. Classic presentation is a painful, swollen joint that exhibits pain even with slightest amount of motion (e.g., tenderness with micromotion). The hip is most commonly affected in younger children, whereas the knee is commonly affected in older children. Complications include avascular necrosis and cartilaginous damage.

PPx: N/A

MoD: Hematogenous seeding of the synovial space. Less often, it can be the result of direct inoculation or extension from a contiguous focus. *Staphylococcus aureus* and *Streptococcus pyogenes* are the most common organisms. *Neisseria gonorrhoeae* may cause septic arthritis in adolescents. *Kingella kingae* common in children below age 5.

Dx:
1. PE
2. CBC
3. ESR/CRP
4. Blood culture (positive in 30%–50% of cases)
5. Synovial fluid aspiration and culture (organisms and elevated WBC count
6. Ultrasound may show fluid in joint

Tx/Mgmt:
1. Joint aspiration (often daily for 1–2 days)
2. Empiric IV antibiotics that cover gram-positive organisms for 4–6 weeks

Osteomyelitis

Buzz Words: Fever + recent injury in which skin was penetrated (e.g., stepped on a nail) + XR/magnetic resonance imaging (MRI) show lesions of the bone → osteomyelitis

Osteomyelitis + sickle cell anemia → *Salmonella*

Osteomyelitis + stepped on a nail → *Pseudomonas*

Clinical Presentation: Osteomyelitis is a bacterial infection of bone. It can present as fever, bone pain, erythema, swelling, and induration. It may manifest as refusal to move the involved limb in younger children or painful limp in older children.

PPx: N/A

MoD: Hematogenous seeding versus implanted hardware versus recent surgically reduced fracture. *S. aureus* and *S. pyogenes* are the most common organisms. *Salmonella* in the case of sickle cell anemia. *Pseudomonas aeruginosa* in children who step on a nail.

Dx:
1. PE
2. CBC
3. ESR/CRP
4. XR
5. MRI

99 AR

Osteomyelitis video

6. Blood cultures
7. Wound culture

Tx/Mgmt:
1. IV or high-dose oral antibiotics given for 4–6 weeks (broad-spectrum antistaphylococcal agents and vancomycin for methicillin-resistant *Staphyloccus aureus* (MRSA)
2. Surgical debridement

Neoplasms

Benign Neoplasms

Osteoid Osteoma

Buzz Words: Older teen + bone pain that is worse at night + relieved by aspirin + small round lucency with sclerotic margin on XR → osteoid osteoma

Clinical Presentation: Osteoid osteoma is a benign bone tumor of osteoblasts that presents as progressive bone pain worse at night and relieved by aspirin. Boys more common than girls. Most often affects the proximal femur and tibia; vertebral lesions can cause scoliosis. Palpation of the area does not alter the discomfort.

PPx: N/A

MoD: Benign bone-forming tumor that produces high levels of prostaglandins

Dx:
1. PE
2. XR of affected bone → shows a small round lucency with a sclerotic margin

Tx/Mgmt:
1. NSAIDs/salicylates
2. Percutaneous radiofrequency ablation
3. Surgical resection/curettage

Osteoblastoma

Buzz Words: Older teen with chronic bone pain + does not respond to aspirin + lytic lesion with radiolucent nidus → osteoblastoma

Clinical Presentation: More aggressive version of osteoid osteoma. Presents with insidious onset of dull aching pain. Predilection for the vertebrae. Unlike an osteoid osteoma, this lesion is not self-limited and may produce symptoms of cord compression if in the vertebrae.

PPx: N/A

MoD: Benign bone-producing tumor

Dx:
1. PE
2. XR

3. CT
4. Bone scan

Tx/Mgmt:
1. Surgical removal of the tumor (curettage/marginal excision with bone grafting)
   - Untreated osteoblastoma will continue to enlarge and may damage bone and adjacent tissues.

Osteochondroma

Buzz Words: Older teen + hard painless mass that has not changed in years + sessile or pedunculated lesion on surface of bone → osteochondroma

Clinical Presentation: Osteochondromas are neoplasms of cartilage and the most common benign bone tumor. Presents as painless mass near a joint or painful mass related to local trauma. One of the most common benign bone tumors in children.

PPx: N/A

MoD: Occur spontaneously but have been reported following radiotherapy. Bony spur with a cartilaginous cap that overlies it and is the source of growth.

Dx:
1. PE
2. XR
3. CT/MRI

Tx/Mgmt:
1. Observation
2. Surgical resection

> **FOR THE WARDS**
> Multiple osteochondromas = multiple hereditary exostosis → can impair limb-growth, requiring close monitoring during growth.

Enchondroma

Buzz Words: Older teen + discovery of bone mass after fracture + lucent, central medullary lesions on XR → enchondroma

Clinical Presentation: Enchondromas are tumors composed of hyaline cartilage that commonly affect the hands. Most enchondromas are discovered incidentally and are asymptomatic unless a fracture is present. When symptomatic, there may be widening of the bone, deformity, and limb-length discrepancy. **Ollier syndrome** presents with multiple enchondromas; malignant transformation occurs in 10%–25% of cases. **Maffucci syndrome** presents with multiple enchondromas, soft tissue hemangiomas; malignant transformation to chondrosarcoma occurs in nearly 100% of cases.

PPx: N/A

MoD: Benign lesion of hyaline cartilage that occurs centrally in the bone

Dx:
1. PE
2. XR (oval, well-circumscribed, central lucent lesion, with or without matrix calcifications)
3. Bone scan
4. MRI
5. Core needle-biopsy to r/o chondrosarcoma

Tx/Mgmt:
1. Observation w/ XR f/u at 6 and 12 months
2. Surgical removal (e.g., curettage and bone grafting) if symptomatic or if in association with Ollier/Mafucci syndrome

Malignant Neoplasms of Bone and Muscle

Osteosarcoma

Buzz Words: Male adolescent + palpable, painful mass + history of retinoblastoma + sunburst appearance on imaging → osteosarcoma

Clinical Presentation: Osteosarcoma is a malignant tumor of osteoblastic proliferation. Nighttime pain and localized swelling without systemic manifestations. Most frequent in adolescents. Most common locations: distal femur, proximal tibia, and proximal humerus, mainly involving the metaphysis of these long bones. There may be limited motion, joint effusion, tenderness, and warmth.

PPx: N/A

MoD: Malignant tumor of the bone-producing mesenchymal stem cells. Associated with previous **retinoblastoma**, Paget disease of bone, Li–Fraumeni syndrome, radiation therapy, and fibrous dysplasia.

Dx:
1. PE
2. XR (sunburst appearance)
3. MRI
4. Biopsy

Tx/Mgmt:
1. Chemotherapy + surgical removal, with amputation or limb-sparing surgery

Ewing Sarcoma

Buzz Words: Male adolescent + pain and localized swelling + systemic manifestations + **onionskin appearance** on imaging → Ewing sarcoma

Clinical Presentation: Ewing sarcoma is a round-cell tumor that has a very characteristic onionskin appearance on XR. Patients present with bone pain, swelling, soft tissue mass, fever, malaise, weight loss, leukocytosis, and elevated ESR. Unlike osteosarcoma, in which long bones are predominantly involved, Ewing sarcoma can affect both flat and long bones.

PPx: N/A

MoD: Unknown, but 95% have a chromosomal translocation between chromosomes 11 and 22.

Dx:
1. PE
2. XR (onionskin appearance)
3. MRI
4. Biopsy

Tx/Mgmt:
1. Chemotherapy due to high risk of metastasis, followed by surgical excision.
2. Radiation therapy is used when complete excision is not possible.

Rhabdomyosarcoma

Buzz Words: Child <10 years old + painless enlarging mass on the back of the neck

Clinical Presentation: Rhabdomyosarcoma is a malignant tumor of the striated muscle. Two-thirds occur in children younger than 10 years of age. Most commonly present as a painless soft tissue mass. Symptoms are caused by compression of adjacent structures, which depends on the region it is affecting. Symptoms may include cranial nerve palsies, proptosis, and obstruction of the oropharynx.
- Most common locations: head and neck, genitourinary tract, extremities

PPx: N/A

MoD: Unknown; arises from the same embryonic mesenchyme as striated skeletal muscle. Associated with neurofibromatosis and Li-Fraumeni syndrome.

Dx:
1. PE
2. XR

Tx/Mgmt:
1. Complete surgical resection, if possible, plus radiotherapy and chemotherapy to eradicate metastasis and prevent recurrence

Degenerative Disorders

Patellofemoral Syndrome (Formerly Patellar Chondromalacia)

Buzz Words: Knee pain + worse when descending stairs + patella in a lateral position

Clinical Presentation: Pain comes from contact of patella with the femur. Presents as knee pain that is difficult to localize, pain is often worse when climbing stairs, squatting, running, or sitting for prolonged periods. Physical examination may show that the patella in a lateral position.

PPx: N/A

MoD: Joint misalignment and excessive use

Dx:

1. PE (medial patellar tenderness or pain with compression of the joint confirms the diagnosis in the absence of a significant effusion and other positive findings)
2. XR
3. MRI

Tx/Mgmt:

1. PT

Legg–Calvé–Perthes Disease

Buzz Words: 4- to 10-year-old boy + insidious hip/knee/groin pain with painful limp → Perthes disease

Clinical Presentation: Legg–Calvé–Perthes disease is idiopathic avascular necrosis of the proximal femoral epiphysis and affects children from 4 to 10 years of age. It can begin painlessly but will progress to a mildly painful limp, usually related to activity. Decreased internal rotation and abduction of the hip. Pain may be referred to the knee or the groin. Has been found to be associated with attention deficit hyperactivity disorder (ADHD) and delayed bone age. High yield for the Pediatrics exam.

PPx: N/A

MoD: Temporary interruption of blood flow to the femoral epiphysis, causing avascular necrosis. Etiology is unknown.

Dx:

1. PE
2. XR: AP and frog-leg lateral views
3. MRI with contrast
4. Arthrogram (if plain films normal)
   - Affected femoral head appears small, shows sclerotic bone and widened joint space. Presence of a crescent-shaped subchondral fracture in the femoral head is termed the **"crescent sign."**

Tx/Mgmt:

1. No weight bearing
2. PT
3. NSAIDs

99 AR

XR of Perthes disease

4. Surgery
   - Principle of treatment is to contain the femoral head within the acetabulum, which prevents deformation of the femoral head.

Osgood-Schlatter Disease

Buzz Words: 12-year-old boy + basketball player + pain over tibial tuberosity

Clinical Presentation: Osgood-Schlatter disease is inflammation of the patellar tendon at the insertion of the tibial tubercle (e.g., apophysitis). Patient presents with swelling of the tibial tuberosity with pain and tenderness over the tibial tubercle that is exacerbated with activity and relieved with rest. Most common in 10- to 15-year-old boys who participate in sports involving repetitive jumping. Usually unilateral but can be bilateral.

PPx: N/A

MoD:
1. Overuse of the extensor mechanism of the patella, causing traction apophysitis at the insertion of the patellar tendon to the proximal tibia.

Dx:
1. Clinical; imaging not necessary unless the patient has unusual complaints.

Tx/Mgmt:
1. Activity modification, rest, ice after exercise.
2. A protective pad can be used over the tibial tubercle to protect it from direct trauma.
3. In severe cases, immobilization of the joint may be necessary.

Spondylolisthesis/Spondylosis (Degenerative)

Buzz Words: Gymnast or wrestler + lower back pain that radiates to the buttocks + worsened by extension of the spine

Clinical Presentation: Spondylolysis is a stress fracture in the pars interarticularis secondary to repetitive hyperextension of the spine. Spondylolisthesis occurs when there is an anterior displacement of the body of the vertebra involved in spondylolysis. May be asymptomatic but usually presents with low back pain that radiates to the buttocks and increases with hyperextension. Spondylolisthesis may present with neurologic symptoms due to compression of the nerve roots.

PPx: N/A

MoD: Can occur secondary to trauma or degeneration or repetitive hyperextension

Dx:
1. PE
2. XR
3. CT

Tx/Mgmt:
1. Activity restrictions
2. NSAIDs
3. Casting or bracing if the pain persists
4. Surgery for chronic back pain refractory to other treatment or for nerve impingement in the case of spondylolisthesis

Traumatic and Mechanical Disorders

Dislocations

Subluxation of the Radial Head (Nursemaid Elbow)

Buzz Words: Child <6 years old + arm pulled by caretaker + pain with flexed elbow

Clinical Presentation: Pain and persistence of elbow flexion even though the patient's hand function is normal. Usually presents after a strong, pulling force is exerted on the arm in patients younger than age 6. Extremely high-yield for the Pediatrics exam.

PPx: N/A

MoD: Sudden, strong, upward pulling of the arm causing rapid extension of the elbow. This causes a dislocation of the annular ligament into the joint and between the radial head and the humerus.

Dx:
1. History and physical (H&P)
   - Radiographs are usually normal because the technician often inadvertently reduces the subluxation while positioning the arm for imaging.

Tx/Mgmt:
1. Supination and flexion with pressure over radial head.
2. Hyperpronation (if supination + flexion unsuccessful).
   - A successful reduction can usually be felt as a click, after which the child recovers movement of the joint and the pain is relieved.

Anterior Dislocation of the Shoulder

Buzz Words: Athlete with severe pain + shoulder "popped" out of place + abduction and external rotation mechanism

Clinical Presentation: Severe pain; patients usually notice that the humeral head is out of place. Some athletes who are prone to this injury are gymnasts, football players, and wrestlers.

PPx: N/A

MoD: Forceful abduction, extension, and external rotation of the shoulder

Dx:

1. PE
2. XR

Tx/Mgmt:

1. Immobilization after closed reduction.
2. Rehabilitation focuses on strengthening the rotator cuff, deltoid, and pericapsular muscles to prevent recurrence, which is very common.

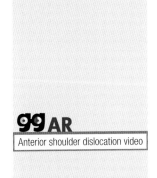

99 AR

Anterior shoulder dislocation video

Fractures

Given that children's bones are more flexible than those of adults, fractures are more common than sprains before adolescence. This structural difference between children and adults is also seen clinically as different types of fractures in children than you would normally see in an adult (Table 14.2). However, one of the most important things to consider is that these fractures may involve the epiphyseal plate, which could potentially cause a deformity. Salter and Harris developed a classification scheme (Table 14.3) that helps establish a prognosis and a treatment plan.

FOR THE WARDS

Salter-Harris mnemonic
SALTER:
 Same (I)
 Above (II)
 Lower (III)
 Through (IV)
 ERasure of the growth plate (V)

Fractures that are suggestive of nonaccidental trauma:

1. Posterior rib fractures
2. Femoral fractures in nonambulatory children
3. Proximal humeral fractures

Scoliosis

99 AR

Adam's forward bend test video

Buzz Words: Asymmetry of the shoulders or iliac crests + bump in the back while bending down

Clinical Presentation: Scoliosis presents as asymmetry of shoulder height, scapular position, and iliac crests. Adam's forward bend test is performed by having the child bend forward from the waist while the examiner looks for a lower back prominence representing posterior displacement of the spine. Scoliosis is typically painless; the presence of pain may indicate an underlying disorder that should be investigated. More common in females than males.

PPx: N/A

MoD: Most cases are idiopathic; however, it can be caused by leg-length discrepancy, neuromuscular disorders, vertebral anomalies, connective tissue disorders, or genetic syndromes.

TABLE 14.2 Common Types of Pediatric Fractures

Compression Fracture (Torus/ Buckle)	Incomplete Fracture (Greenstick)	Complete Fractures
Usually happens at the junction of the metaphysis and diaphysis. Occurs when the bone cortex suffers a compressive force. Heals in 3–4 weeks after immobilization.	Happens when one side of the bone is fractured but the other one is not. This causes the bone to bend toward the side of the bone that is not fractured, causing plastic deformation of the bone. It is necessary to fracture the concave (nonfractured) side of the bone to prevent further bone angulation.	Propagate completely through the bone. Divided into: • Transverse • Oblique • Spiral • Comminuted

TABLE 14.3 Salter–Harris Classification

Grade	Description of Fracture
I (low risk of growth plate injury)	Physeal separation, no involvement of adjacent bone
II	Extends through the physis and into the metaphysis
III	Extends through the physis and into the epiphysis
IV	Extends through the metaphysis, physis, and epiphysis
V (high risk of growth plate injury)	Crushing of the physis

Dx:
1. PE
2. XR: PA and lateral radiographs of the spine are used to calculate the Cobb angle, which measures the angle between the superior and inferior vertebrae tilted into the curve.

Tx/Mgmt:
1. Bracing
2. Surgery (severe cases)

Flexible Kyphosis and Scheuermann Kyphosis

Buzz Words: Patient brought by family members concerned about "hunched back" + voluntary correction (flexible kyphosis) or stiffness (Scheuermann kyphosis)

Clinical Presentation: Usually detected by family or friends. Flexible kyphosis is benign and can be corrected voluntarily, while Scheuermann kyphosis is structural and stiff.

PPx: N/A

MoD: Idiopathic

Dx:

1. Clinical for flexible scoliosis. Scheuermann disease is defined by wedging greater than 5 degrees of three or more consecutive vertebral bodies, so standing lateral spine radiographs are necessary for the diagnosis

Tx/Mgmt:

1. Flexible kyphosis does not require treatment
2. Scheuermann kyphosis can be treated with strengthening and stretching exercises, analgesics, and avoidance of precipitants
3. Bracing or surgical correction if the pain persists or if the kyphosis is greater than 90 degrees

Slipped Capital Femoral Epiphysis

Buzz Words: Overweight 12-year-old + dull pain in the hip that worsens with physical activity

Clinical Presentation: Nonradiating dull, aching pain in the hip, groin, thigh, or knee that causes an altered gait. Internal rotation, flexion, and abduction are usually decreased in the affected hip. Pain is usually increased with physical activity. Risk factors include obesity, hypothyroidism, hypopituitarism, and renal osteodystrophy. More common in African American males. Very high-yield for the Pediatrics exam.

PPx: N/A

MoD: Likely a combination of mechanical and endocrine factors

Dx:

1. PE
2. AP and frog-leg lateral radiographs reveal posterior displacement of the femoral epiphysis. Earliest changes include widening and irregularity of the physis, with thinning of the proximal epiphysis.

Tx/Mgmt:

1. Placement of large screw to pin the epiphysis, which stabilizes the physis and prevents progression. Osteonecrosis and chondrolysis are the two most serious complications

Brachial Plexus Injury (Erb Palsy/Klumpke Palsy)

Buzz Words: Neonate + asymmetric Moro reflex + claw hand (Klumpke palsy) or adducted arm with internal rotation (Erb palsy)

Clinical Presentation: Erb palsy presents with flaccid arm held in internal rotation, elbow extension, forearm pronation, and wrist flexion. Klumpke palsy presents with a claw hand and possible Horner syndrome if there is damage to the sympathetic fibers.

PPx: Avoid excessive traction of the neonate's head, neck, or arm during birth.

MoD: Birth trauma. Damage to C5 and C6 nerve roots causes Erb palsy, while damage to nerve roots C7 and C8 causes Klumpke palsy. Common risk factors include shoulder dystocia or birth weight greater than 4 kg.

Dx:

1. Based on history and physical examination. Radiograph and electromyography (EMG) can be considered to evaluate for fracture or neuropathy, respectively.

Tx/Mgmt:

1. Conservative management with monthly follow-up; surgical intervention may be necessary if the condition does not improve by 3 months of age, although this is not usually required. Partial immobilization and appropriate positioning are used to prevent development of contractures.

Congenital Disorders

Achondroplasia/Dwarfism

Buzz Words: Large head + short arms and legs

Clinical Presentation: Disproportionate short stature with proximal limb shortening. Kyphoscoliosis and lumbar lordosis may be pronounced. Homozygotes have increased susceptibility to pulmonary complications and compression of brain stem and spinal cord.

PPx: N/A

MoD: **Autosomal dominant** mutation in the *FGFR3* gene

Dx:

1. Based on clinical findings. Radiologic findings and molecular testing can confirm the diagnosis.

Tx/Mgmt:

1. Goal is to maximize functional capacity and to monitor and prevent potential complications.

Developmental Dysplasia of the Hip

Buzz Words: Joint laxity/clicking + breech delivery + positive Barlow and Ortolani maneuvers

Clinical Presentation: Asymptomatic in infants, careful examination will reveal hip dislocation using Ortolani and

Barlow maneuvers. In infants greater than 3 months of age, the dislocation can become relatively fixed, and the Galeazzi test should be used. Increased risk in the newborn with breech presentation, positive family history, females, and first-born children.

PPx: The typical physical examination of the newborn includes the use of Ortolani and Barlow maneuvers, because an earlier detection of this condition leads to a better clinical outcome

MoD: Abnormality in stability or shape of the femoral head and acetabulum

Dx:

1. Physical examination demonstrating hip instability, asymmetry, or limited abduction.
2. Imaging may be helpful to confirm the diagnosis; ultrasound is used for infants younger than 6 months of age because the hip and pelvis are not yet ossified at that age.
3. AP radiographs may be used in infants greater than 6 months of age.

Tx/Mgmt:

1. Infants younger than 6 months: Pavlik harness, 6 months to 2 years: closed reduction in OR ± arthrogram.
2. Monitoring is necessary, with regular hip radiographs until the child is skeletally mature.

Leg Deformities

Tibia Vara (Blount Disease)

Buzz Words: Overweight 3-year-old African American girl + bowlegs + lateral thrust with gait

Clinical Presentation: Risk factors include African American females, being overweight, starting to walk early in life, and having an affected family member. Presents as progressive unilateral bowing or persistent bowing after 2 years of age.

PPx: N/A

MoD: Abnormal endochondral ossification of the medial aspect of the proximal tibial physis

Dx:

1. Weight-bearing AP and lateral views of the lower extremities should be obtained.

Tx/Mgmt:

1. Brace treatment for 1 year should be started by 3 years of age.
2. If the deformity does not resolve with bracing, surgical therapy is required. Surgical intervention should

be performed before 4 years of age to reduce risk of recurrence. In the case of adolescent Blount disease, surgical management is the preferred treatment.

Foot Deformities

Metatarsus Adductus

Buzz Words: First-born child + C-shaped foot that can be straightened by manipulation

Clinical Presentation: Presents as medial curvature of the midfoot that can be straightened to a certain degree. Incidence is higher in first-borns and twins. Commonly bilateral, but affects the left leg more commonly than the right in unilateral cases.

PPx: N/A

MoD: Usually caused by intrauterine constraint

Dx:

1. PE

Tx/Mgmt:

1. Observation
2. Passive stretching exercises are recommended in moderate cases.
3. Corrective casting is required in severe cases that cannot be passively corrected to the midline.
4. Can be associated with hip pathology (e.g., developmental dysplasia of the hip).

> **MNEMONIC**
> CAVE: Forefoot (Cavus, Adductus), Hindfoot (Varus, Equinus)

Talipes Equinovarus (Club Foot)

Buzz Words: Chromosomal syndrome + rigid ankle fixed in plantarflexion

Clinical Presentation: Plantarflexion and inversion of the ankle with a medially curved forefoot. It is usually rigid, with little range of motion and calf atrophy.

PPx: N/A

MoD: Multifactorial, frequently associated with myelodysplasia, arthrogryposis, trisomy 18, 22q11 deletion syndromes.

Dx:

1. PE
2. XR

Tx/Mgmt:

1. Serial casting
2. Surgery (typically between 3 and 12 months of age)

Osteogenesis Imperfecta

Buzz Words: Blue sclera + fractures with minimal trauma + deafness

Clinical Presentation: Presents with bone fragility, short stature, blue sclera, scoliosis, hearing loss, teeth that wear quickly, and easy bruising. May be confused with child abuse.

PPx: N/A

MoD: Most commonly caused by autosomal dominant mutations in genes encoding type I collagen (COL1A1 and COL1A2). Classified into different subtypes based on the genetic, radiographic, and clinical characteristics.

Dx:
1. Usually obtained clinically. Abnormality in either quantity or quality of type I collagen can be observed using a small skin biopsy.

Tx/Mgmt:
1. Activity restriction and surgical correction of misalignments.
2. Bisphosphonates may be given to reduce the risk of fractures.

Muscular Dystrophy (Duchenne and Becker)

Buzz Words: 4-year-old boy + enlarged calves + trouble catching up with his friends + family history of a muscular disease

Muscular dystrophy video

Clinical Presentation: Slow, progressive weakness of the proximal muscles, which may present with Gower sign. **Duchenne muscular dystrophy (DMD) has an earlier onset and is more severe than Becker muscular dystrophy (BMD).** Patients with DMD lose the ability to walk by 10 years of age, while patients with BMD are usually able to walk until they are 20 years old. Patients also present with pseudohypertrophy of the calves, caused by replacement of muscular tissue with lipids.

PPx: N/A

MoD: X-linked disorder caused by mutation of the dystrophin gene.

Dx:
1. PE
2. EMG with small muscle potential with normal nerve conduction
3. Elevated creatine kinase (CK) levels
4. DNA testing reveals gene deletion, and decreased dystrophin on immunochemistry or Western blot may make the diagnosis.
5. Muscle biopsy is performed to confirm the diagnosis if the genetic studies are negative.

Tx/Mgmt:
1. Oral steroids can improve muscle strength in the early stages.

2. Physical therapy and respiratory support when needed.
3. Routine echocardiography to screen for cardiomyopathy.

GUNNER PRACTICE

1. A 26-month-old female presents to the pediatrician's office with her mother. The child was noted to be limping by day care staff around 10 days earlier, and her unusual gait has persisted and progressed. However, she has not complained of any discomfort and has otherwise maintained her normal, cheerful disposition. Her past medical history is notable only for a fracture of the right fibula 7 months earlier and an umbilical hernia that has begun to close spontaneously. Her family history is notable for hypertension in her father and vitiligo in her mother. She is at the 46th percentile for height and 35th percentile for weight, and has gained a pound since her last visit 2 months ago. The child's vital signs are T 98.7°F, HR 110, RR 25, SpO$_2$ 98% on room air. On examination, she is a calm, playful child. Her right knee is significantly larger and warmer to the touch than her left knee, and her ranges of motion in flexion and extension are mildly decreased. The right knee joint space is also mildly tender. Initial laboratory values reveal a normal CBC, ESR 57, normal CRP, and a positive antinuclear antibody. Lyme disease serologies are negative. Of the following, what is the most likely diagnosis?
   A. Osgood-Schlatter disease
   B. Systemic juvenile idiopathic arthritis
   C. Transient synovitis
   D. Patellar fracture
   E. Oligoarticular juvenile idiopathic arthritis

2. An 11-year-old male presents to his pediatrician's office with his mother. She complains that he has seemed ill for several weeks, but they live in a remote, rural area and have not been able to make an appointment until now. Her son has been complaining of left hip pain and "lightning pains" down his left thigh for nearly 3 months. He has experienced fevers for over a month, and has often woken up at night drenched in sweat. He has also developed a dry cough and has seemed "winded" for the previous 2 weeks. He has no known medical history, but he is up to date on his vaccinations. His mother has type II diabetes mellitus. In the office, his vital signs are T 99.4°F, HR

89, BP 105/71, RR 20, SpO$_2$ 98% on room air. He is 3 pounds lighter than at his last visit 7 months prior. He is ill-appearing. Examination yields moderate to severe tenderness to palpation of the left anterosuperior iliac spine and pain with passive flexion of the thigh at the hip. Pelvic XR reveals a large, "motheaten" bony lesion, and chest CT shows a mass in the left lung. Biopsy of the pelvic lesion yields sheets of small round blue cells with areas of necrosis. What is the most likely diagnosis?

A. Osteosarcoma
B. Ewing sarcoma
C. Osteoid osteoma
D. Osteomyelitis
E. Giant cell tumor of bone

3. A 13-year-old male is brought to the emergency department by his father for severe hip pain. The child had been complaining of mild aching of his left hip for the previous 2 weeks and had been limping intermittently during this time. At his basketball game this evening, he appeared to land awkwardly after an open layup and was unable to get up. His medical history is notable for mild persistent asthma, and his family history is notable for osteosarcoma in his father. His vital signs are T 98.5°F, HR 98, BP 110/75, RR 18, SpO$_2$ 98% on room air. Examination yields a short, externally rotated left lower extremity and severe pain with passive motion. XR of the hip is shown below. What is the best next step in management?

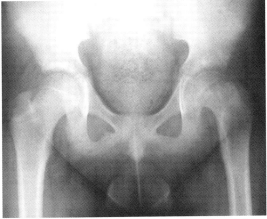

Slipped capital femoral epiphysis. (Iwinski HJ. *Essential Orthopedics*, Chapter 221, 909–911.)

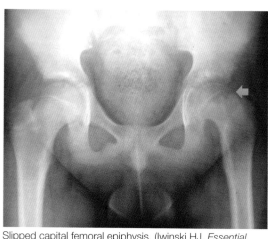

Slipped capital femoral epiphysis. (Iwinski HJ. *Essential Orthopedics*, Chapter 221, 909–911.)

A. Operative stabilization
B. Intravenous vancomycin
C. Operative lavage of the left acetabulofemoral joint
D. Hip replacement
E. Staging bone scan

Notes

ANSWERS: What Would Gunner Jess/Jim Do?

1. WWGJD? A 26-month-old female is brought to the pediatrician's office by her mother. The child was noted to be limping by daycare staff around 10 days ago, and her unusual gait has persisted and progressed. However, she has not complained of any discomfort and has otherwise had her normal, cheerful disposition. Her past medical history is notable only for a right fibula fracture 7 months ago and an umbilical hernia that has begun to close spontaneously. Her family history is notable for hypertension in her father and vitiligo in her mother. She is at the 46th percentile for height and 35th percentile for weight, and has gained a pound since her last visit 2 months ago. The child's vital signs are T 98.7°F, HR 110, RR 25, SpO$_2$ 98% on room air. On examination, she is a calm, playful child. Her right knee is significantly larger and warmer to the touch than her left knee, and her ranges of motion in flexion and extension are mildly decreased. The right knee joint space is also mildly tender. Initial laboratory values reveal a normal CBC, ESR 57, normal CRP, and a positive anti-nuclear antibody. Lyme disease serologies are negative. Of the following, what is the most likely diagnosis?

Answer: E, Oligoarticular juvenile idiopathic arthritis

Explanation: This question assesses your ability to recognize the differential diagnosis of a toddler with a limp. This child has a subacute, relatively painless gait abnormality, and overall appears largely well (as opposed to more severely "sick," based on her vital signs and normal recent development). The physical exam demonstrates the presence of arthritis, as she has a warm, tender joint space with decreased range of motion. Her labs reveal a positive ANA and mildly elevated ESR. This is a classic presentation of oligoarticular juvenile idiopathic arthritis, or JIA. The number of joints involved delineates JIA subtypes and the level of systemic inflammation observed in the patient.

A. Osgood-Schlatter disease → Incorrect. This disorder, which denotes osteochondritis of the tibial tubercle, occurs at the insertion of the patellar tendon in young teenagers experiencing a "growth spurt." The physical exam will yield tenderness to palpation at the tibial tubercle and not in the joint space of the knee, as with this patient.

B. Systemic juvenile idiopathic arthritis → Incorrect. Previously known as Still disease, this disorder is

characterized by high intermittent fevers, ill appearance, an evanescent salmon-colored macular rash, and arthritis as well as many other possible presentations of systemic inflammation.
C. Transient synovitis → Incorrect. The patient with transient synovitis classically presents with inflammation of the hip joint shortly after a viral illness. This painful episode generally subsides with NSAIDs and expectant management. In addition, patients with transient synovitis would not be expected to have an elevated ESR (should be less than 57). The question refers to a patient with relatively painless knee inflammation.
D. Patellar fracture → Incorrect. We are provided with no history of trauma, and the patient is not in severe pain. The physical exam is also inconsistent with this diagnosis.

2. WWGJD? An 11-year-old male is brought to the pediatrician's office by his mother. She complains that he has seemed ill for several weeks now, but they live in a remote, rural area and have not been able to make an appointment until now. Her son has been complaining of left hip pain, and "lightning pains" down his left thigh, for nearly 3 months. He has experienced fevers for over a month, and he has been waking up at night drenched in sweat frequently. He has also developed a dry cough and has seemed "winded" for the previous 2 weeks. He has no known medical history, but he is up to date on his vaccinations. His mother has type II diabetes mellitus. In the office, his vital signs are T 99.4°F, HR 89, BP 105/71, RR 20, SpO_2 98% on room air. He is 3 pounds lighter than at his last visit, 7 months prior. He is ill-appearing. Examination yields moderate to severe tenderness to palpation of the left anterior superior iliac spine and pain with passive flexion of the thigh at the hip. Pelvic XR reveals a large, "moth-eaten" bony lesion, and chest CT shows a mass in the left lung. Biopsy of the pelvic lesion yields sheets of small round blue cells with areas of necrosis. What is the most likely diagnosis?
Answer: B, Ewing sarcoma
   Explanation: This question tests your ability to distinguish between commonly tested bone tumors. The presentation of young male—with progressive hip pain, compressive symptoms, systemic "B" symptoms, and new cough and dyspnea—should raise concern for a metastatic malignant process. The

classic imaging findings and biopsy result indicate that this is Ewing sarcoma. It can be hard to distinguish between the several kinds of bone tumors. Remember, Ewing sarcoma commonly presents in flat bones (pelvis and ribs) as well as long bones, metastasizes frequently, and looks like a neuroendocrine or neuroectodermal type of tumor.

A. Osteosarcoma → Incorrect. This malignancy generally presents with pain in long bones without the systemic symptoms noted by this patient. Additionally, the XR will reveal a lesion with a "sunburst" pattern, and the histology often shows cells producing some type of matrix or stroma.

C. Osteoid osteoma → Incorrect. This is a benign bone tumor characterized by a lytic lesion causing aching pain at night that resolves with NSAIDs.

D. Osteomyelitis → Incorrect. While osteomyelitis should be on the differential diagnosis with Ewing sarcoma, the presence of a lung mass, the description of the XR, and the histology of the tumor indicate that this patient does not have osteomyelitis.

E. Giant cell tumor of bone → Incorrect. Although this (largely) benign tumor can present with a lytic lesion, the patient will not likely complain of systemic symptoms, histology will not appear as described, and the risk of metastasis is low.

3. WWGJD? A 13-year-old male is brought to the emergency department by his father for severe hip pain. The child had been complaining of mild aching of his left hip for the past two weeks, and had been limping intermittently during this time period. However, at his basketball game this evening, he appeared to land awkwardly after an open layup and was unable to get up. His medical history is notable for mild persistent asthma, and his family history is notable for osteosarcoma in his father. His vital signs are T 98.5°F, HR 98, BP 110/75, RR 18, SpO2 98% on room air. Examination yields a short, externally rotated left lower extremity and severe pain with passive motion. XR of the hip is shown below. What is the best next step in management?

Answer: A, Operative stabilization

Explanation: This question tests your ability to recognize a common cause of hip pain in adolescents. This is a classic acute presentation of slipped capital femoral epiphysis (SCFE). Patients are usually young teenagers, often obese, and may have chronic or acute complaints related to hip, thigh, or knee pain. Acutely, SCFE can even present similarly to a hip fracture. A plain radiograph will show the SCFE, which makes the femoral head appear as though an ice cream scoop had fallen off the cone. In an acute setting like this, the patient should be stopped from weight bearing and the bone should be screwed into place.

B. Intravenous vancomycin → Incorrect. This patient is not presenting with a septic arthritis.

C. Operative lavage of the left acetabulofemoral joint → Incorrect. See answer for B.

D. Hip replacement → Incorrect. This is a consideration for patients with avascular necrosis of the hip.

E. Staging bone scan → Incorrect. This is not a neoplastic process.

Endocrine and Metabolic Disorders

15

Leo Wang, Sierra Centkowski, Marissa J. Kilberg, Hao-Hua Wu, and Rebecca Tenney-Soeiro

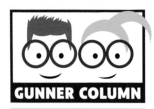

GUNNER COLUMN

Introduction

Endocrine and metabolic disorders make up 5–10 questions on the Pediatrics exam, primarily focusing on congenital disorders in children and disorders that affect teenagers. In both age groups, shifts in hormone levels can bring about dramatic changes in development and anatomic growth. An imbalance of sex steroids at birth, for instance, can lead to ambiguous genitalia. Lack of important hormones in a teenager can delay maturation through puberty, leading to virilization, amenorrhea, or challenges in development.

There are many concepts in this chapter that overlap with step 1. If you learned your lysosomal storage disorders or inborn errors of metabolism (IEM) well, you can use those same buzz words to identify answers on the exam. Luckily, given the broad range of topics that could be tested, from diabetes to congenital hypothyroidism, you will not be tested on hard-to-memorize minutiae (e.g., enzyme deficiencies due to IEM). Anticipate spending 4–6 hours perusing this material.

This chapter is divided into the following sections: (1) Diabetes and Hyperinsulinism, (2) Thyroid and Parathyroid Disorders, (3) Adrenal Disorders, (4) Growth and Pituitary Disorders, (5) Congenital Disorders, (6) Metabolic Disorders, and (7) Gunner Practice (Fig. 15.1).

Below is a high-yield chart of how male and female reproductive systems develop. Make sure to know key steps of disruption, such as presence/absence of the *SRY* gene, presence of testosterone, and so on that can lead to characteristic disease states. Default pathway is female!

Diabetes and Hyperinsulinism

Diabetes is the second most common disease of childhood, affecting approximately 1 in every 500 children, with boys being affected twice as often as girls. There are two types of diabetes: type 1 and type 2. Type 1 diabetes is insulin-dependent. It is characterized by lymphocytic,

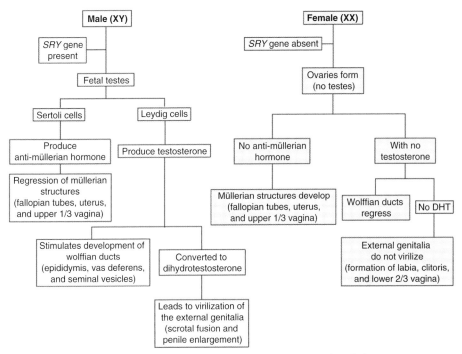

FIG. 15.1 Embryonic development, fetal maturation, and perinatal changes.

autoimmune destruction of the pancreatic islet cells that create insulin. Type 2 diabetes actually has an even stronger genetic component and is caused by peripheral tissue insulin resistance. Complications of diabetes include retinopathy, nephropathy, and diabetic ketoacidosis.

In pediatrics, the opposite phenomenon of hyperinsulinism is also observed in neonates.

Type I Diabetes

Buzz Words: Polyuria/polydipsia/nocturia + fatigue/weight loss

Clinical Presentation: More common form of childhood diabetes. These patients present with typical findings like polyuria and polydipsia, sometimes with enuresis.

Prophylactic (PPx): N/A

Mechanism of Disease (MoD): Autoimmune, lymphocytic destruction of pancreatic islet cells leads to deficient production of insulin.

Diagnostic Steps (Dx):

1. Fasting glucose greater than 126 g/dL
2. Blood sugar—random blood sugar greater than 200 g/dL with symptoms
3. HbA1c greater than 6.5%

QUICK TIPS

Many patients will have a transient decrease in insulin requirements ("honeymoon" period) after initiating insulin therapy, related to increased activity of the remaining beta cells. This occurs soon after initial treatment and lasts up to 1 year.

QUICK TIPS

Two theories for morning hyperglycemia exist:

Somogyi effect describes morning hyperglycemia as a result of too much nighttime insulin.

Theory = Too much insulin at night → hypoglycemia → compensatory mechanisms (glucagon + epinephrine) → hyperglycemia in morning.

Treatment = lower insulin in these patients before bed.

Dawn phenomenon is unrelated to hypoglycemia but rather overnight secretion of growth hormone and the inability of a diabetic patient to increase insulin in response to this.

Treatment and Management Steps (Tx/Mgmt):

1. Insulin—mainstay of therapy
   - Long-acting—glargine/detemir
   - Intermediate-acting—NPH
   - Short-acting—regular
   - Rapid-acting—aspart
2. Every 3 months, check HbA1c (goal <7%).
3. Every year, check urinalysis for microalbuminuria (if positive, start on an angiotensin-converting enzyme inhibitor [ACEI] or angiotensin receptor blocker [ARB]), check serum blood urea nitrogen (BUN) and creatinine (monitor for diabetic nephropathy), eye screening with ophthalmologist (monitor for diabetic retinopathy), and cholesterol levels (if low-density lipoprotein [LDL] >100, start a statin).
4. Every visit, check blood glucose, blood pressure (if >130/80, start ACEI or ARB), and feet (for ulcers).

Type II Diabetes

Buzz Words: Acanthosis nigricans (Fig. 15.2) + obesity + polyuria/polydipsia/nocturia + fatigue/weight loss

Clinical Presentation: Type II diabetes (T2DM) tends to have a less symptomatic onset than type 1 diabetes and is often related to obesity. These patients have peripheral tissue insulin resistance so are typically not started on insulin at the onset of disease. Although this has traditionally been thought of more as a disease that affects only adults, T2DM is becoming more common in the pediatric population owing to rising rates of childhood obesity.

PPx: Diet/exercise + avoidance of high-fructose corn syrup

MoD: Obesity → free fatty acids → peripheral tissue resistance to insulin → pancreatic islet cells secrete more insulin → islet cell dysfunction → reduced insulin → hyperglycemia.

Dx:

1. Fasting glucose greater than 126 g/dL
2. Blood sugar—random blood sugar greater than 200 g/dL with symptoms
3. HbA1c greater than 6.5%

Tx/Mgmt:

1. Diet and exercise
2. Metformin (only oral hypoglycemic medication approved for children). Because there is peripheral resistance, typically start with oral hypoglycemic agents over insulin.
3. Insulin (short acting—lispro, long acting—glargine)

QUICK TIPS

Avoid metformin in renal failure; metformin can cause lactic acidosis.

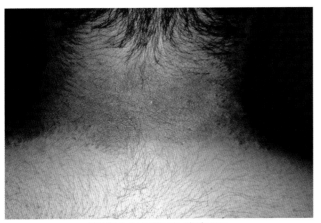

FIG. 15.2 Acanthosis nigricans.

Acute Complications of Diabetes Mellitus

1. Hyperosmolar coma or hyperosmolar hyperglycemic nonketotic syndrome (HHNS)
   a. Most common in T2DM
   b. Symptoms: severe dehydration (low BP, high HR), nausea/vomiting, abdominal pain, polyuria, polydipsia, seizures, and altered mental status
   c. Lab findings: high glucose (usually >900 mg/dL), hyperosmolarity (>320 mOsm/L), normal pH, and high BUN (due to dehydration)
   d. Treatment: IV normal saline and low-dose insulin
2. Hypoglycemic shock
   a. Most common in T1DM, especially in those using insulin. Brain is most at risk during hypoglycemia. Causes include too much insulin (high insulin, low C-peptide in blood), insulinoma, ethanol ingestion, etc.
   b. Symptoms: tremor, palpitations, sweating, altered mental status, seizure, and coma in some cases
   c. Lab findings: low glucose (usually <50 mg/dL)
   d. Treatment: IV dextrose (give glucose!)
3. Diabetic ketoacidosis—*High-yield on the Peds exam!*
   a. Most common in T1DM, but can occur in both T1DM and T2DM. Usually precipitated by stress (illness or trauma) or missed insulin doses.
   b. Symptoms: acute onset of nausea/vomiting, abdominal pain, "fruity" breath (cause by high ketones), rapid and deep breathing (Kussmaul), dehydration, polyuria, polydipsia, and altered mental status
   c. Lab findings: high glucose (usually >450 mg/dL), anion gap metabolic acidosis (pH <7.3 and serum

HCO_3 <15 mEq/L), increased betahydroxybutyrate, **electrolyte abnormalities:**

    i. Hyperkalemia, but decreased total body potassium—acidosis causes release of potassium from the cells

    ii. Pseudohyponatremia—increased osmolarity due to hyperglycemia and water shift into the extracellular compartment

    iii. Hypophosphatemia

    iv. Hypomagnesemia

  d. Treatment: IV normal saline, insulin, and potassium supplementation:

    i. Note: Monitor for anion gap closure as treatment end point.

    ii. Rapid correction of hyperglycemia can cause **cerebral edema.**

QUICK TIPS

Chronic complications of DM such as retinopathy, neuropathy, and nephropathy are not covered here because not covered on the Pediatrics exam. However, these will show up on Medicine.

Hyperinsulinism

Buzz Words: Newborn + jittery + low blood glucose

Clinical Presentation: Infant noticed to be jittery, found to have a low blood glucose. Transient in nature in infant of a diabetic mother, stressful delivery, small for gestational age, preterm neonate. Can be permanent in neonates with other reason for excess insulin secretion (insulinoma, genetic mutation).

PPx: N/A

MoD: Increased insulin secretion → low blood glucose

Dx:

1. Basic metabolic panel (BPM)/complete blood count (CBC)
2. Blood sugar (low blood glucose that persists despite feeding)

Tx/Mgmt:

1. Feed on schedule
2. Provide IV glucose and titrate to maintain Dsticks greater than 70
3. For true, permanent hyperinsulinism, may need diazoxide, octreotide, or even pancreatectomy

Thyroid and Parathyroid Disorders

Hypothyroidism (See Below for Congenital Hypothyroidism)

Buzz Words: Growth deceleration + fatigue+ dry skin + constipation + goiter

Clinical Presentation: Detected in an evaluation of growth due to presence of goiter or in workup for lethargy

PPx: N/A

MoD: Most common in the United States: autoimmune lymphocytic infiltration (Hashimoto) causing decreased thyroid hormone production. In Third World countries, also consider iodine deficiency.

Dx:

1. Thyroid functional tests (T3, T4, TSH → expect to find decreased T3/T4, increased TSH)

Tx/Mgmt:

1. Levothyroxine replacement

Graves Disease

Buzz Words: Exophthalmos + fatigue + tremors + heat intolerance + menstrual irregularities + tachycardia

Clinical Presentation: Gradual development of symptoms. Detected in workup based on exophthalmos, menstrual evaluation, hyperactivity, or fatigability.

PPx: N/A

MoD: Can be caused by thyroid-stimulating immunoglobulin (TSI), thyroid-stimulating hormone (TSH) receptor antibody, antithyroglobulin antibodies, or antimicrosomal antibodies

Dx: Elevated T3/T4, low TSH, elevated antibodies

Tx/Mgmt: Antithyroid medications (propylthiouracil in pediatrics), propranolol (beta blocker to control heart rate), radioactive iodine (ablate the thyroid), thyroidectomy

Thyroid Mass

Buzz Words: History of radiation + palpable nodule

Clinical Presentation: Often incidentally discovered on exam or discovered because of presence of hypo- or hyperthyroidism. Less common in children, but once detected more likely to be malignant.

PPx: N/A

MoD: Thyroid carcinoma, adenoma, papillary carcinoma, medullary carcinoma

Dx:

1. TSH, T3/T4
2. Ultrasound
3. Fine-needle aspiration (FNA)
4. Biopsy or surgical excision

Tx/Mgmt:

1. Monitoring versus resection
2. Definitive treatment depends on etiology

Hyperparathyroidism

Buzz Words: Asymptomatic patient with high calcium on routine labs + family history of hyperparathyroidism

QUICK TIPS

Trisomy 21 is often associated with hypothyroidism.

Clinical Presentation: Patient may present with kidney stones, hypertension (not well controlled with appropriate medical therapy), back pain (due to vertebral compression caused by low bone density). May be related to MEN 1 syndrome, familial hypocalciuric hypercalcemia (FHH).

PPx: (1) Modify risk factors for chronic kidney disease. (2) Maintain healthy vitamin D intake. (3). Genetic testing for MEN 1 syndrome.

MoD: (1) Primary hyperparathyroidism is caused by a problem at the parathyroid, with inappropriate release of parathyroid hormone (PTH), no longer responsive to the calcium levels in the blood (remember, high PTH increases plasma calcium levels up to a point, and then a negative feedback mechanism kicks in, where high calcium signals the parathyroid to stop producing PTH). (2) Secondary hyperparathyroidism is primarily caused by chronic kidney disease, which results in low serum calcium levels (low GFR → low vitamin D → low calcium absorption); the body increases PTH levels in response. Other etiologies include low vitamin D and lithium toxicity.

Hyperparathyroidism due to FHH is caused by an autosomal dominant mutation that results in abnormal calcium-sensing receptors at both the parathyroid cells and renal tubules, so that the feedback mechanism of high calcium does not appropriately suppress PTH release.

Dx:

1. Primary: Normal/high PTH, high serum calcium, and high urine calcium (calciuria)
2. Secondary: High PTH, low/normal serum calcium

Tx/Mgmt:

1. Surgical resection of one or more of the parathyroid glands is first-line. If primary hyperparathyroidism is caused by carcinoma, removal of the ipsilateral thyroid and enlarged lymph nodes is recommended.
2. Medical management includes fluids and possibly furosemide if hypercalcemia is severe. For secondary hyperparathyroidism, treat the underlying cause (i.e., give vitamin D or calcitriol and calcium).

Hypoparathyroidism

Buzz Words: History of neck surgery or radiation + particularly near thyroid + perioral numbness + muscle cramps + hyperreflexia + paresthesias + arrhythmias + prolonged QT interval on electrocardiogram (ECG)

Clinical Presentation: Will typically present with muscle weakness, numbness, and/or tingling. Occurs in setting of history of/treatment for thyroid disease (especially Graves disease), specifically radioiodine ablation or surgical resection of the thyroid.

PPx: N/A

MoD: The most common cause of hypoparathyroidism is removal or damage of parathyroid gland tissue in the course of treatment for thyroid disease.

Dx:
1. Low serum calcium and low PTH, with high serum phosphate

Tx/Mgmt:
1. Calcium and calcitriol supplementation (IV calcium gluconate if severe and in acute hospital setting)

FOR THE WARDS
Calcium supplementation may cause kidney stones. Be careful!

Adrenal Disorders

Primary Adrenal Insufficiency (Addison Disease)

Buzz Words: Hyperpigmentation + hypotension + high potassium + upper-lobe cavitary lesion + syncope

Clinical Presentation: Typically presents with hyperpigmentation, weakness, dizziness. Suspect in setting of tuberculosis (immigrant patient) or history of autoimmune diseases.

PPx: N/A

MoD: The two most common causes of primary adrenal insufficiency are tuberculosis (worldwide), which causes calcifications within the adrenals, and autoimmune adrenalitis (industrialized countries), which involves immune destruction of the adrenals. Other causes of primary adrenal insufficiency include cytomegalovirus (CMV), fungal infections, and postpartum pituitary infarction (see pituitary apoplexy). Destruction of adrenal gland tissue results in decreased cortisol and aldosterone levels (produced in the adrenals), which causes increased levels of adrenocorticotropic hormone (ACTH) and renin (attempting to stimulate the adrenals).

Dx:
1. Low AM cortisol and aldosterone
2. High ACTH and renin
3. Minimal cortisol response to cosyntropin test (synthetic ACTH, which should increase cortisol levels in healthy patients)

Tx/Mgmt:
1. First-line therapy includes oral glucocorticoids and mineralocorticoids.

QUICK TIPS
Adrenal crisis is a medical emergency, during which adrenal insufficiency causes severe hypotension, renal failure, and possibly death if untreated. Admit and treat with IV steroids (hydrocortisone) and fluids and identify underlying cause.

Secondary Adrenal Insufficiency

Buzz Words: Long-term steroid use with abrupt stop + weakness/dizziness

Clinical Presentation: Typically presents with weakness, dizziness; overall, less severe symptoms compared with primary adrenal insufficiency (no hyperpigmentation, no hyperkalemia). Suspect in setting of chronic steroid use, hypopituitarism, autoimmune processes, high-dose progestins.

PPx: Steroid tapering in the setting of long-term steroid use

MoD: Secondary adrenal insufficiency is caused by processes outside the adrenal glands that cause decreased levels of ACTH, resulting in low cortisol and aldosterone; this includes abrupt cessation of long-term steroids, high-dose progestins, and pituitary process causing hypopituitarism (like prolactinoma, craniopharyngioma, etc.).

Dx:
1. Low AM cortisol and ACTH, normal aldosterone and renin
2. Minimal cortisol response to cosyntropin test
3. Brain magnetic resonance imaging (MRI) is also indicated to identify cause

Tx/Mgmt:
1. First-line therapy is glucocorticoids

Cushing Disease

Buzz Words: Hyperpigmentation + weight gain with new abdominal stretch marks and "buffalo hump" + moon facies + hirsutism + type 2 diabetes mellitus

Clinical Presentation: Patient presents with hyperpigmentation, weight gain, stretch marks, menstrual cycle changes, facial hair (women), weakness, depression, and easy bruising related to hormone changes; as in the case of other pituitary masses, bitemporal hemianopsia or headache may occur. Associated with the development of insulin resistance, causing diabetes.

PPx: N/A

MoD: Cushing disease is caused primarily by small pituitary adenomas that increase secretion of ACTH, causing adrenal hyperplasia (from overstimulation), which results in hyperpigmentation, increased cortisol, and aldosterone.

Dx:
1. Low-dose dexamethasone suppression test fails to suppress cortisol (AM cortisol levels >5)
2. High 24-hour urinary free cortisol level

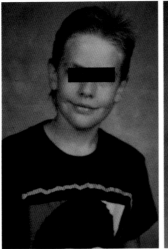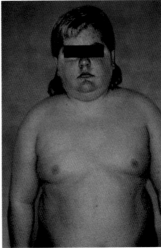

FIG. 15.3 Cushing disease in child.

3. High ACTH → pituitary source or ectopic ACTH production
4. Corticotropin-releasing hormone (CRH) stimulation test that causes increase in ACTH or cortisol indicates Cushing disease
5. Brain MRI

Tx/Mgmt:
1. Surgical resection of pituitary adenoma and bilateral adrenalectomies are first-line (Fig. 15.3).

Cushing Syndrome

Buzz Words: Female patient on steroids or long-term smoker with weight gain (specifically around abdomen) and "buffalo hump," moon facies with acne, and recent development of male features (hirsutism).

Clinical Presentation: Typically presents with weight gain, facial hair (women), changes in menstrual cycle, bone pain (think avascular necrosis of femoral head), hypertension (HTN), muscle weakness, easy bruising. Relevant past history includes chronic steroid use, smoking history, small cell lung cancer, diabetes → especially suspect this in children taking steroids for autoimmune problems.

PPx: Reduce steroid dosages and quit smoking

MoD: Cushing syndrome is caused by increased levels of cortisol in the body, which may be caused by ectopic ACTH production; in children, this is most commonly associated with adrenal tumors. Symptoms include myopathy, high blood pressure, hypokalemia, hypernatremia (with volume overload), and metabolic alkalosis.

Dx:
1. Low-dose dexamethasone suppression test fails to suppress cortisol (AM cortisol levels >5)
2. High 24-hour urinary free cortisol level
3. High ACTH → pituitary source or ectopic ACTH production; low ACTH → adrenal source
4. CRH stimulation test that causes no increase in ACTH or cortisol demonstrates an adrenal or ectopic ACTH source for Cushing syndrome
5. Chest computed tomography (CT) and abdominal CT to identify mass in lung or on adrenals

Tx/Mgmt:
1. Taper glucocorticoid or treat underlying cause (i.e., surgical excision of tumor in lung)

QUICK TIPS
Neuroblastoma – crosses midline; Wilms – does not cross midline

Adrenal Neuroblastoma

Buzz Words: Child <5 years old + abdominal mass **crossing midline** + respiratory distress + Horner + hypertension/ sweating + fever/weight loss

Clinical Presentation: This is a malignant cancer of **neural crest cells** presenting anywhere along the sympathetic ganglion but most commonly in the adrenal medulla. Adrenal neuroblastoma is a common tumor presenting within the first 5 years with 75% in the abdomen and pelvic areas. The chief complaint is usually an abdominal mass, which is found on examination to cross the midline.

PPx: N/A

MoD: Chromosomal abnormalities, deletions and translocations affecting Chr 1, 17, 14, 22; may involve c-Myc.

Dx:
1. Urine VMA/HVA (catecholamine secretion)
2. CT/MRI
3. Technetium-99 bone scan for bone metastasis

Tx/Mgmt:
1. Surgery
2. Chemotherapy
3. Radiation therapy

Pheochromocytoma

Buzz Words: Hypertension + headache, palpitations + "feeling of doom" + anxiety

Clinical Presentation: May have recurrent episodes of headache, sweating, and tachycardia. Occurs in setting of hypertension resistant to medical therapies; family history of MEN 2 syndromes, von Hippel-Lindau syndrome, and neurofibromatosis type 1 (NF1).

PPx: N/A

MoD: Pheochromocytomas are tumors that secrete catecholamines, including epinephrine and norepinephrine, arising primarily from the chromaffin cells in the adrenal medulla. Can be spontaneous or associated with genetic syndromes.

Dx:
1. Twenty-four-hour urine positive for metanephrines (VMA/HVA)
2. Imaging (US, CT, or MRI) to localize tumor

Tx/Mgmt: First-line treatment:
1. Alpha blockers *first* (phenoxybenzamine)
2. Then beta blockers (propranolol) for 2 weeks
3. Followed by surgical resection

Note: Do not start beta blockers before alpha blockers because this may precipitate hypertensive crisis (treat hypertensive crisis with nitroprusside).

Delayed and Precocious Puberty

This is one of the most important concepts on the Pediatrics exam. Some basic concepts: puberty does not begin because the hypothalamus is being inhibited by testosterone and estradiol. When this inhibition goes away, puberty begins and levels of follicle-stimulating hormone (FSH) and luteinizing hormone (LH) increase.

Female puberty occurs between 7 and 13 years of age with breast bud development as the first sign. FSH → estrogen → thelarche. Testosterone → adrenarche. Menarche begins between ages 9 and 15. Male puberty begins between ages 9 and 14. Testicular enlargement is the first sign. FSH stimulates sperm production and LH stimulates androgen production.

Precocious puberty for girls is breast development before age 7 years or menarche before 9 years. For boys, this is penile and testicular enlargement or pubic hair development before 9 years.

Disease	Symptoms	MoD	Dx	Tx/Mgmt
Premature thelarche	Visible + palpable breast tissue in first 2 years of life	N/A	PE	No treatment indicated—but be sure to rule out precocious puberty
Premature adrenarche	Early pubic/axillary hair, more common in girls than boys after age 5	Increase in adrenal hormones—independent of the hypothalamic pituitary gonad axis	PE Labs: DHEAS, consider 17OHP Imaging: Bone age (make sure it is not advanced)	No treatment indicated if simple adrenarche—must rule out congenital adrenal hyperplasia or virilizing tumor
Central precocious puberty	Breast/testicle development, pubic hair, rapid growth early	Early activation of hypothalamus	1. FSH/LH/sex hormones 2. GnRH stimulation test 3. MRI for boys, also evaluate for hypothyroidism, head trauma, brain masses	Treat underlying cause, GnRH analogues
Peripheral precocious puberty	Boys with gynecomastia or premature pubic hair; girls with breast development	Exposure to sex steroids independent of HPG axis, can be caused by adrenal tumors or reproductive tumors	1. FSH/LH/testosterone/beta-HCG 2. Estradiol in girls 3. CNS imaging 4. Rule out exogenous exposure (i.e., mom's oral contraceptive pill)	Treat underlying cause
Delayed puberty	No testicular enlargement by 14 or breast tissue by 13, menarche by 14	Caused by hypogonadotropic (hypothalamus or pituitary failure) or hypergonadotropic hypogonadism (gonad failure)	1. Physical exam 2. Workup for diseases like hypopituitarism (LH/FSH), hypothyroidism (TSH), and genetic syndromes (consider Klinefelter and Turner) 3. Bone age 4. Growth curve	Treat underlying cause Hormone replacement

CNS, Central nervous system; FSH, follicle-stimulating hormone; GnRH, gonadotropin-releasing hormone; HCG, human chorionic gonadotropin; HPG, hypothalamo-pituitary-gonadal; LH, luteinizing hormone; OHP, hydroxyprogesterone; PE, physical examination; TSH, thyroid-stimulating hormone.

Growth and Pituitary Disorders

Acromegaly/Gigantism

Buzz Words: Coarse facial features + increased ring size + large jaw + skin tags + bitemporal hemianopsia (parasellar manifestation)

a. Also associated with aortic regurgitation, hypercalcemia, carpal tunnel syndrome

PPx: N/A

MoD: Excess growth hormone (GH) released by pituitary adenoma causes excess insulin-like growth factor-1 (IGF-1), which leads to excessive growth of bone and soft tissues.

Dx:

1. IGF-1 levels (elevated)
2. Oral glucose suppression test (inadequate GH suppression)
3. MRI of pituitary

Tx/Mgmt:

1. Resection of pituitary adenoma

QUICK TIPS
Most common cause of death in acromegaly: cardiomyopathy (also stroke, colon cancer, renal failure).

Diabetes Insipidus

Buzz Words: Frequent urination, thirst

Types:

1. Central diabetes insipidus (DI): most common
   a. Etiology: Idiopathic (most common), head trauma, surgery
   b. MoD: Low antidiuretic hormone (ADH) secretion
   c. Tx/Mgmt: Desmopressin (DDAVP) is first-line; treat underlying cause
2. Nephrogenic DI: Normal ADH secretion, but renal tubules do not respond
   a. Etiology: Chronic lithium use (most common), hypercalcemia, hereditary
   b. MoD: Resistance to ADH at the level of the renal tubules, normal ADH levels
   c. Tx/Mgmt: Sodium restriction and thiazide diuretics

Dx:

1. Decreased urine osmolality, high serum osmolality (<300); water-deprivation test → no change in urine osmolality; low ADH in central DI, normal/high ADH in nephrogenic DI

Growth Hormone Deficiency

Buzz Words: Short stature (commonly seen in children) + decreased bone density (high rate of fractures)

Clinical Presentation: Idiopathic or occurs secondary to hypopituitarism. Most commonly appears on the shelf as a patient who presents with short stature (see the short stature flow chart).

QUICK TIPS
Short = 2 SDs below average

TABLE 15.1 Using Bone Age in the Differential Diagnosis of Short Stature

Bone Age = Chronologic Age	Bone Age < Chronologic Age
Familial short stature	Constitutional short stature
Intrauterine growth retardation	Hypothyroidism
Turner syndrome	Hypercortisolism
Skeletal dysplasia	Growth hormone deficiency
—	Chronic diseases

PPx: N/A

MoD: Variable. Could be from adjacent mass, idiopathic, etc.

Dx:

1. Low IGF-1 (low growth hormone [GH] in response to a stimulation test can confirm if IGF-1 is borderline).
   - Because growth hormone is secreted in a pulsatile fashion, a one-time value may not be useful.
2. Compare bone age with chronologic age (Table 15.1).

Tx/Mgmt:

1. GH therapy
2. Follow up IGF-1

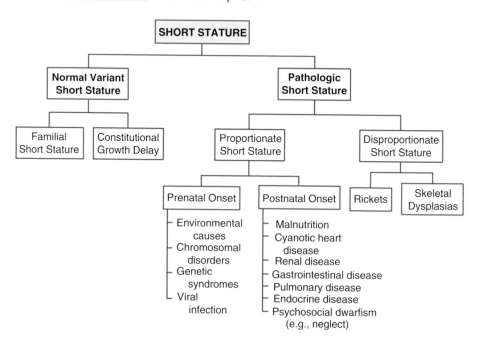

Syndrome of Inappropriate Antidiuretic Hormone Secretion

Buzz Words: Hyponatremia + weakness + lethargy + seizures

Clinical Presentation: In children, this occurs in the setting of severe illness (i.e., intensive care unit [ICU] patients), pneumonia, brain tumors. Can also occur with Rocky Mountain spotted fever.

PPx: Appropriate fluid management in hospitalized patients

MoD: Excess ADH causes increased water retention at the level of the collecting ducts in the renal tubules, resulting in volume expansion and hyponatremia.

Dx:

1. Syndrome of inappropriate antidiuretic hormone secretion (SIADH) is a diagnosis of exclusion, but the following lab values support it: Hyponatremia, hypo-osmolality and concentrated urine (>100 mosmol/kg) with reduced urine volume.
   - BMP/CBC
   - Urinalysis (UA)

Tx/Mgmt:

1. Treat underlying cause and water restrict all patients.
2. For symptomatic patients, normal saline may be used.

QUICK TIPS
Do not correct hyponatremia too quickly or central pontine myelinosis may occur due to rapid flux out of cells into the extracellular fluid space.

Pituitary Adenoma

Buzz Words: Bitemporal hemianopsia + headache

Clinical Presentation: Pituitary adenoma is a neoplasm in the pituitary gland that grows and classically causes loss of peripheral vision due to mass effect on the optic chiasm.

PPx: N/A

MoD: The pathogenesis of these neoplasms is not fully understood, as the mutations that cause them have not been well documented. Pituitary adenomas are usually benign and are most commonly prolactinomas (see below). Symptoms are related to mass effect in the sella (a saddle depression within the skull that houses the pituitary gland). Parasellar symptoms include visual changes (compression of the optic chiasm), headache, and reductions in pituitary hormone release—GH, LH, FSH (compression of the hypothalamic-pituitary stalk). Tumors can also have pituitary hormone hypersecretion, including TSH, ACTH, prolactin, and GH (see respective sections for symptoms specific to each hormone).

Dx:

1. MRI of the brain and pituitary hormone levels, including LH, FSH, prolactin, IGF-1, and 24-hour urine free cortisol

Tx/Mgmt:

1. Surgical resection (transsphenoidal approach) of the adenoma is first-line except in the case of prolactinomas (see below).

Prolactinoma/Hyperprolactinemia

Buzz Words: Bitemporal hemianopsia + headache and galactorrhea in an older male

Clinical Presentation: Very uncommon in children (compared with craniopharyngioma). Symptoms may bring patients into the outpatient office (milder symptoms) or into the ER (changes in vision, severe headache). Treatment will dictate whether they are followed as outpatients or admitted to the hospital. Patients will typically complain of headache, decreased libido, galactorrhea, changes in menstrual cycle (women), and impotence (men).

PPx: N/A

MoD: Unknown

Dx:
1. History
2. Physical exam (with particular focus on the visual field)
3. Brain MRI and hormone levels, including serum prolactin

Tx/Mgmt:
1. Cabergoline or bromocriptine (for pregnant women), both dopamine agonists, are first-line.
2. If symptoms persist or there is not a sufficient reduction in size of the prolactinoma, transsphenoidal surgery may be required.

Craniopharyngioma

Buzz Words: Child falling off the growth curve with headaches or visual changes

Clinical Presentation: Typically presents in children between age 5 and 14. Because craniopharyngiomas grow slowly, patients will likely present in the outpatient setting. Typical chief complaint is growth failure or headache. This is a highly tested concept on the Pediatrics exam. Visual changes may include bitemporal hemianopsia.

PPx: N/A

MoD: Craniopharyngiomas are suprasellar tumors arising from epithelial cells; they are associated with various genetic mutations.

Dx:
1. Brain MRI

Tx/Mgmt:
1. Surgical resection is first line (Fig. 15.4).

Hypogonadism, Primary and Secondary

Buzz Words: Menstrual irregularity or low sperm count + muscle mass and body hair

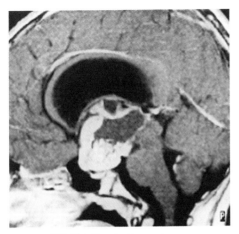

FIG. 15.4 Craniopharyngioma.

Clinical Presentation: Hypogonadism in Pediatrics often manifests as delayed puberty or menstrual irregularity/amenorrhea. Primary hypogonadism occurs with syndromes such as Klinefelter and Turner syndromes. Secondary hypogonadism in Pediatrics tends to be caused by stress, obesity, weight loss (anorexia), athleticism in adolescents, or drug use.

PPx: For secondary hypogonadism, prevent/treat underlying cause.

MoD: In primary hypogonadism, disease—primarily involving the testes—is characterized by low testosterone and high LH and FSH. Infertility (low sperm count caused by decreased spermatogenesis due to low testosterone) in these cases is harder to treat than secondary hypogonadism. In secondary hypogonadism, disease—primarily involving the pituitary or hypothalamus—is characterized by low testosterone, LH, and FSH. Spermatogenesis can be increased (raising sperm count and improving infertility issues) in these patients by increasing LH and FSH.

Dx:
1. History, PE
2. Serum *morning* total testosterone (males), estradiol (females)
3. LH and FSH
4. If secondary hypogonadism is suspected, measure other pituitary hormones as well (TSH, etc.)

Tx/Mgmt:
1. Treat underlying cause
2. Testosterone replacement or estrogen replacement (oral contraceptive pill [OCP])

Multiple Endocrine Neoplasia (MEN₁, MEN₂)

Buzz Words: Personal/family history of endocrine tumors + severe peptic ulcer disease (gastrinomas) + high parathyroid hormone (PTH) + high calcium + thyroid nodule + galactorrhea (MEN 1)

Clinical Presentation: Types:

MEN type 1: Parathyroid hyperplasia, pancreatic islet cell tumor, pituitary tumors; associated with Zollinger-Ellison syndrome (ZES), which produces gastrinomas. (**GC:** MEN type 1 → **PPP** = parathyroid hyperplasia, pancreatic islet cell tumor, pituitary tumors.)

MEN type 2A: Medullary thyroid carcinoma, pheochromocytoma, hyperparathyroidism. (**GC:** MEN type 2A → **MPH** = medullary thyroid carcinoma, pheochromocytoma, hyperparathyroidism.)

MEN type 2B: Medullary thyroid carcinoma, marfanoid habitus (tall and thin, large wing span), pheochromocytoma, neuromas. (**GC:** MEN type 2B → **MMPN** = medullary thyroid carcinoma, marfanoid habitus, pheochromocytoma, neuromas.)

MEN syndromes typically present in older children in outpatient settings, and symptoms at onset are usually mild and related to hypothyroidism. Given the autosomal dominant pattern, many patients will present for screening. Patients are typically asymptomatic initially, as hyperparathyroidism is the presenting manifestation of MEN 1 and 2A syndromes. For MEN 2B, the presenting symptom can be a thyroid nodule. Suspect MEN in the setting of peptic ulcer disease (think ZES), family history of MEN tumors (parathyroid, thyroid, pheochromocytoma, etc.), hypothyroidism.

PPx: Genetic screening prior to symptoms is recommended, as MEN 2A and 2B can progress to medullary thyroid carcinoma. For these patients, prophylactic total thyroidectomy is indicated.

MoD: Autosomal dominant disorder in MEN gene

Dx:

1. Diagnosis is based on the presence of two or more of the tumors specific to one of the MEN syndromes.
2. Supported by genetic testing for RET proto-oncogene germline mutation.
3. Labs indicating normal/high PTH and high calcium (MEN 1 and 2A).

Tx/Mgmt:

1. For patients who are positive for the RET proto-oncogene, total thyroidectomy is indicated to prevent medullary thyroid carcinoma.

2. Surgery is also indicated for pheochromocytomas (MEN 2A and 2B).
3. For mild hyperparathyroidism, surgery is not indicated and observation is recommended.
4. For symptomatic hyperparathyroidism (bone loss, kidney stones, etc.), surgery is indicated.

Congenital Disorders

Congenital Adrenal Hyperplasia

Stem clues: Infant with ambiguous external genitalia + infant presenting in shock with electrolyte abnormalities

Clinical Presentation: Early-onset congenital adrenal hyperplasia (CAH) is more severe, presenting in infancy, while late-onset CAH may present later in childhood. Typically identified from neonatal screening at birth or when associated with poor growth or even severe dehydration and electrolyte abnormalities. Patients will present with failure to thrive, dehydration, early virilization (males) or hirsutism/menstrual irregularities (females), or ambiguous external genitalia but normal female ovaries and uterus in infants. Autosomal recessive disorder, so look for a family history that does not favor males or females and is not present in every generation. CAH is the MOST COMMON cause of ambiguous genitalia and should be the first thing suspected.

PPx: Newborns are routinely screened for 21-hydroxylase deficiency.

MoD: Most cases are due to 21-hydroxylase deficiency, with a smaller percentage due to 11-hydroxylase deficiency. Both enzymes are involved in the production of hormones within the adrenal gland, including aldosterone, cortisol, and epinephrine. Most severe is the salt-wasting phenotype, which can cause vomiting, dehydration, and shock within the first few weeks of life.

Dx:

1. High concentration of 17-hydroxyprogesterone (substrate for the 21-hydroxylase enzyme), decreased cortisol and aldosterone. Electrolyte abnormalities: hyponatremia, hyperkalemia, hypoglycemia.
2. High concentration of 11-deoxycortisol (substrated for 11-beta-hydroxylase).

Tx/Mgmt:

1. Glucocorticoids (dexamethasone) for excess androgens

> **QUICK TIPS**
>
> 21-Hydroxylase: Salt wasting + ambiguous genitalia
>
> 11-Beta-hydroxylase: Ambiguous genitalia + hypertension and hypokalemia

2. Mineralocorticoids (fludrocortisone) to treat electrolyte abnormalities, blood pressure changes, and extracellular fluid changes

Androgen Insensitivity Syndrome

Buzz Words: Child with breast bud (seeming female) presenting for delayed menarche + discovery of growth in abdomen/groin (testicles)

Clinical Presentation: Genetically XY person is resistant to male hormones (androgens) and has physical traits of a woman. Divided into complete versus incomplete androgen insensitivity syndrome (AIS):

Complete: Prevents penis and other male body parts from developing. Patient looks like a girl. Infertility.

Incomplete: Patient looks like a boy but may have failure of testes to descend or hypospadias. Infertility.

These kids may have breast bud development and a vagina but no uterus.

DDX for undervirilized male (XY, ambiguous genitalia):
1. Inborn errors of testosterone (T) synthesis
2. Partial androgen sensitivity
3. 5-Alpha reductase deficiency
4. If internal structures are combo of male + female:
   - Mixed gonadal dysgenesis
   - True hermaphroditism

DDX for virilized female (XX, ambiguous genitalia):
1. Congenital adrenal hyperplasia
2. Virilization during pregnancy (mom with polycystic ovarian syndrome [PCOS], androgen exposure, androgen-secreting tumor, placental aromatase deficiency)
3. Virilizing tumor

PPx: N/A

MoD: Genetic mutations → inherited qualitative or quantitative deficiency to testosterone receptor

Tx/Mgmt:
1. Sex reassignment
2. Dilation therapy
3. Gonadectomy
4. Hormone replacement

99 AR
Grading androgen insensitivity

Congenital Hypothyroidism

Stem clues: Puffy-faced neonate with trouble feeding + umbilical hernia + jaundice + large posterior fontanelle + constipation + failure to thrive → congenital hypothyroidism

Clinical Presentation: Patients with congenital hypothyroidism can present with umbilical hernia, jaundice, and trouble feeding. Other clues may include cleft palate, microphallus, and undescended testes. Can also be associated with autoimmune disorders such as T1DM, musculoskeletal (MSK) disorders such as SCFE, or genetic disorders such as trisomy 21 and Turner syndrome. This topic is high-yield on the Pediatrics exam due to its broad range of associations.

PPx: Routine newborn screening takes place in all 52 states.

MoD: Most cases of congenital hypothyroidism are due to sporadic mutations, which result in poor thyroid development and decreased levels of thyroid hormones (T3 and T4).

Dx:
1. Newborn screening that shows high TSH, low T3 and low T4

Tx/Mgmt:
1. First-line therapy is to start levothyroxine. Treatment must be initiated early in order to prevent poor growth and cognitive decline.

Metabolic Disorders

You do not need to memorize these as in depth as you did for step 1. If you *were* asked about a metabolic disorder, such as Pompe disease, it will be obvious and only the buzz words would be tested. Rarely will mechanism of disease be tested (e.g., acid maltase deficiency leading to Pompe). Instead, since this chapter comprises only 5–10 questions, many of them will be on diabetes and congenital adrenal disorders. Extra details of each disease will be low yield. Learn instead how to differentiate one disease from another in the question stem (Fig. 15.5).

Inborn Errors of Metabolism

Buzz Words: Lethargy/coma + failure to thrive + seizures + unusual odor + developmental delay + family history

Clinical Presentation: IEM should be suspected in children who are acutely ill and not responding to therapy. Whereas knowledge of the unique clinical presentations of each IEM is not needed to succeed on the Pediatrics exam, being able to recognize them in general is important. BMPs will usually demonstrate abnormal values, and failure to thrive (FTT) is one of the biggest keys. A few key associations are below:

Mousy/musty odor: Phenylketonuria

Sweet maple syrup: Maple syrup urine disease

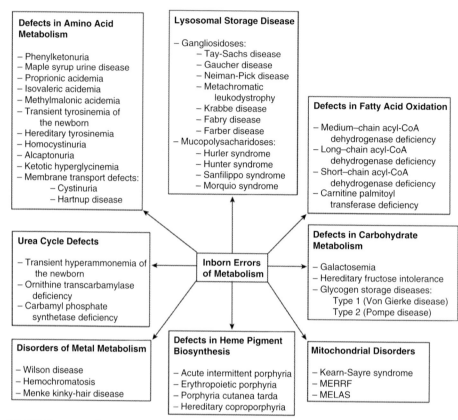

Defects in Amino Acid Metabolism

- Phenylketonuria
- Maple syrup urine disease
- Proprionic acidemia
- Isovaleric acidemia
- Methylmalonic acidemia
- Transient tyrosinemia of the newborn
- Hereditary tyrosinemia
- Homocystinuria
- Alcaptonuria
- Ketotic hyperglycinemia
- Membrane transport defects:
  - Cystinuria
  - Hartnup disease

Lysosomal Storage Disease

- Gangliosidoses:
  - Tay-Sachs disease
  - Gaucher disease
  - Neiman-Pick disease
  - Metachromatic leukodystrophy
  - Krabbe disease
  - Fabry disease
  - Farber disease
- Mucopolysacharidoses:
  - Hurler syndrome
  - Hunter syndrome
  - Sanfilippo syndrome
  - Morquio syndrome

Defects in Fatty Acid Oxidation

- Medium–chain acyl-CoA dehydrogenase deficiency
- Long–chain acyl-CoA dehydrogenase deficiency
- Short–chain acyl-CoA dehydrogenase deficiency
- Carnitine palmitoyl transferase deficiency

Urea Cycle Defects

- Transient hyperammonemia of the newborn
- Ornithine transcarbamylase deficiency
- Carbamyl phosphate synthetase deficiency

Inborn Errors of Metabolism

Defects in Carbohydrate Metabolism

- Galactosemia
- Hereditary fructose intolerance
- Glycogen storage diseases:
  Type 1 (Von Gierke disease)
  Type 2 (Pompe disease)

Disorders of Metal Metabolism

- Wilson disease
- Hemochromatosis
- Menke kinky-hair disease

Defects in Heme Pigment Biosynthesis

- Acute intermittent porphyria
- Erythropoietic porphyria
- Porphyria cutanea tarda
- Hereditary coproporphyria

Mitochondrial Disorders

- Kearn-Sayre syndrome
- MERRF
- MELAS

FIG. 15.5 Summary chart of inborn errors of metabolism. *MELAS*, Mitochondrial encephalopathy, lactic acidosis, and stroke-like episodes; *MERRF*, myoclonic epilepsy and ragged-red fibers.

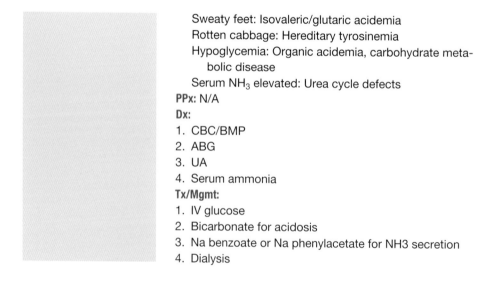

Sweaty feet: Isovaleric/glutaric acidemia
Rotten cabbage: Hereditary tyrosinemia
Hypoglycemia: Organic acidemia, carbohydrate metabolic disease
Serum NH_3 elevated: Urea cycle defects

PPx: N/A

Dx:

1. CBC/BMP
2. ABG
3. UA
4. Serum ammonia

Tx/Mgmt:

1. IV glucose
2. Bicarbonate for acidosis
3. Na benzoate or Na phenylacetate for NH3 secretion
4. Dialysis

Galactosemia

Buzz Words: Hepatomegaly + hypoglycemia after breast-feeding + reducing substance in urine → galactosemia

Galactosemia + fever → *Escherichia coli* sepsis because kids with galactosemia are susceptible to *E. coli* infection

Clinical Presentation: A newborn with galactosemia cannot break down galactose, leading to very characteristic findings such as hypoglycemia after breastfeeding. A neonate can also present with vomiting, diarrhea, FTT, cataracts, renal tubular acidosis (RTA), and seizures/mental retardation due to lack of glucose.

PPx: Prenatal/newborn screening (reducing substance in urine)

MoD: AR, deficiency in galactose-1-phosphate uridyltransferase → deficient G1p-uridyltransferase w/ accumulation in brain, liver, kidney → no breastfeeding and no lactose for life

Dx:
1. Bilirubin (elevated direct bilirubin)
2. Urine test for galactose (quantitative erythrocyte galactose-1-phosphate uridyltransferase [GALT] analysis is the gold standard)

Tx/Mgmt:
1. Galactose-free diet

Hereditary Fructose Intolerance

Buzz Words: Vomiting, diarrhea, FTT + hypoglycemia after fruit juice + severe seizures

Clinical Presentation: Vomiting, diarrhea, FTT

PPx: N/A

MoD: Fructose-1-phosphate aldolase B deficiency

Dx:
1. Urine test for fructose

Tx/Mgmt:
1. Fructose-, sucrose-, sorbitol-free diet

Glycogen Storage Disorders

Disease	Buzz Words	MoD
Type I (Von Gierke)	Hypoglycemia + **hepatomegaly** + gout/short stature + **enlarged kidneys**	G6-phosphatase (G6P) deficiency
Type II (Pompe)	Hypotonia + **heart failure** + enlarged tongue → death by age 2	Acid maltase deficiency

99 AR

Only glycogen storage disease to increase risk of hepatocellular carcinoma → Von Gierke

Disease	Buzz Words	MoD
Type III (Cori/ Forbe)	Hypoglycemia + **hepatomegaly** + muscle weakness/**cardiac involvement**, milder version of type I	Debranching enzyme deficiency
Type IV (Andersen)	Hepatosplenomegaly + cirrhosis + hypotonia + **nervous system involvement**	Branching enzyme deficiency
Type V (McArdle)	Muscle weakness/ cramps	Muscle phosphorylase deficiency

PPx: N/A
MoD: See above
Dx:
1. CBC/BMP
2. UA (ketonuria → type III)
3. CK (elevated → type V)
4. Aspartate aminotransferase (AST)/alanine aminotransferase (ALT) (elevated → type IV)
5. Liver biopsy (type I)

Tx/Mgmt:
1. Correct hypoglycemia
2. Diet management
3. Gene therapy (type II)
4. Liver transplant (type IV)

Fatty Acid Oxidation Defects

Buzz Words: Nonketotic hypoglycemia + hyperammonemia + myopathy + fasting/illness/stress

Clinical Presentation: Presents only during illness or fasting when FAs are required as an energy source. These patients cannot oxidize FAs into energy. Most common is **medium-chain acyl-CoA dehydrogenase deficiency.**

MoD: Deficiency in enzyme required for fatty acid oxidation

Dx:
1. Tandem mass spec for FAs

Tx/Mgmt:
1. High-carb/low-fat diet
2. Carnitine supplementation

Lysosomal Storage Disorders

Buzz Words:
Peripheral neuropathy, angiokeratoma, hypohidrosis →
Fabry
Hepatosplenomegaly, osteoporosis/aseptic necrosis,
tissue-paper macrophages → Gaucher
Neurodegeneration, hepatosplenomegaly, "cherry red"
spot → Niemann–Pick
Neurodegeneration, "cherry red" spot, foam cells →
Tay–Sachs
Neuropathy, optic atrophy, developmental delay → Krabbe
disease
Dementia, ataxia → metachromatic leukodystrophy
Developmental delay, gargoylism, airway obstruction,
corneal clouding, hepatosplenomegaly → Hurler
Hurler + aggressive behavior with no corneal clouding →
Hunter syndrome

Clinical Presentation: Lysosomal storage disorders cause
accumulation of undesirable metabolites in different
organs. Recognize the buzz words, as you are unlikely
to be tested on diagnosis and treatment unless otherwise mentioned.

PPx: N/A

MoD:

Category	Disease	Protein Abnormalities
Lipidoses	Fabry	α-Galactosidase A
	Farber	acid ceramidase
	Gaucher (types 1, 2, and 3)	β-Glucosidase
	GM$_1$ gangliosidosis	β-Galactosidase
	GM$_2$ gangliosidosis	β-Hexosaminidase A
	Tay–Sachs	β-Hexosaminidase A
	Sandhoff	and B
	Metachromatic leukodystrophy	Arylsulfatase A
	Niemann-Pick	??
	Types A and B	Acid sphingomyelinase
	Type C	??
	Type 1	NPC1
	Type 2	NPC2/HE1
	Wolman disease (cholesterol ester storage disease)	Acid lipase
Mucopolysaccharidoses	MPS I (Hurler and Scheie)	α-Iduronidase
	MPS II (Hunter)	Iduronidase sulfatase

Source: Schuchman et al., *Lysosomal Storage Diseases*. Elsevier.

Dx:
1. Urine levels of metabolites or enzyme activity assays
Tx/Mgmt:
1. Enzyme replacement for Gaucher
2. BMT for Hurler/Hunter

GUNNER PRACTICE

1. A 6-year-old female is brought to the pediatrician's office by her mother. She has been complaining of abdominal pain and been vomiting with increasing frequency over the past few days. She has also appeared fatigued and thirsty and now seems less alert than usual. Her mother also notes that she has been "breathing different" since this morning. She has no significant past medical history and has received all required vaccinations. Her vital signs are T 98.7°F, HR 120, BP 81/50, RR 34, SpO$_2$ 98% on room air. On examination, the child is ill-appearing and lethargic. Her capillary refill is approximately 3 seconds, and her respirations are exceptionally deep. There is a fruity odor to her breath. What is the most likely diagnosis?
   A. Viral gastroenteritis
   B. Bacterial pneumonia
   C. Type 1 diabetes mellitus
   D. Hyponatremia
   E. Pulmonary hypertension

2. A 3-week-old male is brought to the pediatrician's office by his mother. She claims that he has been difficult to feed and take care of, and that something might be "wrong with him." The infant was born at 38 weeks, 1 day via an uncomplicated spontaneous vaginal delivery at home. He had routine newborn screening tests done. His mother was called about a follow-up appointment at 9 days, but she does not remember the subject matter and could not find time to go. The infant's vital signs are T 96.1°F, HR 122, RR 34, SpO$_2$ 98% on room air. His length is at the 36th percentile, weight is at the 64th percentile, and head circumference is at the 83rd percentile. On examination, he appears lethargic and mildly jaundiced. Further examination reveals macroglossia, a large umbilical hernia covered by a residual umbilical cord stump, and dry skin. What is the most likely diagnosis and the best next step in management?
   A. Kernicterus; expectant management
   B. Galactosemia; lactose-free diet
   C. Thyroid dysgenesis; thyroid hormone replacement

D. Trisomy 18; expectant management

E. Congenital adrenal hyperplasia; hydrocortisone and fludrocortisone replacement

3. A 13-year-old male is brought to the pediatrician's office by his father. The parent asserts that his son is "too short for his age" and there must be "something we can do." His son, an excellent athlete, has been cut from all of his after-school sports teams due to his stature. His past medical history is notable for multiple episodes of sinusitis and acute otitis media prior to starting kindergarten. His father relates that he himself was "6 feet tall by the age of 14," although he believes the boy's mother didn't begin puberty until age 13 or so. The father is 74 inches tall and the mother is 65 inches tall. The patient's growth charts reveal that his growth in length and weight slowed more than expected during his first year of life, and he has been around the 2nd percentile for height and 4th percentile for weight ever since. Head circumference is 22nd percentile. His vital signs are T 98.5°F, HR 82, BP 104/70, RR 18 SpO$_2$ 98% on room air. Examination reveals no abnormalities, and the patient is Tanner stage 1 with 5-mL testes. A plain radiograph of the hand is read as a skeletal age of 10. What is the most likely diagnosis?

A. Familial short stature

B. Idiopathic short stature

C. Constitutional delay of growth and puberty

D. Cystic fibrosis

E. Growth hormone deficiency

ANSWERS: What Would Gunner Jess/Jim Do?

1. WWGJD?

A 6-year-old female is brought to the pediatrician's office by her mother. She has been complaining of abdominal pain and vomiting with increasing frequency over the past few days. She has also appeared fatigued and thirsty, and now seems less alert than usual. Her mother also notes that she has been "breathing different" since this morning. She has no significant past medical history and has received all required vaccinations. Her vital signs are T 98.7°F, HR 120, BP 81/50, RR 34, SpO$_2$ 98% on room air. On examination, the child is ill-appearing and lethargic. Her capillary refill is approximately 3 seconds, and her respirations are exceptionally deep. There is a fruity odor to her breath. What is the most likely diagnosis?

Answer: C, Type 1 diabetes mellitus

Explanation: This is a basic question to assess your recognition of a common presentation of a common disorder. This young female with fatigue, abdominal pain, and vomiting can initially generate a wide differential. Her ill appearance and lethargy should raise concern, and her vital signs and delayed capillary refill should alert the reader that she has poor perfusion, in this case due to hypovolemia. The history of polydipsia, as well as the fruity smell of her breath and the Kussmaul respirations (deep, fast respirations that compensate for metabolic acidosis) indicate that she likely has diabetic ketoacidosis. The presentation of type 1 diabetes mellitus in children can sound nonspecific, so keep your eyes open for small hints and subtle buzz words when this is an answer choice.

A. Viral gastroenteritis → Incorrect. This patient without loose stools or diarrhea is unlikely to have viral gastroenteritis. Additionally, the fruity breath odor is inconsistent with this diagnosis.

B. Bacterial pneumonia → Incorrect. This patient is afebrile and is neither coughing nor hypoxemic. The breath odor is not explained by this choice either.

D. Hyponatremia → Incorrect. It is reasonable to consider hyponatremia in a patient with reported polydipsia, GI losses, and lethargy. However, this would not easily explain her Kussmaul respirations or breath odor.

E. Pulmonary hypertension → Incorrect. This would not explain many of the patient's symptoms. Additionally, the patient is not hypoxemic.

2. WWGJD? A 3-week-old male is brought to the pediatrician's office by his mother. She claims that he has been difficult to feed and take care of, and that something might be "wrong with him." The infant was born at 38 weeks, 1 day via an uncomplicated spontaneous vaginal delivery at home. He had routine newborn screening tests done. His mother was called about a follow-up appointment at 9 days, but she does not remember the subject matter and could not find time to go. The infant's vital signs are T 96.1°F, HR 122, RR 34, SpO$_2$ 98% on room air. His length is at the 36th percentile, weight is at the 64th percentile, and head circumference is at the 83rd percentile. On examination, he appears lethargic and mildly jaundiced. Further examination reveals macroglossia, a large umbilical hernia covered by a residual umbilical cord stump, and dry skin. What are the most likely diagnosis and the best next step in management?

Answer: C, Thyroid dysgenesis; thyroid hormone replacement

Explanation: This question assesses your recognition of common conditions that can be screened for or caught in the neonatal period. This infant with low temperature, large head circumference, lethargy, feeding difficulties, jaundice, macroglossia, dry skin, umbilical hernia, and delayed umbilical stump separation has many of the common signs and symptoms of congenital hypothyroidism. Congenital hypothyroidism occurs frequently (and is most often caused by thyroid dysgenesis), but it is usually noted by newborn screening and corrected as quickly as possible. The appointment made for him was likely a follow-up for confirmatory testing and initiation of treatment. Timely treatment is extremely important in hypothyroidism, as the longer these infants go without hormone replacement, the lower their IQs will be.

A. Kernicterus; expectant management → Incorrect. This patient displays classic features of hypothyroidism, one of which is jaundice.

B. Galactosemia; lactose-free diet → Incorrect. While galactosemia may cause some of the less specific findings in this infant (like lethargy and jaundice), it cannot explain all of the findings.

D. Trisomy 18; expectant management → Incorrect. A patient with trisomy 18 can have diverse presentations, but he or she will usually be described as a small infant with micrognathia, a heart murmur, and fists closed with peculiarly overlapping fingers.

E. Congenital adrenal hyperplasia; hydrocortisone and fludrocortisone replacement → Incorrect. We are not given any information regarding ambiguous genitalia, sodium and potassium balance, or blood pressure.

3. WWGJD? A 13-year-old male is brought to the pediatrician's office by his father. The parent asserts that his son is "too short for his age" and there must be "something we can do." His son, an excellent athlete, has been cut from all of his after-school sports teams due to his stature. His past medical history is notable for multiple episodes of sinusitis and acute otitis media prior to starting kindergarten. His father relays that he was "6 feet tall by the age of 14," though he believes the boy's mother didn't begin puberty until age 13 or so. The father is 74 inches tall, and the mother is 65 inches tall. The patient's growth charts reveal that his growth in length and weight slowed more than expected during his first year of life, and he has been around the 2nd percentile for height and 4th percentile for weight ever since. Head circumference is 22nd percentile. His vital signs are T 98.5°F, HR 82, BP 104/70, RR 18, SpO$_2$ 98% on room air. Examination reveals no abnormalities, and the patient is Tanner stage 1 with 5 mL testes. A plain radiograph of the hand is read as a skeletal age of 10. What is the most likely diagnosis?

Answer: C, Constitutional delay of growth and puberty

Explanation: This question tests your recognition of the differential diagnosis of a common complaint in pediatric endocrinology. This is a 13-year-old male with short stature. He has been short for almost all of his life, since a longer-than-average decrease in height velocity as an infant, but height has become more important as his peers have reached puberty. He is prepubescent, with a family history of delayed puberty. He has no other health-related complaints, physical exam is otherwise unremarkable, and his bone age is estimated at multiple years younger than his chronological age. This is the presentation of constitutional delay of growth and puberty (CDGP), a normal growth variant. This patient, whose mother was a "late bloomer," will likely also be one. Not only is this family history important but the lack of pubescent features and the young skeletal age also increase the likelihood that he will "catch up" as he ages. Many pathologic disorders can lead to growth failure, so it is important to watch out for signs of failure to thrive (FTT), genetic syndromes, and pituitary disorders, among other things. However, this non-sick patient has remained stable at a low height and weight percentile, which is less concerning than a child who is losing weight or failing to grow at all.

A. Familial short stature → Incorrect. Neither of the patient's parents have short stature.

B. Idiopathic short stature → Incorrect. This patient's young skeletal age and family history of growth and pubertal delay (with both parents finishing growth in the normal height range) make it more likely that he will "catch up."

D. Cystic fibrosis → Incorrect. While it is reasonable to be initially suspicious due to the history of sinusitis and ear infections, this patient does not have FTT and has no ongoing sinorespiratory complaints.

E. Growth hormone deficiency → Incorrect. This patient's history, physical exam, and imaging make CDGP most likely. He has no signs of symptoms of any pituitary pathology either.

Gunner Jim's Guide to Exam Day Success

Hao-Hua Wu, Leo Wang, and Rebecca Tenney-Soeiro

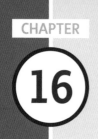

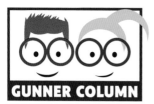

GUNNER COLUMN

Do these three things to perform well on any shelf:
1. Master one review book
2. Do as many quality questions as you can
3. Excel like a Gunner

"Master One Review Book"

The Pediatrics clerkship rotation ranges from 4 to 8 weeks (typically 6). That is not enough time to peruse multiple review books. The most important thing you can do prior to the start of your rotation is to identify the resource that best covers the material of the Pediatrics shelf, such as *Gunner Goggles Pediatrics*. Once you have picked something, stick with it. The point of using a review book is so that you can get familiarized with the scope of the exam.

Most of your learning occurs when you complete questions, so do not be discouraged if you cannot memorize every word of your review book like you did for step 1. Instead, use this review book as a point of reference and annotate the margins.

If you see one topic come up on multiple chapters (or maybe even multiple clinical subject exams), make sure to write down the page numbers where it appears and flip to those pages every time you review. The more connections you make between topics, for example, thinking of syphilis as a disease process that can present as a dermatologic complaint (painless ulcer, palm/sole rash, gummas) and a neurologic complaint (neurosyphilis), the more you will master.

In addition, highlight themes that keep coming up. For instance, anytime patients in the question recently change their medication regimen, suspect the medication change as the cause of their symptoms until proven otherwise. These organizing principles transcend individual topics and can help you do well on any clinical subject exam test question.

"Do As Many Quality Questions As You Can"

The key to success is practicing in an environment that simulates the pressure of test day. And nothing simulates that pressure better than taking practice questions under stringent time constraints.

After you identify your review book, select as many authoritative question banks as you can. We recommend Gunner Practice, UWorld, and NBME Clinical Science practice exams. Do at least 10 questions a day under timed conditions (1.5 minutes a question), starting on the first day of your rotation.

Remember, you can complete the same question multiple times in the course of study! In fact, it is recommended that you retry the questions you got wrong in the first place, just so that you know you would get it right on the test.

It is also important that the questions you complete are of high quality. This means that the length and content of the question stems reflect what you would actually see on test day. Many question bank resources are too easy (giving you a false sense of confidence) or ask about material that would not show up on the exam (wasting your time).

Once you have selected your question bank resources, count the total number of questions and divide it by the number of days you have available to study. Then make sure you set a study plan where you can make at least two passes through your questions. The first pass is completion of all available questions. The second pass is completion of all the questions you got wrong or made a lucky guess for during your first pass. Seeing how many of the second pass questions you get correct should be a nice confidence boost leading into exam day.

As you do questions, jot down patterns associated with the chief complaint. NBME question writers are instructed to write questions with a chief complaint that can plausibly be associated with at least five different diseases. Sharpen your differential after you read a question's first sentence and then use Buzz Words to narrow down your diagnosis. Once you reach your diagnosis, you will either be done with the question or have to draw upon knowledge of PPx, MoD, Dx and Tx/Mgmt.

"Excel Like a Gunner"

How you take notes for the questions you complete is imperative to success.

The most effective strategy is to pick **one** take home point for every question you complete and record it on an Excel spreadsheet specific for your clinical rotation.

For instance, if you answer a question incorrectly about the treatment of Kawasaki's, write "Tx of Kawasaki's" in column A of your spreadsheet and then "aspirin" in column B of your spreadsheet. This allows you to create an immediate, pseudo flashcard. When you review this material the following week, you can put your cursor over column A, say the answer out loud, and check your answer by shifting your cursor to column B. This saves time and emphasizes the most important takeaway is for each question. You can also make your own flash cards on the Gunner Goggles iOS app.

If you understand everything in the question and answer choices, don't record it in the Excel spreadsheet.

If you do not understand multiple things in the question and answer choices, record the most important takeaway point and move on. For test day, it is better to be confident in what you know well than to undermine your confidence by fixating on what you are weak at.

By test day, you should have one Excel spreadsheet that contains one important take home point from every question you were unsure about. The tabs on the bottom should be organized by question bank resource. This spreadsheet would ideally only take 3–4 hours to review, and is something you would go over the day before the exam.

Last but not least, **trust the process**. Students often enter test day anxious and overwhelmed, which can cause them to second-guess their answer choices. Trust the process—trust that you will have covered everything in leading up to the clinical subject exam and have some faith in your answer selections; for these reasons, don't second-guess yourself. Your first instinct is usually right.

In summary: Read, Apply and Review. And prepare for success on test day!

Index

Note: Page numbers followed by "b", "f", and "t" indicate boxes, figures, and tables, respectively.